MAXIM JAKUBOWSKI was born in England but educated in France. Following a career in publishing, he opened London's famous MURDER ONE bookshop. He has published over 70 books, won the Anthony and Karel Awards and is a connoisseur of genre fiction in all its forms. His recent books include ten volumes in *The Mammoth Book of Erotica* series, as well as *The Mammoth Book of Pulp Fiction* and more recently *The Mammoth Book of Pulp Action*. Other well-received anthologies include: *London Noir*, three volumes of *Fresh Blood*, *Past Poisons*, *Chronicles of Crime* and *Murder Through the Ages*. A regular broadcaster, he is the crime columnist for the *Guardian*. His fiction includes *Life in the World of Women*, *It's you that I want to Kiss*, *Because She Thought She Loved Me*, *The State of Montana*, *On Tenderness Express*, *Kiss me Sadly* and *Confessions of a Romantic Pornographer*. He lives in London.

Also available

The Mammoth Book of Awesome Comic Fantasy
The Mammoth Book of Best New Erotica 3
The Mammoth Book of Best New Horror 14
The Mammoth Book of Climbing Adventures
The Mammoth Book of Comic Crime
The Mammoth Book of Egyptian Whodunnits
The Mammoth Book of Elite Forces
The Mammoth Book of Endurance and Adventure
The Mammoth Book of Explorers
The Mammoth Book of Eyewitness America
The Mammoth Book of Eyewitness Battles
The Mammoth Book of Eyewitness Everest
The Mammoth Book of Fantasy
The Mammoth Book of Fighter Pilots
The Mammoth Book of Future Cops
The Mammoth Book of Great Detective Stories
The Mammoth Book of Haunted House Stories
The Mammoth Book of Heroes
The Mammoth Book of Heroic and Outrageous Women
The Mammoth Book of Historical Whodunnits
The Mammoth Book of Humor
The Mammoth Book of Illustrated Crime
The Mammoth Book of Journalism
The Mammoth Book of Legal Thrillers
The Mammoth Book of Literary Anecdotes
The Mammoth Book of Locked-Room Mysteries and Impossible Crimes
The Mammoth Book of Maneaters
The Mammoth Book of Men O'War
The Mammoth Book of Mountain Disasters
The Mammoth Book of Murder and Science
The Mammoth Book of Native Americans
The Mammoth Book of Private Eye Stories
The Mammoth Book of Prophecies
The Mammoth Book of Pulp Action
The Mammoth Book of Roaring Twenties Whodunnits
The Mammoth Book of Roman Whodunnits
The Mammoth Book of Science Fiction
The Mammoth Book of Sea Battles
The Mammoth Book of Sex, Drugs and Rock 'n' Roll
The Mammoth Book of Short Erotic Novels
The Mammoth Book of Tales from the Road
The Mammoth Book of the Titanic
The Mammoth Book of UFOs
The Mammoth Book of Vampires
The Mammoth Book of Vampire Stories by Women
The Mammoth Book of War Correspondents
The Mammoth Book of Women Who Kill

The Mammoth Book of

Sex diaries

EDITED BY MAXIM JAKUBOWSKI

CARROLL & GRAF PUBLISHERS
New York

Carroll & Graf Publishers
An imprint of Avalon Publishing Group, Inc.
245 W. 17th Street
New York
NY 10011-5300
www.carrollandgraf.com

AVALON
publishing group incorporated

First published in the UK by Robinson,
an imprint of Constable & Robinson Ltd 2005

First Carroll & Graf edition 2005

Selection and editorial material
copyright © Maxim Jakubowski 2005

Individual journals are © respective authors

ISBN 0–7867-1497-2

Printed and bound in the EU

Contents

INTRODUCTION   Maxim Jakubowski   vii

JUST ONE BITE   1

MISTRESS MATISSE   26

SASSY LITTLE PUNKIN   55

LOVE SONGS FOR UNDERDOGS   78

LETICIA MCKENZIE   104

NAKED LOFT PARTY   133

LAURA'S WINDOW OR MY LIFE AS A
  FORMER PROSTITUTE   161

GEEKSLUT   188

YOU SILLY LITTLE GIRL: LITTLE EXORCISMS   208

TWIDDLY BITS   231

SWEETNESS FOLLOWS   267

MODEL MISBEHAVIOR   293

KILLBUNNIE23   318

DIARY OF A NYMPHO   347

CAPTIVE HEART   369

COCK UNDER LOCK   395

NEWLYWED SATISFACTION   424

SUBMISSIVE REFLECTIONS   450

RED WHORE   474

TASTY TRIXIE OR THE WANDERING
   WEBWHORE   498

CUMWHORE DIARY   526

PEEP SHOW STORIES   549

Introduction

Maxim Jakubowski

People have written diaries ever since people began writing, I think. There is a compulsion in many to narrate the day to day events of one's life, to explain, to plead, to try and understand what surrounds them. Some intimate diaries are meant for cathartic, personal reasons, while others are for public consumption, albeit often at a later stage. And it is a democratic art: the average man and woman on the street can keep a diary as well as famous artists or personalities.

And, as human beings, we have an unerring curiosity to read what goes on in others' minds. How often have we wondered what a close acquaintance might be writing in his or her diary? About you? About others you know? About events which both of you might have been involved in, of a public or private nature?

Unending grounds for fascination.

And so it has always been, from Samuel Pepys to Anaïs Nin and, no doubt, half the people you cross in the street every day!

However, the Internet has changed all that, or at any rate added some interesting variations: this has now become the decade of the blog.

A blog is strictly speaking a web log. A diary or journal that anyone can write and publish online, and which is therefore visible to all and sundry who know how to locate it, or can wrestle victoriously with a Search Engine.

There are already millions of blogs out there in cyberspace. Many occupy themselves with politics, offering comment, observations, opinions, slander, speculation and conspiracy theories by the dozen. It's a medium which is already becoming both powerful and invaluable. During the Coalition's invasion of Iraq, the most valuable information to come out of Baghdad emanated from a local blogger, for instance, and many independent journalists busy themselves with blogs where they can write without the restrictions of corporate editorial control. There are even wonderful literary blogs (including my favourite, Jenna Crispin's "bookslut.com") which offer a different view of the scene than we get from newspapers and magazines' book review pages. Every subject under the sun can and does become the object of people's blogs. If only there were more hours in the day to keep abreast of such an avalanche of writing!

And then, of course, there are sex blogs.

I first became aware of this new medium when, early in 2004, the Belle de Jour controversy broke in the UK. Belle is the pseudonym for an alleged high-class British call girl who had begun a blog detailing her professional encounters. Needless to say, she was quickly signed up by a publisher, which led to a flurry of speculation as to her identity. Was it a scam by an established writer? Was it really a woman? Was it all true? To cut a long story short, various writers were accused, whom I patently knew were innocent. Then, at a crime writers' award ceremony, I overheard a group of critics and authors within hearing distance actually speculating that Belle could actually be me! Ah, the sins of being an erotic writer . . . The following weekend I, for the first time, went online and actually read the Belle de Jour blog. It was amusing, at times quite witty, moderately sexy, but I was somehow underwhelmed following all the brouhaha. But, I noted that Belle linked to a dozen or so other web sites with clearly interesting names.

Thus began an exploration, following links in every conceivable direction through the Internet, that led to my discovering that there existed out there a veritable universe, a sub-culture of blogs of a sexual nature. And so many of them were so much more interesting than Belle's pioneering effort (although who came first is a moot point).

This is what this book is about.

These are real people and they write about their lives, their sex lives, with total abandon. No taboos, no restrictions by the so-called rules of polite society. And by doing so, they illuminate our understanding of human nature. These are men and women we can identify with.

Some work in the sex industry: a former call girl, a dominatrix, a strip club dancer, web cam girls, and their insights are both hilarious and touching. These are born writers who deserve their own book. And then there are people like you and me, with a fearless intelligence and talent to convey the reality of their sex lives: couples engaged in submission and domination, swingers, women who maybe wrongly call themselves sluts or nymphomaniacs, a newlywed embarking on a great new adventure, a high school student with a wicked sense of humour and an acute sense of observation who is still to cross the sexual Rubicon, an AIDS-infected gay man, lonely souls for whom the call of lust comes or sometimes evades them. All human life is here: the emptiness and the joy of sex, the empty rooms, the silence in the heart of the night as well as the crumpled sheets. Never have I seen people's feelings so nakedly exposed.

Sex diaries have come a long way from Casanova and Frank Harris and I, for one, am happy that modern technology has made these blogs possible. I feel I know many of these writers intimately, despite their necessary anonymity, and they have become my secret friends.

I think they will "talk" to you too.

Maxim Jakubowski

JUST ONE BITE

Eden

http://justonebite.com

Smile pretty for the camera
Sunday 18 May 2003

True story

Heath contacted me online a year ago, referred by a trusted fuckbuddy who said I'd be just his type. He pursued me aggressively and sent many photos and videos of what he had to offer: a scrumptious 9.5″ cock attached to a tall, muscular, attractive guy. He was an exhibitionist and specifically said he'd like to film us playing together and share videos that didn't show my face, but gave me the option to say, "No cameras."

Why on earth would I do that?

He came to my hotel room. I was dressed as he had requested, in four-inch heels, stockings, a garter belt under my dress. We kissed. He was arousing, charming, in control. He took a few posed photos of me in various states of near-nudity and with some props, then switched over to video mode as I put my lips on his cock. It turned me on to hear him talking up the action for the camera. After a few minutes of teasing, he mounted the camera on a tripod, checked the lighting and position, slid on a condom, and pressed the thick head of his cock against my pussy. Even though I was soaked, he was thicker than I had expected and I cried out.

He felt great inside me but wasn't a particularly talented lover. Still, I rode on a massive adrenaline wave as we shifted from position to position, rearranging the camera as needed. We were both very vocal; I usually am, anyway, but the knowledge that others would be hearing me was an encouragement. Heath indulged his kinky side occasionally. He shoved an enormous dildo into me as I squirmed and begged, relieved when it was replaced with his comparatively slender shaft. We fucked for a very long time, taking breaks so he could move the camera, switch to handheld, or simply prolong his climax. I faked an orgasm along the way because he was mistaking my exhibitionist thrill for a reaction to his sexual prowess, but that didn't lessen the sheer nasty pleasure of what we were doing.

Finally Heath lay on the bed and filmed me as I gave him a blow-job and finished him off. We relaxed and talked. He threatened that next time, he'd take my ass (which he did . . . but that's another story).

He soon posted the videos online. It was hot, yet a little embarrassing, to see people discussing the scenes of me being fucked. It reawakened the exhibitionist in me, the same internal imp who continues to do her mischief, who hoped someone would see me sucking my friend's cock last week, be jealous of the look of pleasure on his face, and jerk off to the memory later. The one who loves you reading and sharing my stories.

I drove home yesterday
Tuesday 20 May 2003

Relationships

I drove home yesterday going too fast, radio too loud, overcharged with such a voracious appetite that I envisioned myself eating a thick steak with my hands. I wasn't hungry. Rather, I was still in the aftershocks of a brain-percolating orgasm, the work of my friend and his talented fingers. Ten hours later my pussy is still sore and my knees less sturdy than they should be.

So: Love and sex.

If you've been reading my stories, you know I've fucked many men to whom I had no emotional attachment whatsoever. There have been some I wouldn't have kissed or slept beside if you paid me, but we still had fun sex. On the other hand, I haven't posted many stories of making love, of being one body, mind, and heart, but I've done more than my share. What I find challenging is the space between.

Most men have fallen into this area. With some, we acknowledged at the beginning that we would let ourselves become infatuated, burn off the adrenaline, then calm down and be friends again. Others simply became true lovers as we played, having no fear of passion and affection. We cared deeply, in some cases loved each other, but never shared a primary romantic relationship. I'd walk through fire for those guys, months and years later.

There have also been several in this treacherous middle ground who misinterpreted, who thought I wanted more than I did. For some that was wishful thinking. For others with worse fear of commitment than mine, it was terrifying. They tried to "handle" me – it's infuriating to see that behavior from someone less smart and far less subtle than I am. My heart is not made of ice. Sometimes I've fallen in love when I shouldn't have – haven't we all? – but I take responsibility for my emotions. I'm also very gentle to any man who has chosen to give me his heart, even if I cannot accept it.

One man devastates me every time he gets me off by being overwhelmingly tender and protective as I come. He may have just been calling me a nasty slut, but as I climax he tells me everything is ok, wraps me in his arms, croons that he loves me. And I bawl. I weep like a baby. I drench his chest in my tears as he strokes my sweaty hair. Why? Because, as in control as I can be about getting the pleasure I want, when and how I want it, I desire to be treasured as much as anyone does. I want to love and be loved.

Why is this relevant today? Because what makes the fun I've been having with my friend even better is the knowledge that I really care about him, that I'd be upset if he were hurt, that I'd help him if he needed me. It's been a while since I've had someone in that middle ground for whom I could feel the warmth of true affection surrounding the white-hot peaks of lust. I like this.

See? There's a soft side to me after all.

Never as good as the first time
Thursday 22 May 2003

True story

I think I'll call the friend I've been playing around with for a couple weeks Dante. It doesn't quite suit him, but it's close . . .

Last night: the privacy and space of my house rather than the interior of a car, good music, a fruity Chilean wine. Clothes strewn about the family room. Then, a nice chianti, different good music, the remainder of clothing on the bedroom floor. And . . .

Wet, salty, hot, slippery, hard, sticky, mind-blowing, soft, sweaty. Oh my God. Wave after wave of orgasm, mouths and hands playing, exploring, taking delight in pulling gasps and moans from each other. Feeling him inside me, straddling and riding him, holding his hands down the way I love to be taken. Grasping the headboard to keep from falling off the bed when he pushes his fingers into me again. Again?!? Giggle fits as we lay together afterwards, trying to remember when either of us had an evening like that.

Wow.

Oye mamacita!
Tuesday 3 June 2003

Relationships

I had another mediocre date on Saturday with a guy I dated several times last year. He's very cute, very young, not very bright. I date men older than me by a decade or more all the time, yet it still feels strange to play with a boy in his early twenties. The sex is energetic and without any lasting impression. We fucked on his bed while his housemates watched *Jackass the Movie* in the next room. One of them called me "chica" as we passed by. I felt old . . . but I defy any 21-year-old to give a blow-job as heart-stopping as mine.

I've been longing for more lately. I want a man with whom I can make real sexual magic, passion, steamy sweaty lovemaking and furious fucking. Dante is fantastic but he doesn't count; he's not mine, he's borrowed. I want someone who can sit with me in the dark and let me breathe his breath, just millimeters away from letting our lips touch. Someone who is as comfortable with silence as he is with gasps and moans. A man who can laugh while he's inside me, a playmate and friend. One who wants to explore the world and live deeply, taking every ascent and plunge of this wonderful roller coaster of life with eyes open and hands in the air, one entwined with mine. Someone who curls into my arms when he needs comfort, but is strong enough for the times I need him.

. . . and if he could be at least six feet tall, slightly rough around the edges, an occasional smoker, with sensuous lips and an accent, no inhibitions yet excellent manners, an IQ over 155, a good haircut, a bank balance to make Bill Gates tip his hat in admiration, sensitive nipples, and a beautiful and responsive cock, that would be swell.

Might as well ask for the whole package while I'm spinning fantasies.

Let's do lunch
Friday 6 June 2003

True story

Yesterday, Dante and I teased each other online as usual. He stopped by my desk and I went wet immediately, eyes irresistibly drawn to his lips. We were in a meeting and my body trembled with electricity every time we touched. Most men I've been with haven't understood the word "foreplay". Dante engages in it with me for hours each day.

So it's no surprise that, when we snuck off to a parking lot after work and he lunged at me like a famished lion, I surrendered to desire. No small talk. I wanted him. I walk around wanting him. I wake in the middle of the night wanting him. I realize during pastoral weekend drives that yes, I want him.

We kissed ravenously and then his jeans were open. Yesssssss. His fingers, my fingers, my lips, my tongue. Dante watched me; I watched him. We took him to the edge and back off, slightly, only to rush to the precipice again. He exploded into my mouth and I took care not to swallow but to stay there until he was spent.

I leaned back into my seat with a smile, then melted into him as we kissed, exchanging his taste, trading it back and forth on our tongues, both of us reveling in the continued wave of sensations. It turns me on that he's not squeamish about something that I so joyfully take into my mouth, that he'll steal his taste from my lips just as I suck mine from his fingertips. And our flavours combined? Yes. Oh yes please yes more yes.

We talked for a long while afterwards and when he left to go home to his wife and guests, I was warm and content. He pulled away, and I started my car.

Or rather, I tried to.

An asthmatic little wheeze, but no ignition.

Great.

I called Dante on his mobile and asked if he could come back and jumpstart my car. He played the hero. I, as the distressed damsel, kissed him as he handed back the cables. He rode off into the twilight on his mighty steed. Well, OK . . . we actually drove away in our respective SUVs. For the suburbs, that's a sexy ending.

Why Americans like big cars
Tuesday 10 June 2003

True story

Fooling around in vehicles is getting a little played out. With the arrival of warmer weather, it quickly gets hot and sticky . . . and not in a good way. Dante finds my sweaty hair sexy; I find it uncomfortable. Luckily, the logistical complications that have kept us from playing at my place will soon come to an end.

After work today we parked and took turns making each other come. Dante told me how he'd been fantasizing for hours about lifting my skirt and fucking me from behind, and I spasmed around his fingers just as his teeth closed on my nipple. He makes me come hard and fast, but not very deeply – no vision-blurring, giggle-inducing, aftershocks for minutes, curled in a ball and *please don't touch me yet every nerve on my body is too sensitive* orgasms. I look forward to the chance for him go slowly.

Following my climax I relaxed for a few minutes and rubbed him through his jeans while he sucked my taste off his fingers. Then, on my knees in the driver's seat, ass pointed at the side window, I leaned over and wrapped my lips around him. With enough practice, the position is almost comfortable. I only regret that my approach is from the side, putting my tongue at a less than optimal angle and making it more difficult to look up and see him watching me. Still, it never takes more than a few minutes before he fills my mouth. I love that so much.

We kissed and chatted comfortably, talking about former lovers, other people we find attractive, and wild days in our past. It's not a bad little affair so far. Nope, not bad at all.

Maudlin, but honest
Saturday 14 June 2003

A Mouthful of Lies

I don't love you.

When you bounced around the room on your thirtieth birthday, hair spiked, wearing a suit jacket with your jeans and Docs, screaming "My Way" along with Sid Vicious, I didn't adore you.

When we dragged the kiddies through Harrods, and I took the girls to the loo while you and the boy bought sweets to surprise us later, and on the way home your daughter climbed onto my lap in the cab and fell asleep with her blonde curls resting on my breasts, I wasn't in love with all four of you.

When your weeping woke me again, and I knew my words would not make a difference so I wrapped my body around you, protective, wishing I could shield you from the world but even more from the demons in your own mind, my feeling of overwhelming helplessness wasn't because I loved you so much that I would have given my life to ease your pain.

When I opened my eyes to find you looking at me in wonder, as if you had never seen a sleeping woman, and you leaned forward to kiss my hair, I didn't feel a thing.

When you told me you were moving, and I held myself together on the telephone and didn't let my voice break, because you didn't belong to me and I had no right to make you feel guilty for making the right choice for your family, and then you sent me an e-mail reminding me that I will always be your precious girl, I didn't sob because you filled my heart.

When we looked at three-hundred-year-old schools and warehouses, dreaming of converting them into a home for our family, and you glanced at the necklace you had given me when you proposed, I didn't truly believe that we would have a wonderful life together.

When I think of you now, I don't ache with limitless, undying love.

When you strode through the store purposefully as I struggled to keep up, and you noticed, slowed down, and slipped your strong hand around mine, the rest of the world didn't fade leaving just you and I floating across the industrial tiles and down the rows of merchandise.

When I stood up to my mother publicly for the first time when she was being abusive to you, and I fought for you and for my independence in front of my entire extended family, it wasn't because you made me feel strong and beloved enough to be safe.

When we did something dirtier, kinkier, than I had done with anyone before, and you gathered me into your arms afterwards, redeeming me, smothering me in kisses, tears welling in your eyes because of how completely I had given myself to you, the look on my face wasn't unconditional love.

When I heard that you had died, a part of me didn't die along with you, leaving my heart raw and bleeding for years before I could start to patch the damage.

No, I don't love any of you, and I never did.

I'm just a girl
Thursday 19 June 2003

Relationships

I'm always slightly surprised when someone writes that it would be "exciting but nerve-racking/agonizing/heartbreaking" to be in a relationship with a woman like me. Usually that comment seems tied to sexual possessiveness. That a man would be uncomfortable with his girlfriend or wife fucking other men/women isn't a shock to me, and I sound like a stereotypical cheating husband when I try to explain that it's just sex, not love. I've loved a handful of men. I've fucked a couple of busloads of them. (Wait; how many people can you fit on a bus?) There's a difference, though it's not always a relevant one for monogamous-minded folk. I don't cheat out of cruelty; in fact, I prefer not to *cheat*, but to have a relationship that can stretch to encompass some sexual freedom.

Otherwise, I'm not that different from other women you might date, I suppose. Sex is more available and of a wider variety with me. I've been told I'm less clingy – I like my personal space and I'm not threatened by "boys' night out" and such. I love deeply though I'm ready to bolt at any time. I don't suffer fools gladly or otherwise. Parents like me. I cook and bake well and am a good hostess. I like presents and romantic dates. Really, I'm just a girl.

(Are you rolling with laughter now? You should be . . .)

Because yes, I *am* all those things, but I'm also the woman who will wake you with my tongue in the middle of the night and beg you to fuck me up the ass. I'll stare brazenly at someone across the room and tell you the sexual scenario I'm envisioning. I'll see through your bullshit, even if I don't let you know that I can. I will drag you on road trips to nowhere. I will challenge you. I may only let you see my outer layers, though you think you know me to my core. I will feel you up in inappropriate places. I will love you when you hate yourself. I will curse chain restaurants yet frequent Starbucks. I will crave the comfort and security of wrapping myself in your arms, but freeze up if you try to take care of me. Some days I will scare you. Some days I will bore you. Some days I will not rest until I have drained every last drop from you. I will let you talk for hours and offer nothing meaningful of myself. I will take up a hobby of finding ways to make you smile or get you hard. And yes, I will play around with other men and women, but I will do my best to be respectful of the rules we agree on . . . until I'm very turned on and my pussy takes control, that is. But, I will return to you.

Really, I'm such a ~~wonderful girlfriend horrible cunt typical slut~~ tease.

Into the abyss
Thursday 3 July 2003

Potpourri

Putting your cock into a woman's mouth must be a triumph of lust over fear. When else do you knowingly place your treasured staff into a food grinder? I have sharp incisors lurking behind my full, soft lips. Do you dare? Is the warm wetness of my tongue worth it? When you can feel the sensitive head of your cock grasped in the back of my mouth, if the light glints off a pointed eye tooth, can you hold back?

I bit the inside of my mouth yesterday as I was having my

lunchtime salad. My mouth filled with blood and I moaned in pain. How easy it is to catch some skin while chewing. Last year, a lover scolded me for putting a good-sized gash in the side of his cock during an enthusiastic blow-job. I didn't believe I had done it but, if I even bite myself, I can't deny that accidents happen.

A couple of lovers have singled out my tongue for praise, not only for what I can do with it, but for its velvet texture and embracing width. I like that I can narrow it into a point to focus my attention on a sensitive spot, or wrap it around your cock, wide and thick and strong and wet.

Vocalize your reactions; tell me what works best for you through the sounds you make, let me learn your preferences. Sometimes I'll ignore them in order to tease you. I'll give you what you want for a while, then pull back and lick you like a dripping ice cream cone or blow cool air across your hardness. I'll tempt you with tiny little licks then suddenly swallow you deep, taking you in full-length plunges. Tell me when you're ready to come. Maybe I'll be ready to let you.

Maybe not.

As the novelty fades
Friday 4 July 2003

True story

Dante came over after work yesterday. We sat around and relaxed, chatting, drinking a decent Cab Sauv as we wound down from the day. I got up to put on some music and, like a raptor sensing movement, Dante swooped across the room to kiss and caress.

We moved into the bedroom. Clothing was removed piece by piece. Eventually I found myself with one foot on the headboard, another sprawled in the middle of the bed, my hand on his cock, and his fingers and mouth probing my pussy and ass. I decided not to hurry my orgasm along, but to enjoy every touch, every lick, every time that a finger deeply invaded me. The sensations built slowly, layer on layer.

And then it started. Dante was overloading my senses with so much simultaneous, amazing stimulation, and when he stopped doing everything at once, my orgasm started to creep up. As he simply licked me, I started to come. It was a hollow feeling, a superficial clitoral orgasm that strangely dragged on and on, waiting for more. Ten or twenty seconds may have elapsed, and then he slid his fingers back into me and my nerves went on high alert. I erupted. Mt Vesuvius couldn't compare. I writhed on the bed, bucking and yelling and muttering nonsense and burying myself under the comforter. I curled into a near fetal position and tried to hold back most of the tears that threatened to pour down my face from the physical release. Dante sat back with a triumphant smile as I continued to drift on the aftershocks. Oh. My. God.

We sipped some wine as I came back to earth, then I urged him to relax as I took his cock into my mouth. He took a long time to come; many, many minutes in my mouth, my hand, a few strokes in my pussy as I straddled him. I would have gladly taken all night. His cock is just the right size for my mouth; I can take him all the way in and use the back of my throat, a technique that few men seem to have experienced. Someday I need to explore beyond his cock, learning what works on the rest of his body, but I enjoy playing with it so much. With some men I get annoyed if a blow-job takes too long, if my nose is running and eyes tearing from effort but he still hasn't come. Not with Dante; perhaps because I enjoy giving him every sensation along the way.

He finished, partially in my mouth and partially on my face. I lay there as he trembled, rubbing his cock over my slick, come-covered lips and cheeks. Damn, I love that!

We sat on the bed and talked for a long while afterwards, naked, sipping wine, listening to Recoil. It was good. We've clearly moved on from the first stage, where every touch was a small miracle, and now that we don't have to play in our cars anymore, some of the spontaneous naughtiness is gone, too. It will be interesting to watch the affair mature, and see whether two novelty junkies such as us can keep it stimulating.

The G Man
Thursday 10 July 2003

True story

The first time Adam made me come was on the floor of my family room. I was lying near the fireplace on my back and he was between my legs, licking and probing with his tongue. He slid one finger, then two, inside me. I was very wet. I usually am.

Adam pressed various places inside until he found one that made me squirm. He asked how it felt. I said it felt strange, not good-strange, and perhaps even bad-strange. He continued to stroke that spot as he licked me.

When my climax began to approach, I nearly lost my concentration in surprise. It was bubbling up from somewhere inside me I didn't know existed, setting different nerves aflame as it passed. I came hard, clenching on Adam's hand and bucking up into his teeth. I babbled nonsense, I cried, I giggled, and I curled up in a ball and didn't want to be disturbed for many long minutes.

"See?" he grinned.

It became something of a routine for us. We never fucked – his kink, not mine – but we'd use our hands and mouths. Adam always came first, usually straddling my tits, using my mouth and jerking off onto my face. Then he'd slip down between my thighs and insist on making me come, even if I told him not to bother and it took me a while to become interested in what he was doing. Sometimes he'd make me tell him in exquisite detail what a dirty whore I was. He'd make me describe how it felt to lay there with his sticky come drying on my face, burning pink alkaline streaks into my sensitive skin. He'd keep control while bringing me pleasure; it was an extension of his dominance, not an act of service.

I never faked an orgasm with Adam. It wasn't simply that I didn't have to, but that I trusted and respected him enough that I never wanted to. I knew that if I let him try, and then told him that I simply couldn't come that evening, he wouldn't take it personally. He takes great pleasure in having introduced a few women to their own G-spots or even their first orgasms. Not something one can add to his curriculum vitae, but I'd write Adam a letter of recommendation any day. In a way, I suppose I just did.

Company business
Monday 21 July 2003

True story

It all blurs together now: writhing bodies, fingers, tongues, lips. His hardness rubbing against my wet wet pussy. Watching him stroke his cock while I expectantly urged him on. Feeling his fingers hit just the right spot inside. Falling asleep sweaty, sore, and blissful. I can't give you a "he did this, then I did that" narrative, as I only remember moments. Flashes. Feelings. If you want to sculpt a masturbation fantasy from today's post, picture going on a business trip with the guy/girl from the office who you daydream about, and having this be the way you spend your nights.

Other moments outside of bed are indelible. I sat next to him in a long meeting, inhaling his scent and growing moist and hungry. We watched a restaurant close around us when we were out together one night on one of the best dates I've had in ages. (Why do I squirm inside when calling that a date?) Time slipped by when we talked; we would lie in his bed talking for hours before a kiss would launch us into sexplay.

One of my friends thinks I'm falling in love with him. I disagree, though I might agree that I love him in the way I love my close friends. My Master thinks I need to be wary of his wife; but he is also cheating on *his* wife every time he's with me, so I can appreciate the source of his concern. I simply think it's a relationship unlike any I've had, one that spans friendship, partnership at work, affection, and sex.

Dante isn't perfect, but I don't expect him to be. The relationship isn't perfect, even within its limitations. It's pretty damn good though. I'm at a point where my sex life has been vigorous and fun, but my love life has been miserable because of fear and bad luck. This affair chases some of my blues away without scaring me into petrifaction. I deserve that. This relationship won't stop me from keeping an open mind about finding a partner of my own. My ears still perk up when an interesting single man is mentioned. It won't stop me from finding other playmates, either, though it has made me eager to find some that Dante and I can share.

Truth, though? Back in my own bed, on my own pillow, I didn't sleep as well as I did when I could feel him next to me, naked, his skin brushing my skin, the scent of our sex and sweat heavy in the air.

BDSM & Me: Part Two
Sunday 29 June 2003

Mind & Body BDSM & Me

This is how it feels. Forgive any frilly language; you know I usually choose a forthright style, but these concepts will be hard for me to convey without letting emotion and sensation into my words.

My submissive response is one of mind and body. When I am with someone I trust and with whom I can relax, and he takes charge, I physically melt. There is a sinking feeling, my chest dives into my stomach and continues downward into my womb. My breath catches. My head tilts back, baring my neck as my eyes shut. It is very difficult for me to speak and I have no desire to do so. To compare this *subspace* to being aroused in a vanilla way is to compare heroin to aspirin.

Inside my head, my range of thought narrows and I become fuzzy. Free will takes a holiday. I am focused on sensations and obedience, moving as directed, reacting rather than acting. I would argue that when I am deep in subspace, I can take no responsibility for myself or my actions; it is an altered state. Therein is much danger, to be discussed another time. I have only released that far with a handful of men, and even then, not every time. It is a lot of power to give to someone and not all are capable of accepting it.

When I take charge, it is sheer power. There is a wicked mischief that fills me. I want to play with my partner like a science project: if I press here, what happens? What about here? I want to give pleasure, but more than that I want to lead him/her on a journey of self-discovery, even if it doesn't feel pleasant all the time. And, I want to please myself. When I am submissive, my orgasm doesn't matter. When I'm dominant, I *will* be satisfied.

When I switch, it's almost always playful and erotic. Intense, but not in the same way; I skim the surface of sub and Domme but spend most of the time somewhere in between.

About half of my sexual partners have shared D/S or BDSM with me on some level, though it was often window dressing: a blindfold, lightly tied wrists – no real intent to exchange power, just to control experiences. I've had some excellent sex that didn't involve any of this, but after a while the craving starts. I want to be held down. I want my hair pulled. I want to be taken in the middle of the night when I'm barely awake. I want to see the marks on my skin the next day and feel it all again.

The one with the largest breasts
Thursday 28 August 2003

True story

Dante and I traveled with a number of co-workers on this trip, but primarily our good friend Michael. Michael is gay and has enough of a checkered past that we all get along brilliantly and our conversations are unrestrained. He doesn't quite know all of my whorish traits, but he has a good inkling, especially now.

The first night, I joined Dante in his room. We kissed and talked and spent the night fitting ourselves together like puzzle pieces as we slept. It was lovely. Even without anything sexual, I enjoyed the feel of his body against mine and the musky scent of his skin.

We've been working with some colleagues long distance for several months. We spent the next day working with them face-to-face, culminating in a lengthy, thoroughly enjoyable dinner. Dante and Michael and I sat amongst them, comparing backgrounds and downing pinot noir as if it was never to be produced again. Hours passed, other people left, and finally it was down to four of us alone at the table – we three and one of our local counterparts, Rick. We sipped glasses of scotch and finally decided to continue chatting back at the hotel.

I suppose I flirted a little on the walk there, mostly by making references to my breasts (and to flashing them to get us a cab if the walk proved longer than promised). We settled into the empty lounge with more wine and our state of inebriation began to show as inhibitions lifted. We bitched about work and talked about sexual preferences and relationships – I was the only single person in the group. At one point Rick put his hand on the back of my hair and let it rest there a moment before slowly slipping down, but that was the extent of any suggestive behavior between us. Rick is smart and interesting and sensitive; his appeal is below the skin, but I found him charming.

Glasses emptied and it was suggested that we head to our rooms. We asked Rick if he'd be taking a cab home (hoping he wasn't intending to drive) and he said that he wasn't going there. Oh? "No," he said, "I'm staying with one of you." Some confusion arose, since all of us sleep with men and we weren't sure if he was indicating that he wanted me, the only woman in the group, or our gay friend Michael, or Dante, who is bi but hadn't really been obvious about it.

"Well, OK then," I said. "Which one of us?"

"Which one of you has the largest breasts?" he replied.

"All right, guess it's me," I smiled. There was some discussion, since none of us wanted to push a drunken man into the street, but the men were trying to protect my reputation, I suppose. Dante whispered, "If you need a backup plan . . ." and I nodded. My thinking at the time was that we'd probably go back to my room, fondle a little, and then fall asleep. No big deal.

We all went upstairs. I stopped in my bathroom to brush my teeth, which were feeling disgusting after dinner and booze, and when I came out Rick was lying on the bed in his T-shirt and boxers. I pulled a satin nightgown from my closet as the phone rang. It was Michael, checking to see if I was really OK with the situation, offering to pay for a room for Rick, and being such a gentleman. I told him I was fine but promised to call if there was a problem. Rick got up and tried to call his house, but we were both too drunk to figure out the complicated phone.

In the mostly dark room, I slipped out of my clothes and into the short, soft nightgown. What followed is a jumble in my memory. Rick and I talked and kissed. He wanted to kiss a lot; he loved to kiss and was good at it. He wanted to know what I wanted to get out of the evening. I told him that I wanted to have a little bit of fun with no regrets, to still be able to smile at each other the next day. (I should mention that Rick has friends who are executives in my chain of management, so the possibility of fucking up my career if things went badly was never far from my thoughts.) I asked what he wanted. "Kisses and to make you feel good."

Which started a theme. I wouldn't let him lick or fuck me, which he wanted to do. Why? Well, I didn't have a condom, so intercourse was out. I also just didn't want things to get that complicated. We may never see each other again, but we'll have to work together at a distance (and he's a pal of my boss's boss's boss's boss, part of my mind kept saying), and I wanted to keep things light and fun.

We wrestled on the bed, my nightgown fallen to my waist, playing tug-of-war with my panties, laughing and kissing and groping. I begged him to just let me suck his cock. He said, "After I come, I'll be going home to my wife and child – is that really OK with you?" "No," I joked. "We just met today, I expect a lifelong commitment!" and I kissed him again. He sucked and twisted my nipples hard, pinned me down while kissing me, swatted me on the ass when I was being a brat, pulled my hair . . . and I was aroused and having a wonderful time. He whined that he wanted to make me come, and I repeatedly assured him that I would get an incredible amount of pleasure from *his* pleasure, something he couldn't quite wrap his head around. I promised him he could make me come if he came to visit my office.

But his clothes came off, we twisted around and kissed some more, then I finally got my mouth on his cock. He asked me to put my finger up his ass and I gladly did, wetting it in my mouth and then slipping it inside him as I teased his cock with my tongue and pulled it deep into my mouth. He moaned. After a couple minutes he asked me to stop, pushed me onto my back, and stood over me on the bed as he stroked his cock. I began to get dizzy in anticipation, especially when he warned me that it would be a large load of come (something he seemed to think I would find unpleasant – made me wonder if he hadn't had sex in a while or if his wife was squeamish about his fluids). My thighs clenched, and when I felt him start to climax, his come splashing my lips, cheeks, neck, and breasts, I squirmed in pleasure and my orgasm suddenly surged forward without any additional stimulation. I cried out and trembled, riding the waves of sensation as I licked his incredibly sweet come from my lips, then broke into post-orgasmic giggles.

We lay there for a minute, catching our breath. He kissed me and then wiped the come that smeared onto his face from mine, apologizing again for the quantity. I got up to wash and when I came back out he was nearly dressed. I helped him make the final adjustments: untucking his pant leg from his sock, untwisting his belt, fixing his collar. I told him I wanted him to look respectable if anyone woke up when he got home. "Oh, someone will be awake and pissed off," he muttered. We hugged and kissed one more time and out he went.

I ran to the phone and called Dante. "Can I come sleep with you?" I asked. "Of course." I put clothes over my nightgown and raced to his bed. We cuddled and talked and I told him what had happened with Rick. Knowing about his friendships with our execs, Dante laughed that I had "taken one for the team", but also told me that I was a sweet, wonderful woman (for reasons I really can't explain without giving away too much information). I felt so accepted, warm, and happy, and fell asleep listening to him breathe.

In the morning, I assured Michael that everything had been OK, that we had "negotiated what would and would not happen, and I had sent him home to his family before long." True, just not the full truth. Unfortunately, Rick was a bit stiff around me the next day. I'm hoping that wears off as we continue to work together at a distance, because I like the guy and don't want to complicate things. Ah, the risks of fucking co-workers. It did amuse me to sit between him and Dante at a meeting, though, acting all prim and proper. Ha!

A dull year, overall
Saturday 6 September 2003

Relationships

I want to complain about my sex life, but it was just ten days ago that I was sucking off one of my colleagues before climbing into bed with another one, so I guess I don't have much to whine about.

This has been a quiet year for me, sexually. If I pull up the detabase (yes, I keep a list of my lovers and a few relevant stats – it's the only way that some of them are memorable), I only see two new playmates in 2003, compared with nine new ones in 2002. There was plenty of carry-over to this year, which I suppose is why I haven't been on the prowl, plus I can't deny that health problems and a longing for something more have cut into my bed-hopping.

In most parts of my life, I crave balance. Since late 2001 my sex/love life has been off-kilter: I've fucked around plenty, but there has been little emotional involvement. I love my Master, I've had crushes, I adore Dante . . . but I haven't been in love since Adam. After a while, that takes some of the fun out of my romps. I need fulfillment on more levels than having my innate sluttiness satisfied with adrenaline rushes and a couple of orgasms.

A slight rekindling
Wednesday 1 October 2003

Relationships

I don't believe that things are ever as supercharged as at the beginning of a relationship, when experiences are fresh and you're just discovering each other. Dante and I burned white hot for a month or two, then things cooled off and we were primarily pals, both of us sick and stressed by other issues. Now we're flirting again, stealing kisses in inappropriate places, and telling each other how much we long to do more.

To me, that's the rhythm that makes a relationship last. I know too many people who panic at that first cooling phase, thinking it's a sign that things are going horribly wrong, that someone is cheating, that there isn't any passion. Nonsense. Nature operates in cycles; why should lust be exempt?

Golden moments
Sunday 9 November 2003

True story

I'm about to tell you a lengthy true story that involves Adam, my dear Adam, who I've mentioned many times. Before I write it, I'd like to tell you a little more about him.

Of all the men I've dated or played with, Adam is the least comfortable with his sexuality. Part of the reason is certainly because he suffers from severe and untreated bipolar disorder. He goes into black pits of self-loathing that I cannot comprehend, battling insomnia, bouts of weeping, and such deep internal hatred that he is frequently suicidal. In between, he is an energetic joker who loves punk music and smart, curvaceous women with angelic faces. My heart aches when I think of him, not because I miss him romantically, but because he is too good a soul to be tortured as he is.

Adam is more of a feminist than I am, a fact that may be questioned when you read the story. Any dimestore psychiatrist could say that during sex, he is showing the feelings toward women that he has internalized. I would argue that during sex, Adam "punishes" his partner for the one sin he can never accept: loving him.

Living halfway around the world from each other and being very sexual creatures, Adam and I had developed a strong shared fantasy life. Our phone sex and letters kept pushing each other further, spiraling down into some very dark places to see if we liked what we found. Sometimes we didn't, and laughed afterwards. Other times, we took the fantasies we had wrapped our minds around and placed them on the shelf to act out later.

The few times we visited each other, we never had intercourse. Adam's strong facial fetish meant that most times, he would straddle my face and jerk off onto it after I had gotten him aroused, then he would finger and lick me until I came. Orgasms on both sides were easy and plentiful.

We talked each other through hooker fantasies often. We day-dreamed about meeting in a bar, going out into the alley where he would fuck my mouth, come on my face and dress, and toss $5 on the dirty sidewalk as he turned his back. We considered setting up a bukkake session where I would be dressed in office attire, then forced to sit, my tits pulled out of my silk blouse, as a group of men watched some of my home sex videos and jerked off, finishing on my face, tits, and hair as Adam coached them to aim for "the whore's pretty face".

Verbal humiliation and the embarrassment of being covered in come were huge turn-ons for us both. He'd growl filthy things to me while he rubbed my clit, his slick come drying on my lips and cheeks, knowing it would get me off even harder. He'd make me beg for him to jerk off on me, pinning my arms and making me take every drop.

It's no surprise that after a while, we went to a darker place than that. I had told him the details of my worst rape and he knew that it was still troubling me. So, when the idea of him pissing on me instead of just showering me with come came up, I was the one who put it into words, though we had both been thinking about it for some time. We talked it through as a fantasy over and over. I could imagine the revulsion I would feel, but knew that my submissive heart would swell to obey him if he commanded such a thing.

One night he was in my bed and I was horny and playful. I wouldn't let the poor man sleep; I wanted to touch, rub, and tease him until he had to come. He warned me several times. He said that if I continued, I'd have to be punished . . . and I knew what that meant. With slight hesitation, I kept teasing him.

Adam grabbed my hair and told me that he wanted me on my knees in the shower. I was shaking as I crossed the room, excited and scared, but sure that he wouldn't really do it. He came after me with my digital camera in his hand. The fierce scowl that he often wore during sex filled his face and I couldn't meet his gaze. I huddled on the cold tub floor, my arms self-consciously wrapped around my body. He began to berate me for being such a horny bitch, such a dirty little whore, that I deserved such punishment.

My cheeks flushed and I scrunched my eyes closed. Adam commanded me to beg him to piss on me. I couldn't. He grew more insistent, and I stammered, nervous, barely whispering, as I begged in a tiny voice, "Please . . . please piss on me." He roared for me to ask louder. A tear rolled down my cheek as I forced out the words again.

Silent moments felt like minutes. I was sure he wouldn't do it, but he would leave me there suffering until he felt I had learned my lesson. As I whimpered, I felt the first stream hit my breasts, hotter than I expected. The smell and the feel made my head spin; I was overwhelmingly embarrassed that I was allowing such a thing. He moved the stream higher, up my chest and my neck. And yes, ultimately he continued, growling the whole time that I was a dirty slut who deserved to have a man piss right on her pretty face, as he did. Adam shot a couple of photographs, insisting I tilt my face up so the camera could witness my degradation.

I sat there dripping when he was done, shaking in humiliation. I could hear him as he stroked his cock, and within a minute he had added a layer of come to my wet face. The camera flashed again. I was in the deepest depths of subspace, rolled up inside myself, obedient and compliant, enduring whatever he wished. I hated it, but I loved the feeling of giving myself willingly and completely.

Adam stepped into the tub with me, turned on the water, and gathered me up into his arms. He kissed my messy face without hesitation, praised me for being such a good girl for him. He washed me as I remained speechless, stunned, but resurrected in his strong embrace. By the time we were both clean, I was able to kiss him back.

He dried us both and led me to bed, where he settled between my thighs and brought me to a screaming orgasm. We slept curled together as we rarely did, reassuring each other that the place we had gone was OK, because we had gone there together.

We re-enacted that scene a couple more times with equal potency. Each time brought us closer together in a way we didn't understand but didn't question. And, while I am in no hurry to ever do that with anyone else, sometimes, when I'm playing with myself, I'll remember the flood of conflicting emotions that he brought out in me, and I'll tumble through them in my mind again, always ending with a gut-tightening climax.

Master and commander
Thursday 4 December 2003

Relationships

My Master and I have gotten back in touch, which led me to ponder my hierarchy of affection. Master, Brian, Dante, friends, playmates, former lovers – they all have places in my heart, rarely overlapping yet not encroaching. My feelings toward each of them are distinct. I think it's time to tell you a little more about my Master; you've heard plenty about the others, yet this is probably the most unusual relationship of them all.

Ah, my Master! We barely communicate for months yet he can instantly move me, and vice versa. I love him in a submissive, somewhat daughterly way and also enjoy him as a friend and confidante. He called me a bitch for teasing him today when I sent some recent photos, and that made me shudder with impish pride at causing his arousal. He called me a good girl for giving him my new phone number and times to call, and I purred in delight. I can't wait to see him again. He established certain rules for me almost two and a half years ago and though we haven't been in touch recently, I have still kept within them. Why? Though he would never know of my transgressions, it simply wouldn't feel right to disobey him. He is my Master. I have released my responsibility for some decisions to him, and I thank him for taking that control through my obedience and eagerness to please. I trust him to act in my best interests, a trust he has earned, and not to damage my relationships with others. In the same way, I would never think of doing anything to interfere in the rest of his life. When we are together, he has treated me as both a princess and a whore – HIS princess and HIS whore – and I have felt sublime pleasure.

My Master is married and a father. He lives a couple thousand miles from me and is far less experienced in BDSM than I am, though he is naturally dominant with sadistic tendencies. Coincidentally, we hold very similar jobs, a topic upon which we have often commiserated. He is several years older than I am, well dressed, worldly, and strangely compelling. Even if he were not my Master, I would like him very much as a friend.

Ours is not a romantic relationship. I don't want him for my own, though if he were available and interested, I would certainly reconsider. What I feel with him cannot be compared to what I feel for others; it is in a different realm, neither higher or lower but utterly removed. I respond to my Master with my soul and my pussy more than my intellect and my heart. This isn't to say we don't have emotional and mental connections, but that he pulls the other parts of me like the moon pulls the tides. He makes me want things I never wanted, need things I never needed.

Can someone vanilla possibly understand this? I don't know. It is so hard to put into words, knowing that most of you will not be able to relate to what I write.

This man has brought me to tears of pain and humiliation for his pleasure. He has crooned words of support in my ear when my heart was breaking over another man. He has insisted I do things I hated and deny myself pleasures that I craved, never on a whim, but as a means of shaping me. He has fucked me, beaten me, kissed me, wined and dined me, and listened to endless rants about my job, love life, and family. He relishes my sexuality; I am not his slave or his sub, I am his slut, and he values me as such.

It occurs to me now that my Master's love feels closer to

unconditional than any of the others. I know that even if I broke his rules and disappointed him, there would be a chance for punishment, atonement, and acceptance. Ah hah! Oh, that makes so much sense, doesn't it? It is a role more paternal or godlike than that of a lover or boyfriend – though what transcendence is achieved when the heart and mind also come into play! Most "rules" aren't clear in vanilla relationships and if one of them is broken, there is no straightforward way for the aggrieved to get satisfaction or the transgressor to perform penance. With my Master, when I once broke his rules he took a day to determine my punishment. It was firm and pushed the boundary of what I considered fair, but though I wept in humiliation at the deed I had to perform, he did not relent until he was satisfied. When he was, the sin was erased. I was forgiven. I was back in his loving embrace, his good girl, once again with a blank slate.

I wonder if there is a way to bring the best of that into a relationship that involves less overt, or almost no, D/S. How relieved I would be to know, for example, that if I fell off the wagon and sucked a cock or two or eight when I was supposed to be monogamous, my husband would inflict a severe but reasonable consequence, after which my slip would never be mentioned or held against me again. Perhaps that's not possible. It is something I will consider, though.

My Master and I are writing to each other again, he plans to call me as soon as he can, and there was mention of a potential visit. My heart, mind, body, and spirit all are being nurtured now, through relationships with several wonderful men. It may not be perfect, but it's closer to complete than where I have been. I feel like a wilted flower that has been given the sunlight, water, and nutrients of which it was deprived, slowly lifting its head and tentatively opening its petals.

I don't care what we do
Friday 11 June 2004

Relationships

Today I found out that Dante is definitely moving away. That possibility has had me mildly upset for weeks, but it was still hard to blink back the tears when he told me it was certain. A couple days ago I provided a reference for his new job and was tempted to tell horrible lies so they would rescind the offer. Dante sighed when I told him and said he almost wished I had, so that he wouldn't have had to make the decision. But, much more money, a good quality of life, a promotion into an interesting and powerful job, and an escape from the hellpit that is our company proved too much to turn down.

The only solace I have right now is that he and his wife have lots of people in this area to come back and visit. I love the guy and I'm going to miss him so much. I did offer to go along as a maid, but I suppose his wife might object. Maybe if I threw in yardwork?

Excuse me while I go curl up in a bottle of chianti and get these tears out of my system.

Mistress Matisse

7/4/04

Today was a day where I really enjoyed myself at work. Two clients, both excellent regulars. The first of them was a very sweet man, over fifty, who has an infectious laugh and blue eyes that sort of twinkle when he's having fun. He's relatively new to me – meaning, less than a year – and I'm the first professional dominatrix he's seen. But he's taken to it like a duck to water and he's become a fan of rope bondage. That makes me happy, because I like doing it, and I don't get to so very often.

So he was laughing that unmistakable "wow, I'm really endorphin-high" laugh while I'm tying him up in various positions, and it made me laugh, too. I'm sure that if you asked some random person to describe what a session between a pro dom and her client might be like, they most likely wouldn't say, "Well, they'd probably laugh a lot." But it's not unusual. I like people who laugh when I'm playing with them, although my favorite thing is when I make them sort of laugh and wince at the same time.

My second client I've known for several years and, while he's also over fifty, he's kind of a health-and-fitness nut like I am, and he's so springy and muscular I think if you dropped him off a four-story building, he'd probably bounce. And he'd smile, because he's an unsinkably cheerful guy.

He likes intense sensation (pain, for those of you not up on this lingo) and we did some play with sounds. I'll now explain what "sounds" are, but if you squick easily, you should skip this next paragraph.

A sound is a medical instrument, a long slender metal rod that's designed to be inserted into the male urethra. (This is advanced play; please don't do this unless you've been taught by someone knowledgeable, or you could really damage someone's body.)

So there I was, sliding this metal rod into his dick, thinking, "What a magical thing this is." And that's how it seems to me when I'm playing – like it's magic. Like I'm magic. Like I'm magic. I love that I can do these intense things to people's bodies, and somehow, through some alchemical transformation, it's not a bad thing. Instead, it's wonderful. That's where the power comes from, for me. Not in making people endure something nasty – that's just bullying someone. No, the magic is doing fierce things to people and making them like it.

I can do that kind of magic.

15/4/04

The Thirty-Seconds Rule

There's an amusing scene in the 1983 movie *The Big Chill* in which actress Mary Kay Place is talking to Glenn Close about her experiences as a single woman evaluating men as potential boyfriends. She says, "It's gotten so I can tell in the first thirty seconds if there's a chance in the world."

Glenn Close reacts with disbelief, but I know exactly what Ms. Place's character means, because when I get a phone call from a potential client, I can tell in the first thirty seconds if there's a chance in the world.

Of course, some guys make it easy. Consider this fatuous ignoramus . . .

Ring Ring!
Me: Hello?
Caller: Well . . . good evening to you, pretty lady.

The caller is speaking in an extremely contrived "sexy" voice. It's the kind of voice you hear affected by radio DJs on "smooth jazz" stations – rather slow, and as deep and as resonant as he can possibly force it to be. Produces something of an *I'm-a-totally-Caucasian-guy-trying-to-sound-like-Barry-White* effect. I don't like it.

I wait to see if he's going to say something else. He doesn't. We're five seconds into the conversation, and he's off to a bad start. But I try again.

> **Me:** Good evening – can I help you?
> **Caller:** No, you can't. *(meaningful pause)* Because *I* want to be the one who helps *you*.

Now, what the hell am I supposed to say to that? He wants to help me? What is this, State Farm's sexy new telemarketing campaign?

> **Me:** Okaaay . . . So, are you calling about my ad?
> **Caller:** I'm calling because I think you're a beautiful woman, and I want to make something magic happen with you.

Great. It's not State Farm – it's David Copperfield! It's now been ten seconds, and I'm not liking this guy any more than I did five seconds ago. I still don't even know if he's actually a prospective client, or an obscene phone caller who likes to do a little foreplay. So I try the direct approach.

> **Me:** I'm afraid I don't understand: are you calling me because you'd like to see me professionally?
> **Caller:** What I'd like is to get together with you in front of my fireplace, put on some music, open up a bottle of wine, and just talk for a while. I think you and I should *(meaningful pause)* get to know each other. And then, I'd like to just *(meaningful pause)* see what happens.

I smother a snort of laughter, because I have an instant mental image of this guy lying hog-tied on the floor in front of a fireplace while I sit on the couch and drink wine with my feet propped up on his butt. I'd lean over and say to him, "See what happened?" But, as charming a fantasy as that is, I really don't want to do what it would take to make it come true. It's now been twenty seconds, and

I'm quite sure this guy is not client material – at least not for me. It's time to wind this up, so I give him a gentle little tap with Mistress Matisse's clue stick.

> **Me:** You know what, I think you've called the wrong woman. My name is Mistress Matisse, and I'm a dominatrix. It sounds like what you're looking for is an escort.
> **Caller:** No, I'm looking for a lady to *connect* with, and I think you're the one. You're not *afraid* to try something a little different, are you?

Afraid? *Afraid*? Oh – now he's done it. Now he's crossed a line, and now I know, for sure, that he is a complete asshole, and unworthy to be the recipient of my good manners. I really do not like it when people try to manipulate me so blatantly. Of course, I don't like when people try to manipulate me *subtly*, either – but at least it's not such an egregious fucking insult to my intelligence. It's time to mess with this guy's head a little, and his use of the word "afraid" has given me an idea.

> **Me:** (in a sexy voice) Well, now that you mention it . . .
> **Caller:** Yes, pretty lady?
> **Me:** (still in the sexy voice) Can I tell you a secret?
> **Caller:** Oh, yes – you can tell me *all* your secrets.
> **Me:** I **am** afraid. *(speaking louder and faster)* Terribly, terribly afraid. You see, I have a bad case of agoraphobia. I'm afraid to leave my house. I haven't been outside for weeks. It's very sad, and I'm actually very depressed about it. Deeply, intensely depressed. Maybe if I could just talk to you for a while about it, I'd feel better. You see, I think it all started early in my childhood – *(he attempts to break in, but I don't stop talking)* – when my parents made me take ballet lessons instead of tap, but my brother, he got to take tap, and I just felt so –

Click. He's gone.

I laugh.

16/4/04

I was going to post something last night . . . but a pleasant languor came over me, and writing seemed like too much exertion. I had spent several hours with one of my favorite clients, who we'll call Milo. (Not his real name.) I like playing with Milo for all the reasons that I generally like playing with anyone – he trusts me, he's open to new things, and he's got a high tolerance for pain. He's also a physically big guy, and I enjoy that about him. I'm five foot five and I weigh a hundred and twenty pounds, and there's something deeply satisfying about making someone who's at least nine inches taller and ninety pounds heavier than me roar like a lion singing an opera.

But there's more to it than that. Milo is one of a handful of clients with whom I have a certain connection. You see, in my sessions, one of two things can happen. The way it most often goes is that I create an experience for someone that sends them on a physical, emotional and psychological journey. Picture someone para-sailing – with me driving the boat. It's both an erotic and an artistic exercise for me, and I enjoy doing it.

Sometimes, though, it's different. I'm still creating the experience – but something happens along the way – and the wind catches me and whoosh, I'm up in the sky, too.

Last night I hooked my electrical box up to Milo's most sensitive places and stretched out on top of him like he was my own private chaise lounge. And then I turned up the dial until he bellowed.

It's such an amazingly intimate thing, to hold someone close to you while they're writhing and hissing in pain – pain that you are creating. I rubbed my cheek against his as his body shook with the stress of the electricity, and I looked in his eyes and told him how beautiful he was to me. I could have dialed down the intensity. I didn't. Each time the wave of electricity crested over him, his eyes opened wide and his muscles went hard underneath me. I put my face kiss-close to his and sucked the breath from his mouth like it was nitrous oxide.

In other conversations, Milo has told me that he admires my self-discipline. I wonder if he realizes that this is the school in which I learned it. Sadistic pleasure is an intoxicant, and I have taught myself to only take carefully calibrated sips. So before I really want to, I turn the dial back down again. But as soon as he can speak, Milo whispers, "Let's do it again, Mistress."

How could I refuse?

30/4/04

My Least Favorite Phone Call

Ring ring!
Me: Hello?
Caller: *(very irate-sounding female voice)* Who is this?

Oh shit. I really, really hate it when this happens.

Me: Who's calling, please?
Caller: No, tell me who this is, right now!
Me: *(in my very haughtiest tone)* I think you must have the wrong number. Goodbye. *Click.*

She'll call back, though. Ten seconds later –

Ring ring!
Me: Hello?
Caller: Look, I found this phone number on my boyfriend's cell phone and I want to know who this is!
Me: I have no idea who you are or what you're talking about –
Caller: *(interrupts)* His name is John Doe – do you know him? Is he seeing you?

I don't recognize the name, or the number she's calling from, thank God. I'm glad it's not one of my regular boys. It's probably some poor guy who's curious enough to call me, but who got nervous and hung up when I answered. I get a lot of that. But my number got saved in his outgoing-calls log, and she's checking up on him.

Me: *(slowly)* I don't know who you are, I don't know your boyfriend, and I want you to stop calling me.

Caller: Why is your number on his phone? I want to know who this is!

Jesus Christ, she's positively shrieking into the phone. I hold it away from my head to keep my eardrums from being shattered. According to Caller ID, this call is coming from an area code in another state. That's good thing: if this woman was local she'd probably start stalking me or something, the way she's going on.

I know other sex workers also get this type of phone call. Several of them have techniques they swear by for dealing with it. One of them claims to be an insurance agent, another one pretends to work for a car dealership. If this was a call about a client I knew, I'd be more apt to start spinning some kind of folksy, non-threatening yarn, based on trivia I'd picked up about the guy. "Oh, a girlfriend of mine works with Joe down at the real estate office, and she gave me his number. My husband and I are thinking about buying a timeshare in Mexico, and she said ya'll had one. We just wanted to ask – have ya'll had any problems drinking the water down there? Because those salesmen, they won't tell you about stuff like that, and we don't want to be – you know – *having a problem*, especially with the kids and all . . . I'd left Joe a message and he must have tried to call me back."

But, with nothing to build on, trying to concoct a plausible story seems like a real long shot. Besides, I hate lying. The minute you lie to someone, you become emotionally involved with them, and I don't want to get involved with either one of these people.

She continues to harangue me without seeming to draw breath, bouncing back and forth between demands for my identity and telling me what a low-life piece of scum her beloved boyfriend is. After about sixty seconds she notices that I've stopped speaking.

Caller: Hello? Hello?

I say nothing.

Caller: I know you're there! Tell me who this is!

I still say nothing. It seems like the best solution. If I hang up, she'll just call back. I could let it go to voicemail, but that'll give her

more information than I want her to have – like my name, for
starters.

This woman sounds rather young – not as savvy as other
suspicious lovers who've called me. I remember one woman
who called and asked, "Do you do incall or outcall?"

Her flat, hard tone of voice tipped me off. "I'm afraid I don't
know what you're talking about."

She wasn't fooled. "I know what you are. If I find your number
on my phone bill again, I'll call the police and report you."

Report me for what? I thought. Being attractive to your partner?
Lady, if you think the police don't know about me, you're crazy.
They know about everybody. We have ads in the paper, for God's
sake.

It's not that I can't feel some sympathy for a woman who,
underneath the bluster, is scared. But I don't break up couples.
None of my clients who have wives/girlfriends has ever left their
partner for me, and none ever will, because I wouldn't allow any of
them to become emotionally involved with me to the extent where
that would seem like a reasonable idea. I am not the problem in
someone else's relationship, and I'm not willing to take the blame
for someone else's fears, be they based on reality or imagination. If
you're angry with your lover, yell at him, not me.

Are they cheating? Is it infidelity even if one doesn't have sex?
I don't know. I know these boys are keeping their time with me
a secret. They tell me their partners don't share their interest in
BDSM, but they feel it's better to stay in the relationship, and
satisfy their desire for kink elsewhere. I'm polyamorous, so I
understand that, while their partners don't fulfill this particular
need, that doesn't mean they don't love them and want to be
with them. I wish they felt they could be honest, but I have to
respect their right to make their own choices. Who am I to
judge? I haven't been hitched to someone for twenty-plus years,
with kids and a mortgage and 401K and a shitload of shared
history, both good and bad. I have no idea what I'd do in their
circumstances. I'll leave the slick superficial snap-judgments to
Dr Phil.

This caller, though, is sounding more like a candidate for Jerry
Springer. I lay the phone down on my desk and listen as her voice,
rendered tolerable by distance, clicks and hisses on. Gradually it

stops. The display switches from "End" to "Menu", indicating she's hung up. I wait to see if she'll call back.

She doesn't. Thank god. I pick up the phone and save the number into my phone book as: IRATEGF.

But the phone beeps admonishingly at me.

"IRATEGF" ALREADY EXISTS. REPLACE?

Christ. Okay, let's try IRATEGF2.

SAVED.

If only it were just that easy.

28/4/04

A Near Goddess Experience

You know you're a seasoned professional when conversations like this don't throw you.

> *Ring ring!*
> **Me:** Hello?
> **Caller:** Namaste, Beautiful Goddess.

I am deeply suspicious. I've taken yoga classes, so I know what "nah-mah-stay" means. But you see, gentlemen, when a potential new client calls me and we talk, what I'm doing is assessing him to see if he's going to fit smoothly into my system. So when I pick up the phone, and I expect the person on the other end to say hello, and instead they give me a Hindu greeting . . . Well, it makes me wonder in what other ways this person might not be what I expect — or want. The lesson is: do not strive to be unusual in your initial approach to professional ladies like myself. At this stage of the game, your manner should indicate to us that you will be a reassuringly familiar experience. Wait until later to start being unique.

> **Me:** Namaste. Can I help you?
> **Caller:** I have been reading your column and meditating about you for some time, Oh Goddess, and I wish to come to you so that our souls can be one.

Hmmnn, I don't recall "soul uniting" being on my published list of kinky specialties. I don't think this one's going to be a keeper. However, we'll keep an open mind about this for a little while longer. One would hate to throw out the pervert with the bathwater over what might be a purely semantic issue.

> **Me:** Well, I'm not entirely sure what you mean by that. My name is Mistress Matisse. I'm a dominatrix. Is that what you're looking for?
> **Caller:** You are the earthly embodiment of The Supreme Goddess. I wish to serve you.
> **Me:** O-kay . . . So, if I saw you, exactly how is it that you would serve me?
> **Caller:** I would anoint your feet and kiss them clean, Oh Goddess.
> **Me:** That sounds nice. What else?
> **Caller:** I wish to enter into a sacred space with you, Oh Goddess, and be purified by your whip. And then, when I have proved myself worthy, I beseech you to allow our souls to join together in ecstasy.

I consider what he's said. This "Goddess" thing he's into is not my usual style, but I might be able to work with it. There's that bit about souls joining together in ecstasy, though – that's worth clarifying.

> **Me:** You do realize I am not a full-service escort, don't you?
> **Caller:** Yes, Oh Goddess, you who are the source of all power, I know that I am but an unworthy slave who must never raise his eyes above your divine feet.

Well, he's going to have to raise his eyes above my feet at some point, or he may fall down my stairs.

> **Me:** What's your name?
> **Caller:** Clifford, Oh Goddess.

I have to hold the phone away for a moment because I'm giggling. *Clifford?* I mean, it's a perfectly nice name, I just would have expected something like – Ayodhya. Or Jafar. Something a bit more in keeping with this half-Eastern-spirituality, half-Goddess-worship kink he's got going on. But no matter.

Me: So, Clifford, you do know that my fee is 250 dollars for a one-hour session?

There's a pause. *Oh, see, here it comes,* I thought.

Caller: My Goddess, I wish to offer you tribute, but I am very poor.

Figures the religious type would be broke, doesn't it? This guy's problem is that he doesn't have his own television show. He's not the first one to call me and plead poverty in the hopes of a discount. However, this kind of charitable donation is not tax-deductible.

Me: *(in a pleasant but unencouraging tone)* Oh, that's too bad.
Caller: Oh, my Goddess? Your slave would ask you a question.
Me: Go ahead.
Caller: Does the Goddess permit her slaves to make their tribute by credit card?

I toy with telling him he could offer me cattle and casks of wine, just to see what he'd say, but he shows every sign of being dead serious about this Goddess thing, so I skip it. The last thing I need is some guy showing up on my doorstep with a heifer and a couple of cases of chardonnay.

Me: No, the Goddess requires cash.
Caller: Oh Gracious Goddess, would you be willing to allow your slave to visit you for a lesser tribute?

Part of me is strongly tempted to blast him with some Goddess-y indignation. "Offer ME lesser tribute, will you, puny mortal? For that, you shall be chained to a rock so that crows can pluck out your liver! Mwah ha ha ha haaa!"

Jesus, this schtick of his is infectious. Stay focused, Matisse.

Me: No, Clifford, I can't do that, I'm afraid.
Caller: *(makes sound of distress)* Oh Beautiful Goddess, I am forced to delay my visit to pay you homage.
Me: That's a shame. Well, Clifford, call me back when you're ready.
Caller: Oh Goddess, may I meditate about you in the meantime?

Meditate, huh? I've never heard it called *that* before.

1/6/04

How I Met Jae

I've talked about my friend and play partner Jae here before. But I haven't told you the story of how we met, and I should, because it's unusual . . . We met on the job, as it were. A mutual client introduced us.

You see, about eight years ago, I had a client who I think I'll call Mystery Guy, or MG. The reason I call him that is that, although I saw him pretty regularly for several years, I had very little knowledge of who he was. By that I mean: I didn't know what, if anything, he did for a living. I don't think he was married, although I'm not positive. I used to go see him on his yacht, and I think that's where he lived, but I couldn't swear to that, either. Usually you can tell something about someone by their home, but this boat, while luxurious, was so impersonal that it could have been a hotel suite. There was no personal clutter around, no clues as to his interests or hobbies, no pictures of friends or family, nothing. Sort of odd.

MG himself was odder still. He was a nice-enough-looking guy, late forties, tall and with a somewhat imposing presence. His WASPy looks and his to-the-manor-born demeanor, combined with his slightly lock-jawed, *Thurston-Howell-the-III* accent, lead me to believe he came from a wealthy background, probably in the northeast somewhere. But when he took off his clothes, he had several large and pretty nasty-looking scars on his body. Some were quite old, and some were well-healed but clearly newer, and somehow none of them seemed like scars from, say, surgery.

"Wow, what happened to you?" I asked.

He gave me the kind of look Dick Cheney gives to impertinent reporters at White House press conferences. *O-kay*, I thought, *I get the message: don't ask. But I'd hate to see the other guy.*

I wouldn't say I ever really trusted MG – there was just something about him that set off my *don't-turn-your-back-on-this-one* alert. But, session after session, he continued to play by the rules, and his money was certainly green. So I always kept my eyes open, and my wits about me, and we didn't have any problems.

One day he called me up.

"Jamie, babe," he said. (I've had a number of names in my career – Jamie was the one he knew me by.) "Listen, I've got a lady friend, a sweet little submissive girl, and I think she'd like to meet you. And I'd love to see what you do with her. Want to get together?"

"Sure," I replied.

"Great. But Jamie, babe, when you get here, don't tell her you're, you know, *a professional*. We'll just let her think you're a friend of mine, all right?"

"Sure, MG, no problem."

The day of the appointment found me knocking at MG's door. He slid it open.

"Jamie, babe, come on in." I climbed onto the boat and stepped down into the cabin.

Sitting on the couch was a small, fair-skinned girl, with large blue eyes, and red hair of a shade definitely not found anywhere in nature – and not many places outside of it, either. She was wearing a short black dress with a plunging neckline, fishnet stockings and black boots. She had a rather large purse close beside her.

I took exactly one look at her and thought: *Oh, "friend", my ass. She's fucking working, same as I am.*

It's hard to explain how I knew that immediately. I mean, it wasn't like she had the words "call girl" tattooed on her forehead. And she didn't look like the traditional conception of a hooker – not that many prostitutes do. What she looked like was a Capitol Hill chick on her way to go dancing at Re-Bar. But there's just an energy about women in the business that one learns to recognize instinctively.

Why didn't he just tell me he wanted to have another working girl here? I thought. *I wouldn't care.* But it didn't really matter to me. If

MG wanted us to pretend we weren't professionals, I had no objections. And after another look, I thought: *Besides, she's pretty cute.*

"Jamie, this is Jae. Jae, meet my friend Jamie."

She met my eye and smiled, and I saw her look me up and down, and smile even more.

She's clocked me, too, I thought. *And she doesn't care either.*

We made small talk for a few minutes. Jae went downstairs to use the bathroom and MG slipped me an envelope with my fee, which I tucked away into my purse. When she retuned, MG said, in his Martha's-Vineyard drawl, "Jamie, babe, I've been telling Jae here how dominant you are, and she's been all excited to meet you."

Sounds like he's been a regular of hers, too, I thought. Aloud I simply said, "Reeaally . . ." and regarded Jae with an arched eyebrow.

"Oh, yeah," she replied, cocking her head to one side and grinning at me widely. "MG thinks you're pretty good." There was a definite come-and-get-me lilt to her voice.

Huh, this might be more fun than I thought. I believe this girl might genuinely enjoy getting roughed up a little bit. I had come prepared to just do a little light slap and tickle with a nervous wanna-be, but I was reading Jae as ready for a bit more than that. I studied her face for another moment: her eyes were a little dilated. *Oh yeah, this might go just fine.*

We adjourned to the lower cabin, the bedroom. MG stepped into the head, leaving us alone in the room for a moment. Jae slipped off her dress and tossed it carelessly over the back of a chair. The fishnet hose turned out to be an entire fishnet bodysuit – with no crotch, of course. I also slipped off my street clothes, under which I was wearing the traditional black bra, corset and garter-belt outfit. And then, at more or less at the same time, we both opened up our purses and started pulling out the tools of our trade.

We both had small zippered makeup bags stuffed with condoms and a small bottle of lube. Her condoms, I noticed, were the flavored ones. In addition, I had wide leather wrist cuffs, some black-painted clothespins, a leather paddle – fake fur on one side, nickel studs on the other – and a silicone butt plug, all of which I placed on one of the two bedside tables. Then I looked across the bed and watched Jae unpack her bag of tricks. She had two dildos –

one was bubble-gum pink, with silver glitter swirled into it. The other was black, and so improbably large that I could only assume it was a conversation piece – or possibly a bludgeon, if Jae's clients got out of hand. She set in on its base, pointing up, so that it wobbled gently in the air as if seeking a home. She also had a dual control vibrator, with a molded bunny incorporated into it – the kind with the ears that twitch against one's clit. *Good taste in toys. That's nice.*

She finished setting out her paraphernalia and looked across at me, and at the things I'd laid out. We met each other's eye, and then, without saying a word, we both started laughing, because we were both thinking the same thing: *Oh, no, we're not working girls – not at all! We just dress like this and carry this kind of stuff around with us all the time! Doesn't every woman?* Our laughter was redolent with a shared understanding of the absurdity of the situation, in that moment, a connection was made.

And then MG came back, and the three of us got on the bed, and thus began what was quite possibly my worst professional performance in my career to date. Because I put the cuffs on Jae, and I got her on her knees with her ass in the air, and something happened. It was as if some electrical circuit was suddenly completed. I knew exactly what I wanted to do with her, and what's more, I knew how she would respond. There was no hesitation in her, and none in me. As we say in BDSM circles, we just *went there.*

But MG – well, we rather forgot about MG. The chemistry between us was so absorbing that he just faded from our awareness. I wouldn't have thought that was possible. MG definitely wasn't a man around whom I felt I could let down my guard. And, too, I have always taken great pride in the fact that I am very good at what I do. I always give 100 percent to my sessions – anyone who's a client of mine deserves that.

Except – that time I didn't.

I mean, we must have done *something* with him – I can't believe we were so lost to etiquette as to totally ignore our basic responsibilities. (Nor do I believe that MG would have meekly accepted being completely pushed to the side.) But I'm damned if I remember anything about it. However, I have vivid memories of Jae's butt turning redder and redder as I spanked it, of how her cunt felt around my four fingers, and of how hard I had to pull Jae's hair to get her mouth off my clit when it had become too sensitive to be touched.

Afterwards, the two of us got dressed again in a pregnant silence. MG was still lying on the bed, looking a trifle sullen. Jae and I looked at him and exchanged glances, and she gave a half-embarrassed shrug. I mouthed the words *oh, well*. The Goddess of Sex Workers would have to spot us this one dereliction of duty.

We made our farewells to MG and left the boat together. The synchronized click of our high heels on the marina dock echoed off the water as we walked side by side.

"Been seeing him long?" I asked.

"Yeah, a couple of months. You?"

"About a year, maybe a little more."

We were playing with the words, each of us wondering who'd admit to being a professional first. Click, click, click, click.

"So," she said, glancing up at me from under the assertively red fringe of her bangs. "You work for a service or by yourself?"

I laughed at her boldness. "For myself. And so do you."

"How do you know?"

"You didn't get a call-out, and we were there for more than the hour."

"Yeah, you're right. How much do you get for the hour?"

"Two hundred. And you?"

"The same."

"Probably a good thing we got the money up front this time." She gave a small, breathy laugh. "Seriously."

I shrugged. "He'll call back. We can make it up to him."

"I bet he won't do another double with us, though."

"No, I would imagine not."

There was that odd mixture of connection and shyness between us that happens sometimes after one has had an intensely intimate experience with a stranger. As we reached the top of the dock, she pivoted and stood in front of me, leaning one-handed against the marina gate like an old-movie Lothario.

"So —" she began, and then seemed to stumble over what she'd meant to say. "I – uh, I mean, so do you —"

I laughed and pulled out a card case from my bag. "Here's my number. Call me."

"Cool! I mean – yeah, I definitely will."

"Good." I smiled at her and strolled away. As I got into my car and started the engine, my headlights picked her out moving across the parking lot. She turned and waved.

I arrived home and walked through the door to find my lover sitting on the couch. He looked up at me. "Hi honey – everything go okay?"

"Just fine."

"Oh, some girl just called for you a few minutes ago – she said her name was Jae? I didn't recognize her voice, do you know who that is?"

I smiled. "Yes, darlin' – I know *exactly* who that is."

7/5/04

The date says Friday but to me it's still Thursday night . . .

Two good clients today, both regulars – the blue-eyed rope bondage lover with the infectious laugh, and a guy from Vermont with a sweet nature and a very tough ass.

I did a partial suspension with Blue Eyes – a hog-tie on the floor, with lines going to a point in the ceiling. There was a lot of tension on his arms and shoulders, but he just laughed happily. So did I. We always have a good time together.

Vermont is a fairly new client to me – I think this was his third visit. I'm discovering that he's quite delightfully masochistic, with a nice high pain threshold. When I'm with a new person, I'm so used to carefully modulating the level of physical intensity that when I began flogging his ass, it took me a few minutes to trust what I was seeing: that he could really take the heavier blows.

So I traded my soft suede flogger for a heavier, stiffer one. He took a few thumps with that and just smiled and wiggled his butt at me invitingly. *Oh, this is going to be fun*, I thought.

He took half an hour of pretty steady beating with my nastiest, meanest flogger. It's got thick tails made out of rubber instead of the usual leather, and it bites – hard. It usually falls into the category of "Tired Top Toys". A TTT is a toy you get out when you're the top and you're playing with a bottom whose capacity to absorb intense physical sensation (read: pain) is just flat wearing you out. You're sweating, you're panting, your arm is getting sore –

but you don't want to wimp out before the bottom does. Heaven forbid, your reputation as a sadist would be ruined! So you get out the nasty-mean toy – the one that will, after just a few strokes, make them say "Mercy!"

That's all very tongue-in-cheek, of course. I wasn't trying to make Vermont end the scene, I was having far too good a time. I was swinging that whip like Babe Ruth and he just kept smiling and holding his ass out for me.

When I decided his butt had had enough, I lay down on my bondage table and had him take off my high boots, and he kissed and caressed my feet and legs. I could really spend a whole hour just doing that, because having my feet kissed and touched is very high on the list of "Things Mistress Matisse Really, Really Likes". Every foot-kisser has a slightly different style. Vermont did it like a man playing a woodwind instrument – subtle, delicate, with his fingers moving in sensual counterpoints to his mouth.

I love my life.

5/5/04

Sexual Darwinism At Work

Some guys do everything but cut off their own penis to ensure that they will not meet women and have relationships, and perhaps that's a good thing, because then they'll be unable to breed. Consider this example . . .

> *Ring Ring!*
> **Me:** Hello?
> **Caller:** Um, hi, is this Mistress May-**tiss**-ee? (He rhymes the middle syllable with *piss*.)
> **Me:** My name is pronounced Mah-teese.

Makes a good impression right off the bat, doesn't he? I didn't pick this name by accident, you know. I'm fond of old Henri's drawings and paintings, and I like the way the M's and the sibilants flow together, but I also chose it because if you don't know how to pronounce it, that's going to tell me a lot about you immediately.

Caller: So, um, I'm calling about your ad?
Me: Yes, what questions do you have that I can answer for you?
Caller: Well, I don't have very much money.

Great. The Thirty-Seconds Rule proves itself again. He pauses, perhaps waiting for me to launch into the pitch for my May Masochistic Madness Sale. Except I'm not having a May Masochistic Madness sale, or any other kind of sale, ever. So instead I say . . .

Me: That's not a question – that's a statement.
Caller: So what I was really looking for was a relationship. I was wondering if you'd be willing to have a relationship with me.

You know I'm about to slice this guy into bite-sized literary hors d'oeuvres for your bloodthirsty reading pleasure. But, before the filleting begins, I will just pause and acknowledge two things that this person kind of, sort of, almost didn't do wrong.

1. He did, at least, get right to the point without wasting oodles of my time (translation: five minutes) making me believe he might be a viable client.

2. I do believe that if you want something, it's important to put your desire out to the universe. If you keep it all inside and don't acknowledge it out loud, it's much less likely to happen.

Now then: What the *fuck* could possibly have gone through this man's head to make him think that I could possibly have any kind of positive reaction to this question?

Maybe he was thinking that in spite of the fact that men find me attractive enough to give me money for my erotic attentions, I might still be a sad, lonely girl who never gets asked out any dates, and that I would thus be ready to start talking about having a relationship with a total fucking stranger after twenty seconds on the telephone. Especially with someone like him, who is clearly pursuing me for my rich intellectual and spiritual qualities, and who would *never* hit on me just because I'm a hot babe and he'd like me to fulfill his sexual fantasies for free.

But that can't be right, he'd have to be a moron to think that. Oh, wait, now I see how that works. He *is* a moron.

I'm so, well, flabbergasted by this bold-faced stupidity that I just say . . .

Me: No. No, I'm not looking for a relationship.
Caller: Are you sure? I've got a lot to offer.

I swear to God that's what he said. "A lot to offer." To a therapist? Yes, he's probably got a lot to offer. To a comedy writer, definitely. I have no earthly idea what he thinks he's got to offer to me, since we've established that it isn't money, and I'm quite sure that it isn't a keenly analytical mind or rapier-like social sophistication.

Me: *(more firmly)* I am quite sure. Goodbye.
Click.

What's the lesson here? Number one – don't call up sex workers and ask them for (non-professional) dates. It's amazing to me that I would have to tell anyone that.

Number two – and this applies to all socio-sexual situations: don't ask a stranger if they want to have a relationship with you. Ask a stranger if they want to have coffee with you. Or, in the appropriate circumstances, ask them if you can give them a blow-job, or they'll give you a spanking, or whatever else seems to go with the surroundings. But if you go around asking strangers to have a relationship, your sex life is going to be extinct.

10/5/04

I had dinner at Hana with Miss K a few days ago. I don't recall if I've mentioned this, but Miss K is an independent call girl. So whenever we do dinner, it's an opportunity to have a Bitch-About-Work Fiesta. We both like what we do, but sometimes you just have to vent to someone who gets it.

"Okay, who gets to go first?" I asked.

"Oh, I think that would have to be – ME!" she answered

"Ooo, that good, huh? Well, let me have it, baby."

"Fuckin' A, the weirdo I saw this week – you won't believe what he did."

I start laughing a little already, just watching her head do that snakelike swivel of outrage. Miss K has a background in theatre, and it shows: her eyes, her hands, her shoulders – they all eloquently express her total disdain for this man who dared offend her. When all six feet of an irritated Amazon queen gets going, it's better than a floor show. I love having such entertaining friends.

"So, it was a new guy, and he sounded a little weird on the phone, but not scary-weird, just no-social-skills-weird."

I understand this perfectly. It's nice when one gets to see sophisticated men as clients, but frankly, if it weren't for guys with no social skills, there'd be a lot of hungry sex workers in the world.

"He arrives for the appointment ten minutes early." We share a grimace. We hate it when people are early, since we're always flying around getting ready until the last possible moment.

"I have him sit down on the couch in the living room and ask him to wait for a few minutes. I leave the room for, oh, maybe five minutes. When I come back into the room –" she leans forward for emphasis "– he's rearranging all my fucking furniture."

"You're kidding me?"

"I'm serious. He's moved the couch and coffee table, and he's got the edge of the area rug, and he's pulling on it."

I sit there silently for a moment, picturing this. "That's bizarre."

"Oh – and did I mention he's naked?"

I give a whoop of laughter. "No!"

She gestures with her hands to indicate that she can find no words to express her incredulity. I try to stop laughing, not because it offends her – we always play these kinds of incidents for laughs with each other – but because it's so outré that I have to say: "So you asked him what the hell he was doing, right?"

"Oh, yes," she says, with a rising inflection that bodes ill for the nude furniture mover.

"Yes, I asked him what he was doing. And he told me – get ready for this – he told me that *in his fantasy*, the room was arranged differently."

I can hardly speak for laughing. "He – he – he had a fantasy about *your living room furniture*?" I really don't know what the staff at

Hana must make of our conversations. I'm sure they think we are very, very strange.

"Apparently he felt it was important."

"Okay, you win the prize for weirdest person of the week. So what did you do?"

"Well, I just stood there for a minute and gave him a look. And then I told him that he shouldn't have moved my furniture without permission, and he apologized. And then I asked him if the way that *I* looked more or less fit with his fantasy, because I really wasn't interested in having him try to rearrange *me*."

"Oh, good one."

"So he apologized again, and –" she shrugged "– we did the date."

Of course she did because, for all her show of indignation, Miss K has the generosity of spirit to forgive faux pas like these. It's one of the traits that makes her a good friend, and I also consider it essential to being a good sex worker. Yeah, it's great to have a good figure and a pretty face and the technical skills that go along with your particular specialty. But if you don't have some kindness and compassion to give your clients, they'll feel that, and a lot of them won't come back. That's true in any branch of the sex industry – even mine.

8/6/04

Dear Mistress Matisse,
In your blog, you only talk about how nice your clients are and what a good time you have with them. Isn't this a bit unrealistic? I'm a dancer, and I get a lot of asshole customers at my job. Surely you have clients you dislike, or who do things that annoy you?

Not for more than one session, I don't. I've danced myself, so I do know what that's like, and I agree, there's a pretty high asshole ratio there. But it's a whole different situation for me. I can pick and choose who I'm going to see, and I'm good at sussing out who I'd like and enjoy playing with over the phone.

However, there is one type of client who, in the past, has annoyed me – and in one case, seriously pissed me off. It took me longer to learn how to spot them early on. That's because what they do is subtle – they aren't dangerous or blatantly disrespectful, they don't disobey the rules, or try to get me to do things I don't wish to do. They are the guys I call *Mr Defensive*. I've learned not to waste my time with clients like this. It's not that I've met that many of them – just a few, really. But having even one in the regular roster is too many.

Mr Defensive's problem is that he's deeply conflicted about what he's doing. Getting off on being submissive doesn't fit his image of himself, and he's unable to let go of that and just say, "What the fuck – I don't know why, but it makes my dick hard, so I'm just going to do it and enjoy it. It's got nothing to do with who I am in the rest of my life. It's just for fun." Mr Defensive hates himself for his desires. He brings all that self-hatred into the dungeon with him, projects his negative attitudes about what we're doing onto me, and then spends the entire session responding to them. He doesn't seem to be enjoying himself at all, he doesn't believe that I like what I do, and after the session is over I can feel him trying to psychologically distance himself from what he's just done as fast as he can. Usually he'll do that by making disparaging remarks about what freaky weirdoes my other clients must be. The subtext clearly being "*I'm not one of those people*". It's the kind of energy that makes me close the door behind someone and say to myself, "Thank you, *God*, that's over."

I'm always amazed when Mr Defensives call me back for another session, because it's so clear to me that it's *just not working*. But they usually do. The urge is all the stronger for them trying to forbid it to themselves.

Ultimate Mr Defensive moment: there was a client I'd been seeing for a year or so. He was so extremely defensive that it was impossible to have any kind of connection with him. (It was only barely possible to have a conversation with him.) But he kept calling, and I kept doggedly trying to create a scene with him that I, at least, could feel good about. I tried every toy, every type of sensation, every role play I could think of – and that's a lot. It never worked, and every time he left I swore I wouldn't book with him again. But a few weeks would go by, and he'd call, and I'd mentally vacillate for a minute and give in. *He's not a bad guy – maybe he just needs more time to trust me before he can really let go. I'll give him another chance.* Soft-hearted? Maybe – but I also just hate to lose, and admitting I couldn't really get this man to embrace the experience he said he wanted felt like losing.

I was about three-fourths of the way through a session with the Mr Defensive in question. I had him tied down to my bondage table on his back, and I was preparing to do some electrical play with him. He looked up at me and said, "Can I ask you a question?" This was a common ploy of this guy – he would try to try to regain some sense of control by asking me questions like, "Why do you think you like doing this?" It was his way of sabotaging the mood and the flow of the scene, and an attempt to put *me* on the defensive by making me explain myself. Usually I would say, "Let's talk about it later," and just go on with what I was doing.

But that day he said, "So, why do you think you hate men so much?"

I stood there and stared at him for a moment, and then I turned around and walked out of the room. I was so angry that for a moment, I could hardly see. *Why do you hate men so much?* This, when I've been knocking myself out trying to make something happen for this asshole, this is what he gives back to me? I pour my positive energy into these sessions with him, try to give him an experience that's good for him even though he's resisting it all the way, and he has the nerve to tell me I hate men? How dare he? How dare he! *Fuck, I should show him what a scene with someone who hates men would look like.* It was the only time in my career when I was really tempted, just for a second, to hurt someone in a non-consensual way.

I sat on the couch in my reception room and took a deep breath, trying to calm down. *Don't let him get to you,* I told myself. *Don't let him dump his shit on you. Get your boundaries up, girl. What he says, what he thinks – it's got nothing to do with you, and you know it. It's all about the bullshit in his head. Breathe, and let it go.*

Through the curtains into the playroom, I could hear him breathing and stirring restlessly on the table. "Mistress?" he called out.

"Don't talk."

Now, the question was: untie him and kick him out immediately – or finish the session?

My first impulse was to throw him out, pronto. Then I thought, *But then he wins. He's trying to get control by making me lose my cool. He's trying to make himself feel powerful by emotionally manipulating me. I'm not going to let him make me react like that.*

A few more deep breaths, and I walked back into the dungeon. "The Mistress has decided she doesn't like you talking," I announced. "So we'll just fix that right now." I took a large gag and put it into his mouth, and then I went on with the rest of the session I'd planned. I got him out the door without any conversation afterwards. And, the next time he called, I refused to book with him.

18/6/04

Legend In His Own Mind

Ring ring!
Me: hello?
Caller: Is this Mistress Matisse?
Me: Yes, it is.
Caller: I'm calling about your ad, but I'm not a submissive. My name *(dramatic pause)* is Master Ryker Blackstar.

I've met enough pompous twits in my time to know one when I hear one. "Master Ryker Blackstar", my ass. I live to stick pins in people like this.

Me: Are you calling to sell me long-distance service?
Caller: No!
Me: Oh, I'm so sorry, I must have misunderstood. What is it I can help you with?
Caller: I wanted to ask you some questions. How long have you been in business?
Me: Several years.
Caller: And who did you train under?

Who did I train under? Oh, give me a break. I'm really tempted to say something like, "Well, I worked with Ah-nuld on the weight training, but Jane Fonda advised me on my cardiovascular routine."

Me: Why are you asking me this?

Caller: Well, it's just that we've never heard of you.

We've never heard of you? Am I speaking to someone with Multiple Personality Disorder? Great. At least one of his personalities must have heard of me, though. Otherwise, how would he know to call me?

Me: Who is "we"?

Caller: A group of us . . . So, who trained you as Mistress?

Me: No one person trained me; I'd been in the community for years before I became a professional.

Caller: Ah. So you're not affiliated with anyone?

Affiliated with anyone? What am I, a fucking credit union or something? I have no idea where he's going with this.

Me: No – and again, why are you asking me these questions?

Caller: Well, as I said – we've just never heard of you.

Me: Well, I've never heard of you, either, and I still don't understand why you called me. What is it that you want, exactly?

Caller: Do you give tours of your dungeon?

Me: No. *(Not to people who annoy me, anyway.)* Why do you want a tour of my dungeon?

Caller: We're just wondering what kind of facilities you have.

Me: Okay, who is this "we" you keep talking about?

Caller: There's a group of us.

Me: Yes, you said that already. Are you some kind of BDSM organization? Because if you're looking for a dungeon to rent for parties, I don't do that, sorry.

Caller: No, no, no. We're not *that* kind of BDSM organization. We have our own dungeon. You see, I am the head of a very private and selective BDSM house. It's called "The House Of Blackstar".

Ah, so Mr Blackstar is one of those "House of . . ." people. That explains a lot. When someone in the BDSM world says "I'm part of the House Of Somebody", what he means is he's part of a group of leather people who've declared themselves to be something like a family or a small clan. They may or may not actually live together, but they usually have a single authority figure, and they usually have some kind of formal structure and hierarchy. And they're usually a bunch of pretentious, self-important jackasses.

Not always, now, not always. I've met some cool people who had a chosen leather family and who called themselves the "House of . . ." whatever. The "House Of Gord" folks, for example, are great.

But in this case, my sense is that it's sheer self-aggrandizing crap. I'm betting that "The House Of Blackstar" consists of Ryker – whose real name is probably Eugene – his pet iguana, Frodo, and several plump, shy, "cyber-submissive" girls who live in very small towns at least five hundred miles away from here. Call it a hunch.

> **Me:** I'm going ask you one more time – what do you want from me?
> **Caller:** Well, we'd have to check you out more thoroughly. But provided you meet with our standards, I'm prepared to offer you an affiliation with our house.
> **Me:** No, thank you.
> **Caller:** What? But –
> **Me:** I don't want to be affiliated with anyone. So if that's all, then I'll say goodbye.
> **Caller:** Wait a minute, I think you're making a mistake. The House of Blackstar is connected with some of the best Houses in the world.
> **Me:** Really? Like, The White House?
> **Caller:** (huffily) No, I mean some of the best *secret European Houses*!

Oh, God, no – not the "secret European Houses" thing. This story is like the Loch Ness Monster of the BDSM community. The basic storyline of the fable goes something like this: There are secret "Story of O" type places in Europe where mysterious people train eager slaves in some brand of BDSM that's more pure and true than ours. Then they sell these slaves to other members of this secret society, where they have many erotic adventures. (Sounds *just* like a porn novel, doesn't it?) These houses have been in continuous existence since the nineteenth century or even earlier, and lots of famous and important people belong to these secret societies, as Masters and Mistresses. They can do that without fear of exposure, you see, because these houses/societies are very, very secret. Nobody knows about them.

Except, of course, all the pathological liars who claim to be connected with them in order to get laid and look important, and the people they tell their lies to. And, of course, folks like me, who tell other people what a flock of bullshit it is, and laugh at those who try to spin me this story. That all amounts to a pretty large group – so it's hard to imagine how they'd really be much of a secret anymore.

So, just for the record: there ain't no such thing. There are plenty of very kinky people in Europe, there are some great events and organizations there, and I'm sure that there are people forming "Houses" of their own. But there are no ages-old secret European slave-trading societies that train people in some magical method of BDSM. Trust me, I'd know.

> **Caller:** If we were affiliated, we could send you submissives for training. You see, I'm forming my own secret House here.

And he's calling up people he claims not to have heard of to *tell* them about this secret House of his. Hey, it's good that he's getting a head start on this – you don't want to be like the Europeans, they had to wait for a hundred years before people started talking about *their* secret Houses. This is the kind of drive and initiative that makes America great.

> **Me:** No, I don't want to be affiliated with anyone.
> **Caller:** I could really send you a lot of business.

Apparently it's going to be a rather *large* and *busy* secret House. Jesus.

Me: No, I'm not interested. Goodbye.
Click.
I hang up.

I wonder if Europeans talk about "the secret American BDSM Houses"?
I bet not . . .

SASSY LITTLE PUNKIN

Lindsay William-Ross

http://sassylittlepunkin.blogspot.com

29/2/04

A Dialect of Secondary Language

Hidden in a sip of red wine, in a salty bite of a briny olive, there lies an impulse poised, unspoken, but emergent, an inclination passed from mouth to mouth. It is in sighs and murmurs nearly inaudible, it is a case of verbs in action, a study in the language of signs. I understand the meaning of teeth pushing in to the tender flesh of the thumb, the sudden intake of heightened breath, the music of unexpected laughter. I speak in letter less sounds, in silent prayers of gratitude, in tongue. My hips swivel in the vernacular native to my own personal dance floor, and the response is relayed in a beatific smile. In the quiet dawn I curl up in the monologue of your hand resting on my outer thigh. There is the signal of fingertips, the heat of gentle pressing, the welcome of the crook of an elbow, the sweet taste of secret places. And while words are never a struggle, we easily submit to the dialect of our secondary language, consent given with a glance, each statement reciprocated in dialogue, until finally I surrender, whispering "baby, baby," as you lay your head on my heart.

17/11/03

Gravity From Moving Ground

Mitch broke up with me over a plate of nachos on a July afternoon inside a Hawaiian-themed restaurant.

When I look back on that day, a number of questions come to mind. Did I really not see this coming? Why didn't I go with my gut and cause a great big scene? Was he cheating on me? Why did he even bother to order the nachos?

When I first met Mitch I thought he was gay. After all, he dressed well, matched his belt to his shoes, and knew all the punch lines from any given episode of *Absolutely Fabulous*. I loved to tease him, give him a hard time – it was easy to do, since he was barely eighteen, and I was a worldly twenty-one. And, in our mutual world of the educational supply store we worked in, we occupied two different slots in the chain of command: I was his boss.

We started to spend that crucial outside of work time together. I wrote long passages in my diary about how much of a crush I had on him. I quit smoking because I knew he had disdain for the habit. And finally, one early November night, at the end of another long night of him not making a single move on me, I confessed my feelings for him in the parking garage of my apartment building. Mitch was relieved that I was the one who'd had the nerve to speak up about the brewing chemistry between us. He told me: "I'm a dumb guy, you have to spell these things out for me!" After we muddled through the wordplay, it became apparent he really liked me, too. First kisses are always delicious, even inside parking garages.

I was Mitch's first serious girlfriend. When we'd get left at night to work together we'd sneak off to the stockroom to make out for ages and ages behind the shelves of crayons, counting beads and young scientist kits. The lovebirds couldn't keep their hands off each other. Mitch became my everything – I did the horrible absorbed-by-couplehood thing of abandoning my friends in favor of the boy. He lived sixty miles west of me, and work was in between, so we'd bunk together a couple of nights at a time in either direction, though for the first three months our bunking curriculum was on the tame side. Mitch's status as edgy virgin forever dispelled the myth of the over-eager teenaged boy for me. Our nights together were marathon heavy-petting sessions for about the first four months of our relationship. I was fine with that; I could stay up all night making out with him, and we often did just that.

Mitch first told me he loved me in the parking lot outside work. We d only been dating a couple of weeks, and I was just so thrilled to hear it that I didn't bother to see it as a red flag. Sure, looking back it's easy to read it as "too much, too soon", but no one would have dared point that out to me then. Maybe they did, and I just didn't listen.

"I love you" became the password to the relationship. Every phone call had to end with it, or I would jump to the conclusion that something was wrong. Notes scribbled to each other in the Laundromat were peppered with its variations. On the fifth of every month we celebrated our "anniversary", and gave each other cards littered with lines of devotion. The thing was, when I said "I love you" to Mitch, I meant it. I loved him, very much. I loved his intelligence, his warmth, his kindness, his laugh, his ambition, and his quirks. He called me "honey" and "sweetie" and held my hand whenever we were out walking. He cooked me dinner, he sent me emails just to say he loved me. He only flinched a little when I talked about our future together.

It took a great deal of gentle encouragement and the screening of a skin flick late one March night to lure Mitch over to the dark side of sexual experience. Once there, though, and his virginity abandoned to me, I found Mitch to be a happy convert. We became the proverbial rabbits, retreating to the cave of the bedroom at any given opportunity. We were indulgent with each other, we were enthusiastic, and we were sometimes insatiable. I soon began to learn about the role sex played in a serious relationship. How it could enhance the hum-drum routine of a morning shower. How it could add an exclamation point as punctuation on the otherwise maddening sentence of a lover's spat. How it could be the salve to any number of wounds. How it was always better than dessert.

For the first time in my sexual history, I was able to allow myself to be fully present, rather than send myself into an out of body experience as a defense mechanism against the confrontation of physical awareness. Mitch deferred to me a sort of proprietorship of his body, of his parts and their delightful function. I was never afraid, and that security was so intoxicating and so liberating.

We had the perfect high school sweethearts relationship – only we were grown ups. With Mitch I got to indulge in the sentimentality and overkill that most teenage girls get to experience with their teenaged boyfriends. I actually never dated in high school; the classic late bloomer, I hadn't even kissed a boy outside a game of

Truth or Dare until I had graduated, moved out of the house and was loose on the streets of Manhattan – literally. I wasn't then (and, for the record, am not now) the kind of girl who gets dated, asked out, wooed, romanced.

On our six-month anniversary Mitch presented me with a beautiful gold ring with a purple stone. Nothing extravagant – it was just a token to show that he loved me. I felt as though I was a heroine in the movies. I was the luckiest girl in the world.

Ten weeks later I was inside a Hawaiian-themed restaurant, a plate of nachos growing cold between us, and hearing the love of my life tell me he didn't want to be with me anymore. That we didn't have a future. That he wasn't attracted to me.

The world took to motion like the way film in fast-forward blurs the lights of speeding cars whizzing down the highway. It was sickening, spinning, everything-is-wrong and topsy-turvy. I didn't so much want to die, but I didn't so much know how to cope.

Suddenly I felt as though any given stranger could sense my inner, or outer, defects. That I might as well be wearing a T-shirt that read: 'I just got dumped, I am unlovable." Crowds of people got my heart racing, my palms sweating, my thoughts whirling at such a terrifying pace that I'd have to step away and regain composure. I cried out of the blue, and for hours on end. I couldn't listen to any of the songs I d been enjoying just days earlier. Any movie, TV show, book, meal, street name and so on I'd come across I'd link in some way to Mitch, and I would just lose it.

We were in the parking lot, once he'd paid the bill and the untouched pile of congealed cheese, spiced meat and tortilla chips was thankfully cleared away, and he was pulling a box out of his car. It was all my stuff from his house, I realized in a panic. Though we were outside, I could feel walls closing in. "You brought my stuff?" I asked, and he nodded. Things were starting to really sink in. "Can we have one last kiss goodbye?" I asked. He shook his head: "No." I was a wreck. When we parted I just sat in my car, listening to the angry, raspy voice of my favorite chick rocker raging about her own loss of love. I was too stunned to begin the long drive home.

The feelings I experienced in the weeks after Mitch and I broke up were unlike any feelings I d known to that point or any I have known since. I could barely function – couldn't get more than a yogurt down for days, couldn't go more than a couple of hours without crying. But worse than that, I devalued the entire relationship in retrospect. I was convinced the entire relationship had been a scam, that he'd been lying about his feelings, using me, duping me. That he hadn't really loved me, and that no one would love me ever again. How could they? I was unattractive – unattractive even to the one boy who just days ago had made me feel like the most beautiful woman in the world with his words, his eyes, his touch.

Eventually I took myself to a therapist to deal with my emotions. There was little or no quality in my life, and I had been reduced to a quivering pile of insecurities. This was no way to be living. Talking to the therapist helped – with his neutral eye he could ask the questions I needed to be asked, and make the points I needed to hear.

Time, like the merciful nurse she is, healed all my wounds. And I moved on to other relationships, and to feeling a lot better about myself. No breakup has been that traumatic since, thank God. But, by the same token, no relationship has been so dreamy. Life in extremes is never healthy, I suppose.

I still send Mitch a Christmas card every year, and wish him well. I forgave him for hurting me a long time ago but, more importantly . . . I forgave myself.

24/11/03

In Your Room

You'd given the excuse that you wanted to show me the rest of the place. I took my cue like a seasoned actress and followed you down the short and narrow hall towards your bedroom. It was dark, and you fumbled for a light. "This is my room," you said, gesturing vaguely. You pointed out some this-and-that, and I wondered why you were still bothering with the pretense, since we'd successfully and politely left your roommate in the living room.

We sat on the edge of the bed, and you gave me a laundry list of reasons why you didn't want to be in a relationship. I didn't understand you then; I didn't know the way you spoke in broad generalizations and obscure allusions of your personal history. You'd turned out the light; it was too dark to see the red flags you were waving like the color guard captain in his first parade.

It was early February; early enough in for me to still be high on the self-made promises of the New Year. It was fairly early in the evening, though we'd been sitting knee to knee on the love seat for some time. I was just getting over a cold.

I knew my limits, and I wanted to be the kind of girl who could meet a new person and take delight in slowly getting to know one another – peeling the onion. You didn't want a serious girlfriend because you'd been burned in the past. It took me a while to realize "burned" was a stand-in word for "hurt". It meant defenses, and fortress walls around your cynic's heart. It meant cold shoulders and prolonged silences and un-returned phone calls. It meant lies and someone else and things going on too long. "Let's just get to know each other," I offered, that night in your room. Maybe you should have just said "no". Maybe you did.

But you seemed to be interested in me, and you'd been trying to get me to meet you after months of friendly email volleys. We were making each other laugh, we were finding out we had a lot in common. It was nice.

My self-confidence was holding me aloft like the invisible ropes and lines used to fly Peter Pan across a stage. It was breathtaking, it was magic, it was moment after moment of potential and exploration.

I wanted to kiss you. Moreover, I wanted you to kiss me.

We'd stretched out by now, you and I, side by side in the dark and in the cold. Your room was always so cold. But it was comfortable, lying there, with you. Comfortable in that uneasy and new kind of way. I was trying to read every word, breath, silence, motion for clues. If I tilted my head just so, would you read my mind and know to kiss me? So I tilted my head just so. I didn't know how my body could tell your body to do things. Not yet.

You told me you had to work at some ungodly hour, but that you'd like for me to stay with you until you had to go. It was late, it was cold out, it was . . .

Anyhow, we were face to face, and the space between our mouths was small, but just far enough to feel like a canyon that was impossible to cross. That space was alive; it had tension like a rubber band or a pair of magnets, and we pulled with it, and pushed against it, and finally we broke the invisible barrier and kissed and didn't stop kissing for hours, until your alarm clock signaled that time was up.

You were a good kisser. Not the best but, like our relationship, you had potential.

You didn't want me to walk home in the cold and dark, though months later I would make the trek in colder air or torrential rain or burning sun just to crawl into your cave and find that thrilling on-the-precipice feeling of getting to know you, of your arms holding me safe against the wind or noise or sadness, of your punch lines and backrubs and electric touch.

That morning, long before the sun rose and when I could still taste your lips on mine, you drove me to my place, at the other end of your block. It was our block for months to come. It's my block again – it has been for some time now – and I never see you on it. We've hurt each other so profoundly that it's hard to imagine a time when a call from you could make my day, or some Dr Pepper-flavored chapstick and a seductive leaning forward on my part could make you break your fidelity to someone I still consider to be far inferior to me.

When I think about you I like to think about that first kiss; I like to think of us in terms of raw potential, of arms entwined on a winter's night, of getting to know each other, of bursts of genuine but nervous laughter. And I try to think of you as happy with the choices you've made, and happy with where I've found myself in the game of life. And I never regret a single moment we had together. Only sometimes on a cold and dark night like tonight I long to be in your room, so I can solve your mysteries, just one more time.

28/11/03

The Story of (S)Cary Date: Wherein Punkin Finds Herself in a Sticky Situation (A Parable of Love Sex in the Electronic Age)

I have never been one to shy away from Internet dating. I am not ashamed to admit that in the past I have used a number of online dating services to meet "eligible" bachelors. In fact, it is via such services that I met and dated two of my exes, Jack and Simon.

Being an active online dater takes work. Believe it or not, it takes a lot of time and effort. There's the game of logging on to your own profile to see who's viewed it, and to make sure everyone knows you've been "active" in the last x-amount of hours or days. There are the lists of what you like, and what you want. Then, when you start to get inquiries, it becomes a matter of weeding out the weak from the mighty. Then there's the emailing back and forth. Lengthy explanations of who you are and what you are all about. Some witty banter, perhaps. Relevant questions and answers. And so on.

My first Internet dating experiences go back to when I lived in New York City in 1994, when through the miracle of online chatrooms I found myself meeting all sorts of . . . well, characters. There also was a time, a couple of years ago when I had an uncharacteristic amount of free time on my hands, when I was the self-proclaimed queen of online dating. Dozens of replies came in to my inbox daily. Some were short and obscene, some so off-base that I had to laugh, and a slim margin had potential. It was a juggling act; I actually had to keep an index card file. I had never been so popular! I had more dinner-and-a-movie dates than I'd imagined possible. So when Jack and I went on another one of our famous "breaks" one fall, I went back to the old reliable, and signed up to an online dating service. I was a little more skeptical at this point, but somewhat buoyed by the successful match up of my dear friend Judy and the now love of her life.

I had received an incredibly intelligent, flattering and intriguing email from a man named Cary. He seemed to be a pretty together guy – early thirties, a lawyer, with a cute photo of himself posted. I threw caution to the wind and gave him my number. My cell phone rang almost immediately. We chatted for a long while, and the longer we talked, the more I thought I was right on the money about him. This guy seemed great! So when he suggested we meet up later that evening, I agreed.

Now, I m a savvy dater. I get the digits, and make sure a couple of gal pals know exactly where I'm going to be in case of an emergency. I don't let strangers know my address, or have them pick me up in their car. I'm a meet-in-a-public-place kind of gal. Hey, it's Los Angeles in the 21st century – I'm no no fool. So I agreed to meet Cary in the park near his apartment in the posh Mid-Wilshire area.

From the moment we met face to face I knew that this was not going to go well.

His cologne greeted me before he did, and my eyes were drawn to his gold chains and his exposed hairy chest. No handshake for this man – no, he was moving in for the bear hug immediately. But, now, I am a fair person, so I decided to give him a chance. So he didn't look much like his photo – photos can be deceiving! After all, I couldn't just bolt after thirty seconds, no matter how much I desperately wanted to.

We sat down in the park, and made some very small talk. I think it was about eight minutes in when I realized he was staring at me with what had to be love/lust in his eyes. "What are you thinking?" I asked, hiding my amusement.

He moved in for a kiss.

He was denied.

This was getting fun! I had gone from being around Jack, who expressed little or no interest in me, to being around this funny, little, hairy, smelly man, who seemed absolutely enchanted by me. Oh, yes . . . he was complimenting my hair, my clothes, my eyes, my lips. He was making the moves in Olympic record time. It was like when you drive past an accident on the highway; it's so hideous that you just have to stare. This man and this rendezvous had the same grotesque intrigue. I just couldn't pass this encounter by without fully taking it all in.

Being that it was so ridiculously early in our encounter, I knew I just couldn't terminate it then and there. Saying: "Oops, I forgot I had to do ————" just wouldn't fly. It was nine o'clock on a Sunday night, anyhow. He was suggesting options. We could go out to dinner. We could order in food to his apartment. I knew I would sooner eat my own arm than dine out with him. But, I figured, if I opted for the apartment, I could kill some time until I could make a better exit. So we headed up to his bachelor pad, so he could show me his view.

I'll admit . . . he had a nice view. It would have been more enjoyable had he not suctioned himself behind me, and attempted to maul me seductively in the window area. I scolded him, and peeled him off me, saying something like: "Not so fast, OK?" I mean, I'm not a total heartbreaker! But a girl can only stand to feel that hard-on poking her backside through a guy's pants for so long. And I was getting near and nearer to saying "so long".

Cary's idea of a romantic setting was to turn on the TV. *The Practice*, another one of those legal dramas I make it a point to avoid, was on, and when he asked if I was a fan, I told him quite adamantly, "No, I don't watch this show. I don't know anything about it." I perched on the edge of the couch. He draped himself in what I can only imagine he thought was a sexy position to my left. Was this his idea of proper seduction?

And closer to me he crept. His hand wandered to my leg, and with a masterful move he flipped himself over so that he was hovering over me. He started to go to town on my breasts, and I'll admit, I'm a bit of a sucker for that. So I let him play. Not more than a minute or so later I realized he'd worked a free hand down to his fly, and was extracting himself.

Oh, he wanted me to touch him . . . he wanted to kiss my lips, my ears . . . he suggested we go to the bedroom. He suggested I do all sorts of things that there was no way in hell I would do to him. I didn't have more than a few moments to dodge his advancements, when . . .

"Uuuuuuhhhhhh!" He shuddered, and stood upright. What? I asked. Huh?

"Wow," he said, surveying the damage. "I just came on my couch."

I sat right up and made sure none had landed on me. Thank God, I was clear.

What can one possibly say in reply to that?

"I'm gonna change," he said, bounding happily into his bedroom. "Don't you move!"

I took the opportunity to gather my purse, and put on my coat.

Cary re-emerged, having freshly donned some really attractive (note sarcasm) sweat pants.

"I have to go, actually," I told him, playing that early exit card a little too late. "It's later than I thought, and I have to work early . . ."

He walked me to the door, and sent me off with a faint hug, and asked me that I'd promise to call him when I got home, so he would know I was safe and sound. How was it possible that he could think that this date had gone well? Did he seriously think I was going to call him, to encourage further contact?

"OK, sure," I told him, heading out the door.

I never talked to (S)Cary again. Because, really, folks, when you come on the couch a half hour in to the first date . . . what kind of future is there?

11/1/04

She May Get Weary

I'm wondering if it's really true that men just want to date the air-headed blonde bombshells of the world. Women who are so beautiful that it doesn't matter that there are rocks rolling around inside their head in place of brains. "Men don't like smart women," my friend Kelsey told me over dinner last night. "You have to coo and purr over a man and be in awe of him."

Now, when it's time for cooing and purring, I know when to start my motor. And if I'm dating a man who is passionate about an interest or hobby or life pursuit, I will happily listen to them talk about what makes them excited, and I will be a little in awe of their expertise, their dedication, their what have you. But, look, pal, when *Jeopardy* comes on, I'm going to give you a run for your money. 'Cause baby here is smart. And I don't play dumb. Don't even get me started about how witty, playful, interesting, creative or talented I am. I shouldn't have to script a personals ad just to get noticed.

So I'm not an air-headed blonde bombshell. I don't have a butt you'd sell your mama to grab a handful of, I don't have flawless skin and a model perfect figure. But I know what I've got and I know how to use it. I have, as they say, skills. I won't leave you wanting. But unless I get a T-shirt printed up that says, "I know how to keep my man satisfied" no one will give me the time of day. No one's about to buy me dinner to find out if beneath my smarts and less-than-perfect body I have it going on.

Well, guess what: I have it going on.

And if the men out there are so busy looking for someone better, someone perfect, someone invented by the media, well, you're going to miss the fact that there are good – no, great – people right in front of you.

Yeah. That's right. I'm talking about me.

18/12/03

The Lucky Strike-Out

At the end of the night he held her in his arms and she cried on his shoulder. They were leaning against his car at two in the morning, cold, on the street where she lived.

"I'm sorry," he said, a dozen times over.

"Don't be," she said sincerely. "It's just that it's been a really hard year," she tried to explain, but stopped short. The cold and the liquor and the tears were making it hard to think, to see, to feel straight.

He had explained the rules of his game before the night had even begun. But she didn't play by anyone's rules, and so she moved with an exaggerated shimmy dancing to the tunes in the dive bar, she broke out the innuendo, and by her fourth drink in the shiny new hipster bowling alley she was both frankly drunk and frankly frank.

She had started to cry when she found her friend in the restroom – the pretty friend that everyone liked. Her friend held her in her arms and she cried on her shoulder. They'd walked back to the crowd arms about each other, smiling and laughing, and like in any good episode the music was cresting and the credits, by rights, should have been rolling.

But the night wore on, and she checked the score and she was coming in dead last.

He said goodnight to her on the street, but instead of a brief farewell she put her head on his shoulder and started to cry. "It's been a really bad year," she said again, and she thought about the disappointments, the losses, the heartbreaks she'd endured. "I'm so sorry, I'm such a jerk," he said, but it wasn't even him. He'd never broken her heart because she'd never given it to him.

Their relationship had been about tension, never love. It was the tension between their fingertips and in the getting-to-you-know chemistry of their first date, years ago. It was the tension of his giving his virginity to her and the anxiety that accompanied the act. It was the tension of their ceaseless sparring, of her uncanny ability to make him cry. And now it was the tension of the failed evening as she cried in his arms and he offered apologies.

It wasn't until she got home that she realized her strike-out had been a gift. It was the gift of their conversation, of hearing that she was silly to think she wasn't pretty, or interesting or attractive, of hearing that, though he could not play her game tonight, she was still special to him. And she took his apologies as representative of all the boys she'd loved before and since him, because none of them would ever speak to her, none of them could ever offer an apology for the world of actual hurt they'd left her with in their partings. And this boy – this boy had never been one of them, but he spoke for them now when he said, "I'm sorry." So she thanked him, and they pledged friendship, and they said goodnight.

This time the episode was really over, and she made her way slowly down the middle of the dark street, her extra-long green scarf trailing on the cold street, with a smile replacing the tears.

She was home. And the game was over.

16/2/04

Columbus and the Art of Kissing

It was as though the story was writing itself in my mind: under a red lamp, fingers gingerly perched on the stem of a chilled martini glass, he and I leaning in for another kiss.

Words and stories and peals of laughter had tumbled from our mouths all evening, like a ceaselessly spilling bag of marbles. I gathered moments like piles of artfully won treasure, each morsel of each other shared like a weighty, sparkling jewel in the palm of my hand. The space between us was a field of vibrant energy.

My surroundings melted away, and I forgot that I was part of an ever turning world, part of the night's population in a crowded bar just off Hollywood Boulevard. My knees trembled with violent pleasure, we pressed closely together, and I turned my head away and bit my lip. There was infinite solace in his gleaming eyes, comfort in his fingertips laced with mine. This was no story of invention; it was an experience more incredible than anything my writer's mind could craft, save a single word: synchronicity.

Like Christopher Columbus boldly staking claim to a land already discovered, I realized last night that I had just discovered the art of kissing. The action in both theory and practice became utterly redefined to me as the night progressed, as I wondered how I could dare stop, as I became aware of my desire taking on the sound of power lines humming on a sultry summer day.

It began, unexpectedly, on Valentine's Day, and where it goes is as yet to be determined. But like Columbus I have landed on the shores of my wildest imagination – brazen, invigorated, and ready for adventure.

26/9/03

Doing the Time Warp Again: Going Back to my Grounds Zero

I lost myself completely in the re-reading of the journal I kept around ten years ago. It's a silver sparkly lined journal; the pages are crammed with my girlish handwriting in many colors, stickers, notes, drawings, poems, things I wanted to tape inside and save for ever and ever. I found myself transported back to a time when I lived in the most incredible studio apartment at the foot of the Hollywood Hills, in a building that used to be a hotel in the 1920s. It was my first quarter ever enrolled in university, and I was a Theatre major – somewhat irritated that I had to take a class in stagecraft, which meant I had to draft things and know about bolts and sets and things, when I naively thought Theatre majors did nothing but act. I had a part-time job at a bookstore, and I spent all my free time (which I apparently had much of, considering I ditched a lot of school) perched on a stool at the counter of a local coffee house.

Grounds Zero, as it was called, was a tiny little bohemian coffeehouse that was on an odd stretch of space on Sunset Boulevard. This was before there was a Starbucks on every corner, and when going for coffee was more desirable than even maybe going for drinks, but then, I could well have been biased. My friend Laurie had stumbled on the place one night when she was supposed to be knocking on doors raising money for Greenpeace, which was a job we both held. She took me back there with her, and when she eventually moved back East, I moved in to Grounds Zero. I may as well have gotten my mail and phone calls there, because I lived there. I've even slept there . . .

The clientèle was your typical urban artsy Gen-X mêlée, though some of the more aesthetically rough-and-tumble types were actually members of Narcotics Anonymous, and only looked as though they partied hard. It was the kind of café that hosted a fledgling open mic night, had the occasional musical act, and the artwork hanging on the walls was done by the token local eccentric. It was dim, it was cozy, and everyone knew my name. I was there morning, noon and night. I almost never paid for a single iced mocha, cup of Joe, sandwich, cookie or what have you that I ordered. I would get asked to run errands like going to the bank or the market, or to make drinks while the employee on duty played a game of pool. I stayed late to do the dishes. I knew everyone who hung out there like me, inside and out, and same went double for the staff. There was plenty of scandal, intrigue, adventure, flirtation, excitement and romance in the air at any time. And I was in love with about a half dozen people who either worked or hung out there.

This was a most curious time in my life; I was eighteen years old, living on my own, balancing work and school. I'd just had my heart broken by someone whom I'd allowed to be my first intimate. I wrote long, wordy passages about my rapidly beating heart, my desires, my deep despair, my anguish, my early adulthood torment and delight. I had an intense crush on a fellow named Jonas, who worked there, and I'm sure he knew it, everyone knew it, and it tortured me – I was in sheer agony over the fact that we were just pals. If he wasn't in my good graces I turned my affections to any number of other people – some guy named Rick who played pool there, and two other employees, Ethan and Monroe. I'd sit, ever impatient, on my stool at the copper-covered counter, sipping endless sugary drinks, reading novel upon novel, penning furiously in my silver journal, smoking Marlboro Reds that I pulled out of a little pink tin box that served as my purse. I wonder now what made me so appealing to so many men – my diary was full of "so and so made a move on me" – and I didn't want a single one of them – if only I had people making advances on me like that these days! I was fighting them off with sticks, completely naive of how men and women interacted, and amazed that they took an interest in me. Meanwhile I was lusting with unrequited love for men who didn't show a single bit of interest in me. Then, just like now, all I ever want are the ones who don't want me back.

That is, until one October night.

Jonas wasn't giving me the time of day, so I had turned my attention to someone else: Monroe. He lived with his girlfriend. He was much older, maybe six or seven years. He was a poet. How utterly romantic, wouldn't you say? It was a Friday night, and I'd remained behind to help him tidy up. He counted out the register, showed the bug spray man where to spray, and I happily went in back to do the dishes.

Suddenly he was right next to me.

"I'm on to you," he told me. "I've been wanting to take all those hooks you've been hanging out for me, only I don't know how you'd take it. But I know you're flirting with me, all the time. And I think you're cute. And I can totally see us, naked, going at it on that couch there."

I was stunned. I was busted. But, thrill of thrills, he actually liked me back!

"How about I give you a foot massage?" he offered, when the dishes were done.

I said yes, and I stretched out next to him on the couch. He took my foot, and rubbed it, and then slowly worked his way up my bare leg. And then we kissed.

"Do you have a condom?" he asked me.

Of course I did. I retrieved one from (where else?) my little pink tin, and there we were, naked, going at it on the couch, just as he and I had both pictured. It was naughty, it was impetuous, and it was making a cheater out of him.

I was in heaven.

We hooked up every Friday for the next month right there in the cafe – in the backroom, on the couch, and even on the pool table. One night my car was locked in to the back parking lot, and we slept there. His girlfriend showed up in the morning, worried because he hadn't come home. She seemed almost relieved to see me there, because she and I were friendly. She'd go shopping and show me what she bought, or we'd talk about life and smoke cigarettes together. I don't know if she ever had any idea I was sleeping with her live-in boyfriend.

Monroe, well, he was moody; to say the least, and that in turn made me more neurotic. Any thing he said or did would send me into a tailspin, either high or low, but dramatic no matter what. He was unhappy at home. He was not being productive, creatively. He didn't like his job. He said once that he was as able to commit to me as "a dog with fleas", whatever that meant. He'd say he would call so we could go out, and he wouldn't. Time after time I'd be waiting to hear from him, a whole day wasted for me. Then he'd show up at the drop of a hat: "I was in the neighborhood, and thought I'd stop by" or "can I come over to practice giving a full body massage?" I was head over heels in love with this temperamental man – he would read poetry to me in restaurants, rub my neck gently as we drove around, lie with me on the park grass. To him, I'm sure, I was this oddball young thing who complicated his life, but who would drop her drawers at the slightest suggestion. "It's funny," he said one day, "the Sex Monster doesn't bite me when I'm just talking to you. But when I touch you . . ." As soon as I closed the door behind him when he left I picked up my pen and wrote an angsty homage in verse using his very words. I had mistaken what he was offering me as love.

It came to an end in the spring. He'd left his girlfriend and moved into some kind of roommate situation, and when I finally got him on the phone after several attempts, he said, "Hey, me and my roommates are making home-made beer right now. I'll call you tomorrow, okay?"

He never called.

Today, almost ten years later, after I read all these episodes in my diary, I grabbed my books and went in to Hollywood to see what had become of the old place. It's changed owners a few times, and motifs, though the talk in the room today showed me that it still was a spot for urban hipsters, Hollywood wannabees, and "Friends of Bill W." I got a coffee and sat down, and like a good little scholar I did my reading for school. There's different paint on the walls, the couch and pool table are long gone, even the copper counter top is gone, too. But my ghost is in there, the ghost of a kid who lived and breathed with such intensity within those walls. I told the guy at the counter that I used to hang out there, years ago, but that I hadn't been back for ages.

"Did you move out of town?" he asked.

"No," I said, laughing. "I guess I grew up."

Through the miracle of the Internet, I know that Monroe eventually married, and he and his wife and son live just about two miles north of me, of all places, in this small world of a sprawling city. I emailed him several months ago, and, no surprise, he never wrote back. I wonder if he knew just how much I cared for him. I used to always wonder if he really factored me in to his life – if I became an issue with him and his girlfriend, if he even considered being the boyfriend that I'd hoped he would be for me. I suppose I might never know. And I suppose you can't ever go back. Not really.

12/2/04

On the Street Where I Live

"I left you by the house of fun", sings Norah Jones, and I smile and turn the volume up on my car radio dial. Then I remember you said hearing that song made you want to light a candle, "but don't get any ideas," you added as caution. I should have left you then, when you said that, or when you said any of a countless other heartless things, but we were driving, and the forward motion was about all that was holding me aloft, though I'd already fallen. We were always in motion, and even in rest I could sense your movement away from me, the internal sprint to some constructed notion of safety.

I think about the winter night it rained for hours on end, the drops falling heavy in a shroud of steam, and I ran down the block to the warm safety of your room, to the salty sweat of your body, to the familiar mounting tension of your mouth on mine. The humidity was palpable, the heat as delectable inside as out. No candles, no care packages, no long distance flights between you and I, just one short stretch of damp, slick concrete glistening under the night sky. In your house of fun I looked at a trick mirror that let me see past reality, past a framed photo on the bed stand, past a secret stash of notes, past my own trinkets and sundries hidden in some box under your bed. You had me with a trick of the light, a sleight of hand, with the ease of convenience, and I ran to you as quickly as you ran away.

I should have left you for good that rainy night, but we'd left each other long ago so that it was no longer a matter of leaving. I walked home slowly, not minding that the rain was gently washing over me, washing a little of your scent from me, but leaving me with your taste, which lingered like the best morsels of the last supper. I was clean, but far from pure, and full, but far from satisfied; the closest I ever came to leaving was in walking out alone.

30/5/03

First Kiss No. 5

We had been taking turns playing CDs for hours. We'd polished off a bottle of the inexpensive wine with the notorious moniker of Two-Buck Chuck and smoked our fair share of cigarettes. I'd moved from the floor to the couch where he was. The backrub he'd begun early in the evening had never really ended; his fingers had not left my hair, my neck, nor my arms since the first touch. It was late, but that didn't matter. We got up, to change the CD, to stretch, to have a drink of water. He stretched out on my bed. "No more couch?" I asked. "It's more comfortable for two of us on the bed," he said, and so I joined him. I hadn't felt this calm in a long time. I had shivers running up and down my spine from when he gently played with my hair, or tickled my fingertips. I'd been laughing all night as we told each other stories from every category of life.

"Well, I can't sleep, I'm too wide awake!" I said.

"Hmmm, what can we do?" he wondered aloud, with a grin.

"Hmmm, I dunno," I said, playing along.

"Wanna make out?" he asked.

3/2/04

The Last Time

It was warm when I woke up; maybe it was the sun itself filtering through the apartment-issue mini blinds that stirred me from my sleep. We'd managed to pass the night without the expected shared-bed controversy. I kept my word and to my side of the mattress, and he kept, typically, to himself.

This time he remembered that I like to start the day with a cup of coffee, and so he served me a watery cup of Folgers Instant shortly after rising. By character he was thoughtful, though, so I took the act as no sign of romantic interest.

I was the chatterbox in contrast to his routine of silence. Every leaf, stem, petal or shrub was subject to my commentary. It was a gorgeous late-August day in San Francisco's Golden Gate Park – how could I keep from gushing? My lungs were readily drinking in the clean air, my eyes the breathtaking views of the city by the bay. And I was bound and determined for him to see that I'd moved past the hurt of his dissolution of our intimate ties in the haze of early summer. I was hell-bent on my happiness, high on a Katharine Hepburn *joie de vivre*, optimistic and keen on maintaining our friendship. When it was his concern that I would take advantage of the mutual sleeping space scenario, it was my mission to remain staunchly platonic. I promised myself I would under no circumstance initiate a single thing.

His silence was maddening, and as the hours of the day marched on, and our feet marched us through the streets of San Francisco, it became a game of tolerance on my part. As we rode knee to knee on the BART train to Berkeley I realized I no longer felt a shiver of delight buzz through me as we touched. He was tiresome. And so I endured.

The evening was pleasant; I was chatty, animated, conversational, freed from the dumbstruck bonds of infatuation. I could hear my own laughter, sparkling, during the dinner that we ate on plates perched on our laps in the backyard, and then later during a raucous improv show where we saw our mutual friends perform brilliantly. But our last stop on the jam-packed itinerary was to some kind of hipster cowboy bar, where we were to make an appearance at someone's birthday gathering, someone I didn't know. Inside the faux-ranch saloon I was finding myself physically shut out of conversations by people stepping in front of me. I couldn't breathe, I couldn't play the social game. I slid out of the fray and sought refuge outside on a slatted bench. He found me there, a cigarette and a half later, angry at my having left without informing him. He mocked me, he made a show of giving me a hard time in front of some friends of his. But I refused to accept it, so I spat out some retorts.

Finally he asked me: "Do you want to go?" and I asked him: "Why?" He replied: "Because I hate this place and I want to leave."

And I exhaled.

It was cold, dark, and rather late at night. My feet ached from our journeys, my mind was tired of banter. We collapsed on the bed and rehashed the day. "I had a nice time," I told him, and asked if he had, too. "Yes," he replied, "but not the part at the bar." I was too tired to argue, so instead I curled up and closed my eyes. He followed suit, his face just an inch or so from mine, and we lay there, sideways, wrong-ways, on the bed.

It must have been he who started the kiss, but my response was so remarkably instantaneous that it might well be argued that we started at the same time. And so we kissed. Eventually he began to use his hands to steer me towards greater pleasure.

My eyes were heavy, though and, despite my recent satisfaction, I couldn't keep from yawning. I knew sleep was impending, so I insisted we shift to lay right-ways on the bed. I glanced at the clock. It was past one a.m. and so I slept. We slept.

I heard my name being called out in the dark. It was coupled with his exclamation of: "What does it take to get some attention from you?" as well as an errant hand lingering on my body. I peeked at the clock. It was now well past three in the morning. I cited the time, and the fact that I was, or had been, sleeping. But he persisted. It seems he felt I owed him something, that I was selfishly withholding sex from him. And I thought of an old conversation of ours, where he had said in no uncertain terms that he believed firmly that we should never be intimate again. That he felt that I took our sexual relationship to have more meaning than he was ever willing to invest in it. Yet, here I was, awoken in the middle of the night, charged with one count of lack of willingness for reciprocity, one count of being rude for not giving him pleasure.

I didn't know what to do but laugh, and loudly at that. I laughed so much so that I feared I couldn't stop, even as I sputtered, "I'm sorry!" and excused myself to the restroom so that I might splash water on my face and regain my composure.

When I returned he'd burrowed himself in the blankets, like a child, his face to the wall, leaving me nothing to address my words to but an expanse of back swathed in a T-shirt. I asked if he would turn over, which he begrudgingly did, so that I might talk to his face. I reminded him of the time on the digital clock display, of my exhaustion, of the very words he'd said to me on this very topic. He pouted still, and I offered an apology for not expressing gratitude for the attention he'd given me; our kissing had, after all, led to just a tiny bit more activity that was, I gather, geared more towards my satisfaction. And I told him, finally, that quite frankly, I was so confused by the events of the late-late night that I'd hoped to take what remained of the time to see how I felt, and if I was even comfortable with it.

And so we slept, wrapped in each other's arms, and when the morning sun woke us up we lingered in bed, and we both broke our promises to ourselves, and maybe each other, and it this time our actions were geared towards mutual satisfaction.

It was the last time I saw San Francisco. It was the last time I saw him.

11/3/04

Dear Mister Unspecific

An unnamed panic gripped my body on Sunday, and I couldn't shake the shakes. The marathon traffic stalled at a snail's pace, the air heavy with the gloom of false summer. A lesson in the physics of mechanics taught me that explosions only happened in the movies, but I still sensed the rumblings, I trembled with the thought of flame meeting fuel, I joined the crowd of impatient onlookers, resentful for the wait. Scraps of paper bore testament to my fragility, hinting at swimming with Virginia and baking with Sylvia; most words could not escape the swirl of my mind, though, and there they idled, wrestled with the rationale of public face. Like a rocking horse jockey I'd sat astride muscled flanks to the tune of "learn to love yourself," pausing even to remark on its familiarity. Ultimately, the lesson was a reminder, like chalking childhood lines as punishment in numbers seeming infinite. His final childish lines came in the modern epistle; they read as conversational, vague and unspecific. But I refused to address a reply, and instead typed lengthy essays at late hours, fulfilling obligations despite the hampering burden of unqualified withdrawal. I drive with a six-pack of Guinness in my car once intended as a gift; I have a CD I want to return, too, if only to prove that the intangible costs were incalculable.

LOVE SONGS FOR UNDERDOGS

Danor

http://danor.blogspot.com

Craving

One of the three spiritual poisons, according to Zen Buddhism, is craving. (The other two are hatred and ignorance.)

Fathers and teachers, I ponder "What is craving?"

Let us contrast craving with love. Love is generally conceded to be a good thing. Love is appreciation of an object or person for its own nature and for the benefits it can give us. For example, at Thanksgiving dinner, one might say, "I love candied yams." Because one loves eating candied yams, because they taste yummy. Or one might say, "I love my flannel pajamas," because they are soft and comfy and help you sleep. Or one might say, "I love my Dom," because he is sweet and funny and interesting and gives good head and the sound of his voice makes you warm and crinkly all over and he makes you a better person when you are with him, etc, etc.

So love is different from craving. To me, craving is the belief, or at least the feeling, that you cannot be happy or complete or live a good life without the thing you crave. It is often temporary ("I am craving candied yams. Luckily, tomorrow is Thanksgiving") and pretty tongue-in-cheek ("How will I survive while my flannel jammies are in the wash! I NEED THEM!").

However, they can definitely poison you. Suppose you crave a particular person. Then that person leaves you. If your craving doesn't go away, you either remain unhappy and fixated for the rest of your life, or you go to extreme lengths to get the other person back, and neither can really lead to happiness, unless you are a character in a Hollywood romantic comedy where that sort of thing is encouraged.

Or suppose you crave candied yams, and all the yams in the world go away. One can really apply it to any situation.

It amounts not to not wanting things, but to being able to get on without things. Perspective is key. If you cannot have yams, you cannot have yams. This is factual. You will never taste your beloved yams again, and you may reasonably mourn this fact. Craving, however, turns this factual statement into "I will never taste anything good again, and my tastebuds will be a barren wilderness until I die a miserable starving wretch in an attic somewhere, surrounded by broccoli and cauliflower." Which has the unfortunate attribute of depending for its falseness or trueness on whether you believe it or not. Because if you believe it, it will probably come true (well, maybe not the bit about the cauliflower), but if you don't, it almost certainly won't.

Now, take, if you will, the situation I found myself in a couple of months ago. I had been ordered to stimulate my clit every hour on the hour, bringing myself as close to orgasm as possible, and then stop all sensation. Here's what I wrote for Kam after the first four hours:

When I left for class, I was already wobbly, unable even to imagine the total mess I would be by the time you arrived. My clit ached, my pussy was soaking wet. I sat through the first half-hour of class both dreading and longing for one o'clock – longing to touch my throbbing clit, dreading the build-up that would only lead to more frustration.

At one I crossed my legs and leaned forward, pressing the seam of my jeans directly onto my clit. I felt a little faint at the intensity of the sensation . . . rubbed very lightly at first to try to get myself acclimatized, then obediently increased pressure, biting my lower lip fiercely to keep from moaning aloud. I remained on the brink of orgasm for a few more moments, wanting so desperately to come that stopping at that point seemed as though it would be physically impossible, but I stopped. My clit seemed to scream in hysterical protest as I tried to find a comfortable position in my chair, tried to focus on the board.

As two approached I was so torn between the desire for the slightest touch on my clit and my misery that I wouldn't be allowed to come that I felt almost calm. I had done it an hour ago and had gotten through it, this couldn't be too much worse, I thought – until the seam of my jeans again brushed my clit and I realized it was, it was much, much worse. It was as if I had left my desire to simmer and when I took the lid off it exploded all over the kitchen. I didn't orgasm, but if I had started out with harder pressure I might have done so before I knew what was happening. I had to add pressure slowly, cautiously, in terror that I might lose control. I rubbed my clit with a slow ferocious hunger, feeling my juices trickle down to soak the crotch of my jeans. When I stopped, tears filled my eyes, almost spilling over; I blinked them away and tried to breathe.

Walking back from class, I wondered how much longer I would wait. I imagined falling at your feet and begging you, crying, to let me earn an orgasm any way I could; I would suck your cock, lick your shoes, compose an ode in iambic pentameter to your mercy. I thought of crying, how I worry that my tears blackmail you, that they tip the balance of an argument unfairly because you don't like to see me cry and it deflects your anger or annoyance. I wondered how you would respond if I cried to be allowed to orgasm.

It's three now; I'll follow your instructions. Be right back . . .

Jesus, my clit is so swollen it feels like a touch will burst it, spilling orgasm down my thighs. I touched it cautiously with a cold finger, which soothed as well as tormented until it rapidly warmed up. My pussy is wet enough to drown in. I want something in it, anything – cock, fingers, vibrator, hairbrush, cucumber, anything for my aching walls to clench against. Massaging my clit carefully, harder, I know you would want it harder, I will not come, I will not come.

I will not come until you say I may.

I love you, sir.

Danor

He made me continue this build-up without release for more than four more hours, during some of which he licked and spanked my clit, fucked me, and took me out in public with an anal plug in. You can imagine the wreck I was by the end. Craving hardly begins to cover how badly I wanted to orgasm. Nothing else mattered. Release was all I wanted in the world.

Except that's clearly not true, because if it were really all I wanted, there was nothing to stop me from having ten freaking orgasms if I felt like it. Though my entire physical and emotional being was concentrated in the desire to orgasm, my will, my center, wanted something else more: to please Kam with my obedience. Even though everything I felt was about wanting to come, I knew on a deeper level what was important. Craving versus love, and love won.

Kam, of course, deliberately built up this craving in me to highlight exactly that difference. Most conflicts between craving and love are less obvious and more complicated. There's craving to be with a person right now because you love them, but knowing that love requires you to be understanding of his other obligations and not make things harder on him by complaining. There's craving to be with a person who doesn't treat you right, but forgetting to love yourself enough not to put yourself through the shit that entails. The rituals of BDSM, however, often entail exactly this clear-cut choice for the submissive. Our Doms build up the craving – for the pain to stop, for the release to come, for whatever – and then demand that we choose willed obedience over the ultimate craving. And when we do, that's when we achieve subspace – that zone of clarity and peace and freedom from craving (or, as J.D. Salinger put it, "cessation from all hankering") where we feel like we can accomplish anything, because we are really, really fucking strong.

Or maybe that's just me.

Implements

I love the cane. Its deceptive lightness and simplicity. The swooshing sound just before it lands. Those sharp burning lines of pain laid across a raw and stinging ass. Feeling myself so thoroughly striped.

I love the belt. Such a basic tool of intimidation. When he unbuckles it, I never know whether I'm going to be beaten with it or whether he's just taking his pants down to fuck my mouth, pussy or ass. Snapped across my quivering nipples or obediently outthrust buttocks, the crack of tanned and dried skin on burning, living, cringing skin.

I love the paddle. He made me shop for it alone, along with lube, rope and a negligee, dressed skimpily and thoroughly made up, my short shorts barely hiding my bruises from the previous night. It, too, is deceptively light. I now get a Pavlovian frisson when I see people playing Ping-Pong, suddenly imagining a volley of smacks descending as I shriek and try not to writhe away.

I love the hairbrush. I've been missing it lately, its loud unmistakable smacking sounds making it somewhat unsuitable for use in my thin-walled apartment. An innocent household item, suitable for travel, with a wicked flat back and an insertable handle. A lot of my fantasies lately involve being pulled over his lap and spanked with the hairbrush until I think my bottom is going to burst into flame.

I love his hands. Striking, caressing, pinching, scratching, teasing, kneading, clenching, jerking, pushing, pulling, holding, stroking, comforting. Fisted in my hair, working my swollen clit as I sob and beg blindly to be allowed orgasm, slapping sharply, soothing gently. Harsh and loving.

Not a bad girl

I have had my issues with my mom (hey, who hasn't?) but I really can't imagine a better mother for a little kid to have had. She was warm, caring, honest, creative and completely committed to raising my sister and me right.

One thing that stands out for me in retrospect is that she never told either of us that we were bad. She was very good at maintaining the distinction between behavior and nature. We sometimes (often) did bad things, disobeyed, caused trouble; we ourselves, however, were not bad kids. In fact, she scolded me once for saying "Bad dog" to the dog. She told me to say "No" instead.

I know that for a lot of people being called a bad girl, a dirty slut, a filthy worthless cunt, is a good and liberating part of scenespace. It means you can relax into the desires you normally aren't comfortable with, because that's who you are – you're a bad girl. For me, being horny and kinky and craving discipline and everything else I desire are all part of being a good girl. He loves those desires in me, and I love displaying them for him – I beg when I'm allowed to beg, I offer him my craving and my pleasure to enjoy, and he does enjoy them. There's no shame in that.

Kam tells me I'm a good girl, as praise, but he's never told me I was a bad girl. Partly this is because I'm rarely disobedient. But he has had occasion to be quite harsh with me at times, yet he's never told me that I was bad or worthless. This is extremely important to me. It means that he never withdraws his love and respect as a disciplinary tool. It means that even if I need to be severely punished, I am still, essentially, his good and beloved girl.

Secretary and the cane

Unrelated topics. Last things first.

Kam and I watched *Secretary* at last, this afternoon. I was interested to find out whether it was a good movie or just popular among kinksters due to, well, kink.

We both enjoyed it hugely. It was funny, often amusingly apt and sometimes heartbreakingly so, and reminded me in that way of *Kissing Jessica Stein*. An unusually honest (not necessarily realistic, but honest) romantic comedy, I thought, with a good solid message, one I wasn't entirely expecting. And both of the principals were sexy-cute as hell. It had its flaws, but overall, highly recommended. The last scenes particularly affected me, personally, for reasons which I'll probably describe at some point.

In the interests of science, can anyone tell me if you can actually bruise a bottom that visibly with a hand spanking? Kam is a wuss about his hands, prefers implements.

Aha! A segue! Speaking of implements, my ass got thoroughly caned this afternoon, after a warm-up with some stripes and belt whacks to my inner thighs and nipples, and Kam jerking off in front of my face while I moaned and sobbed to be allowed to take him in my mouth. Just to be really cruel, he turned his back to jerk off further and even, once, left my line of sight altogether, which almost brought me to tears. He did kindly fuck my mouth for a while, but stopped without coming and then gave my bottom a good hard palm spanking (a rare occurrence, see above) before bringing out the cane again.

This was, I think, the third prolonged caning I've received, and I think the first two were just getting the hang of things, because this session was FANTASTIC. Kam put on Nine Inch Nails' "The Fragile" (if anyone is ever looking for good scene music, nothing brings out the desire to rhythmically rape and pillage more efficiently) and established a good rhythm early, which helped me relax, and built up the severity of the strokes gradually, not fucking with my head so I didn't tense up. In fact, at first the strokes were light enough that I pushed my bottom up into them, wanting more.

The harshness of the strokes varied, but never hugely from one to the next, and I discovered that there's something about that particular quality of pain that really zones me out. I was completely relaxed, completely at peace . . . it was better than a massage. I think I could have fallen asleep if I'd let myself go completely. I made soft noises to let Kam know I was still there, but I was breathing deeply and regularly, my mind completely blank of anything but the music, the rhythmic burning strokes, and Kam somewhere behind me, calm and in control.

When I expressed all this to Kam (after he stopped, gathered up my limp and dreamy body in his arms, kissed me and praised me for my endurance), he said he could tell I was completely relaxed and asked if I was also aroused. I replied that I had gotten extremely wet, but felt no urgency to climax, though I probably could have if he'd told me to. He said he would have gone much longer, but this was our first experience of this sort of thing and he wanted to check in with me to make sure I was really enjoying it as much as I seemed to be. He hinted that our next session might be upwards of an hour.

I'm not sure why the cane has such a different effect on me than other implements. It might have something to do with noise – I HATE loud noises, and the paddle, the belt, the hairbrush and the hand, when used hard enough to be effective, all make loud smacking noises that startle me every time so that I can't relax (not that this is a bad thing, in most scenes). It might have to do with the quality of the pain; the cane has that blend of sting and thud that somehow just works for me, and it occurs in lines which are manageable increments (rather than, say, large ovals). Whatever it is, when Kam and I finally get to live together, I might beg for a nightly caning, to cleanse me of the day's problems and worries, and send me off to dreamland with my bottom nice and toasty warm.

Saturday 20 December 2003

The courtesy of lovers

It seems like the longer I get to spend with him at a time, the more I miss him after we have to say goodbye.

I don't actually realize until I am away from him (and with others) how much more I feel like myself when I am with Kam. How much freer I am. I enjoy my family, but compared to how I feel when I'm with Kam, I feel strained.

Kam and I are very comfortable with each other – we giggle a lot and play with each other and say silly things and act foolish and tell each other about our crushes and our weirdest sex dreams. We are not polite, in the sense that our interaction is not governed by general social rules.

But we are courteous. We are quick to apologize to each other and eager to bring each other pleasure. We unfailingly show respect for each other, even when we quarrel, and neither of us would deliberately hurt the other. (Except in the good, erotic way.) This courtesy comes not from prescribed social rules or notions of propriety, but from our desire to make each other happy in as many small ways as possible.

I think many BDSM-ers enjoy rituals – prescribed from Gorean novels, borrowed from fellow kinksters, or made up out of whole cloth – because they provide a useful way to express that courtesy between lovers. When there is a special ritual to demonstrate to one's Dom that bringing him a drink is a genuine personal pleasure because it brings him pleasure, or when a Dom can take pleasure in granting his sub some small treat she has to ask permission for, these everyday things are no longer mundane, but as intimate and loving as a kiss.

But anything ritualized can also become meaningless, as any

Catholic will tell you . . . after eighteen hundred repetitions of The Lord's Prayer, one actually has to strain to recall what the syllables mean. Or ask any fifth-grader to paraphrase the Pledge of Allegiance. Parrotted words and gestures can be as empty of meaning as if they were never spoken. It's the spirit behind the ritual, not the ritual itself, that infuses life with a sense of new meaning and erotic excitement – and that spirit is one of courtesy.

This courtesy in no way prevents Kam from calling me a horny little slut or slinging me around by the hair or beating the tar out of me. These, too, are acts of courtesy – of love and intimacy and respect for a very, very deep and important part of my nature – and I receive them as such, and thank him for them, and for the greatest fulfilment of all – offering all my desires to him, and in the act of offering myself, finding that I am satisfying his desires as well.

10 things I love/are fun about being kinky:

1) I am a huge geek, so I love it when I get into something that involves endless trivia, jargon, schools of thought, signature equipment and a circle of Kink Solidarity.

2) Playing "spot the kink" in ostensibly vanilla movies and books.

3) Actually having words for people who are not into what you are. "Vanilla" is my second favorite word for the canaille, next to "Muggles".

4) The fact that Ping-Pong tables, large spoons and tack shops make me wet, and every time I brush my hair, I'm extremely aware of the other uses to which the brush can be put.

5) I'm proud of who I am and what I'm interested in, but I don't think that people whose interests are different are bad or wrong. Because a lot of people think my interests are perverted, I'm more open-minded than I might otherwise be.

6) You never know how strong you are until you're tested. Kam puts me to the test, and I'm usually a lot stronger than I think I am.

7) Wearing a leather dog collar to a party.

8) My strong desire to please is organized and ritualized, so that it doesn't cast a stifling cloud over what is supposed to be a "normal" relationship. I am able to discuss and analyze the aspects of submission and can therefore differentiate between submission and codependency.

9) Knowing that the stuff of my day-to-day life is the stuff of other people's wildest, darkest, most secret fantasies.

10) "You are my good girl and I'm very pleased with you."

Bad to be sexy, or sexy to be bad?

My absolute most despised word in the English language: "Naughty."

Why do I hate this word with a fiery vengeance?

OK. Let's come up with an example. (I'm making this up; any resemblance to weblogs living or dead is purely coincidental.) Let's say you get really horny in a public place, so you go to the restroom and masturbate yourself to orgasm three times. And let's say (God forbid) that you later decide "naughty" is a good word to describe this act, as in "I told Sir what a naughty horny little girl I had been, masturbating in the bathroom like that!"

A thing is either bad (negative, destructive, deceptive, cruel, disloyal) or it is good (positive, constructive, honest, loving, faithful) but it cannot be both things at one and the same time. When you say you were "naughty", you are implying that you were bad in some way. But if you honestly believed you were bad, you would be ashamed of yourself, not using giggly words like "naughty". So either you're using the word incorrectly, or you're internalizing what other people might think about your actions, which I think is a dangerous mental habit.

If a thing is good, it's not "naughty"; it's good. If it's bad, it's not "naughty"; it's bad. If it's good but condemned by society, it's not "naughty"; it's good, and society can go fuck itself. If it's bad but you don't care, it's not "naughty"; you have sociopathic tendencies.

Please, please, please, everyone, stop using this word. It's one of the words, like "selfish", whose current use embodies a very pernicious concept that needs to be eradicated from our society.

Be proud of the constructive, positive, honest, loving things you want and do, sexual and otherwise. Enjoy them, not because they are "naughty", but because they are nice.

Thank you.

In other news, I really, really, really need to be fucked, caned, and snuggled, in that order.

OK, I don't think people got what I was saying in that last post. Let me try once more to explain, and then I'll leave this topic alone. Incidentally, I've been thoroughly fucked and snuggled since I last posted, and Kam's promised me a caning when he gets home from work, so I'm in a much better mood than last time, as well. :-)

It's not the word "naughty" I have a beef with, except as an example of what I do have a beef with, which is the fact that people find activities sexier and more exciting because they are "bad", "naughty", "wicked", "forbidden" or whatever.

I believe that this mindset is wrong and destructive for several reasons.

1) It's immature, a sign of arrested development (unless you are a teenager, in which case it's run-of-the-mill teenage behavior. Like Buffy said when Giles told her she was acting immature, "You know why? I am immature. I'm a teen. I have yet to mature.") Not that mature adults never break rules, but they break them incidentally, because the rules are wrong or unnecessary, not because it's fun to break rules. Children and teens break rules because their lives are normally so structured that it's exhilarating. If adults feel the need to break societal rules just for the sake of it, it's probably a sign that they're paying too much attention to those rules in the first place, which leads me to my second reason:

2) It's just another form of obeying the rules. Kam compared this to an equally pernicious form of feminism – the form that says women must do nothing that the patriarchy might approve of, such as get married, have children or accept domestic discipline from their husbands – even if they would choose it from among equally available options. That's not freedom; it's allowing the system to

dictate how you live, just as much as if you obeyed the system. By getting your pleasure from breaking rules, you're nourishing the existence of those rules and retarding their much-needed abolition. If everyone was open-minded and intelligent, would it deprive you of pleasure? Can you only derive pleasure from a flawed and prejudiced world? Which brings me to my third point:

3) We, as human beings, should always be considering how our activities – all the activities that we intentionally pursue – make us better, happier, more open-minded, more interesting, more focused, more intelligent people, and we can't do that if we think of our actions as "bad", "wicked" or "wrong." Mature people are counterculture only insofar as the culture is wrong, and as such, we need to help turn the culture around if necessary, not accept their evaluation of our direction as "wrong" or "naughty."

Therefore, I believe this mindset – the one that leads people to say things like "forbidden fruit tastes the sweetest" – is wrong, immature and destructive. If you use "naughty" to mean just plain "hot", with no connotations of wrongdoing whatsoever, that's interesting, and certainly possible – Kam calls me his slut with no negative connotations, referring lovingly to my eagerness for sex and my openness to be used by him – and in that case, I don't think it's an example of this mindset, or that there's anything wrong with it.

I hope that makes things a little clearer.

Introduction to Noncontradiction: Or, Submission Is Not Suicide For Wusses

So you identify as submissive. Great. Me too.

So you want to be "owned". You want to be a slave. His only, his forever. Great. Wonderful. Get a lock-on collar, get his name tattooed on your bikini bits, put yourself in the Slave Register, sign a contract in blood transferring your immortal soul into his possession, write an undated suicide note just in case . . . whatever, you know? I'm a libertarian; if you're a legal adult, and you're not infringing on anyone else's basic rights, I don't think there's much you shouldn't be allowed to do.

But.

You cannot give up, hand over, or otherwise immolate your self.

Your right to choose. Your moral sense (by which I don't mean the prurient prudishness that makes quote-unquote "transgression" so titillating; I mean, basically, the judgement you pass on the choices you make. Whether you act in accordance with your own principles for living, or not). Your right to decide what's OK with you and what isn't.

I don't mean you shouldn't, or aren't allowed to, abdicate your self. I mean you actually, factually can not. You can sign a contract saying that a thing can both be and not be in the same respect at the same time, but the laws of logic will take precious little note of your contract. You cannot both consent and not consent in the same respect at the same time. It simply doesn't work.

No matter how deeply you are enslaved, no matter how masterful a master (or mistress) you have – you are either consenting or not. It's the utterly essential difference between BDSM and abuse, rough sex and rape. You can't let that go. You are responsible for your own consent.

And as such, you are responsible for your own actions and for the events of your own life. If your master/dominant tells you to do something, and you do it, the moral responsibility for the action is yours, not his/hers. Likewise, if your dominant fails to provide you with something you feel you need, it is your responsibility – as in any relationship, D/s or vanilla – to either seek it out, or do without. You have the right to wallow and complain all you want, of course, and I certainly do my share of both, but if you think it's anyone's responsibility but your own to get you where you need to be – including headspace – you're fooling yourself. And if you are in a D/s relationship because you can't deal with your own personhood or your own moral responsibilities as a human being, and you think slaves don't have to deal with that sort of thing, well, think again.

Yeah, I feel very strongly about this, although this particular issue is just symptomatic of a larger problem that is really bringing out my homicidal tendencies of late. It seems like everyone and everything is pissing me off on this subject lately, and while the level of rage I'm currently sustaining is probably due to premenstrual hormones, I don't think I'm wrong to violently object to the sheer stupidity being foisted upon me and the world by everyone from people arguing about gay marriage to people arguing about presidential elections to people describing their romantic relationships. It really, really isn't that hard to grasp the basic concept of logic, and it really, really isn't excusable not to. Nobody thinks it's excusable to be ignorant of the laws of physics – it's not considered sane or healthy to jump off a high building because you feel like you can fly – yet everyone seems to think it's fine – nay, laudable and beautiful – to ignore the laws of reason (which are, by and large, a hell of a lot more reliably immutable than the known laws of nature) in favor of how you, personally, feel about any given person or situation.

bashes own brains out against a number of brick walls

stomps off, brains leaking from shattered skull

When I first asked Kam if he'd like to step up our D/s activities to a 24/7, total power exchange lifestyle, he asked me why I wanted that. After some conversation during which I tried to sort that out, he suggested that maybe since I was soon to graduate from college and enter the adult world, I was panicking at the thought of leaving the safety of my parents' control and eager to line up a replacement "parent" in Kam.

I became furious. How dare he question my submissive identity! This was who I was! I was trying to become my fullest self, not hide from it! Clearly Kam had not done sufficient Internet research on the nature of submission!

Of course, I didn't say any of that. I just got upset and shut the conversation down. Later we discussed it again, more calmly, decided to give the TPE a trial run, and eventually decided against continuing it for several reasons of varying levels of bloggability.

Now, reading blogs and other personal accounts of submissive and slaves, I often bless Kam's conscientiousness in making sure that submissiveness did not, and does not, become a crutch for me. Though Kam loves me, cares for me, advises me, and brings me great joy and fulfillment, he has made it clear that only I am ultimately responsible for my own life. Kam doesn't micromanage; he has no interest in picking out my clothes or scheduling my day for me on a regular basis. And when he does give me instructions, though he expects ready obedience, he also expects me to use my own judgement to evaluate those instructions and hold myself responsible for all my actions, undertaken in obedience or otherwise. I may be his girl, his slut, his plaything – but I am also an intelligent and independent adult, and to lose those parts of me would be to lose a great part of what he values in me.

One reason we stopped the 24/7 was that in my constant efforts to be a good submissive, I stopped being the smart-mouthed intellectual equal he loves so much. I believe that ideally, I could be both at the same time. I'm still learning – slowly – that sometimes my responses during a spanking or a scene aren't textbook slave responses, and sometimes it's OK to go with that. Sometimes it's OK to be a little bit talkative during a scene, or squeal with delight when the cane comes out instead of shaking with fear. Disobedience isn't tolerated, but being who I am is downright encouraged. I'm learning that being submissive isn't about conforming to an abstract standard, but releasing the parts of me that flourish in a BDSM context – the gleeful girl who glories in the "toy chest", the slave who is simply desperate to please in any way possible, the slut who will do anything to be touched by his cock, the pain slut who craves the endorphin rush, the emotionally unstable wench who needs an excuse to cry uncontrollably on his shoulder, the grump who needs a caning to get her head back on straight – and more. And the best part is that these parts can joyfully coexist and interact with the feminist, the soapbox ranter, the sarcastic and the silly and the bibliophile and the Christian and the Buffy fanatic. Once I let them all out of their little boxes and into a big padded room where they can stretch their legs and gossip about each other in corners, they're all way more fun.

My point here is, I once believed (without really thinking about it) that in order to be a good submissive, I had to pick some aspects of myself over others. Kam wouldn't allow that. He loves all of me, and part of what he loves is the fact that I am whole without him. I wouldn't want to live without him, but I could, and I would be a whole and (reasonably) well integrated person. He has helped me grow into that person, and he continues to help me develop myself

– sexually, submissively and otherwise – but if I lost him now, I wouldn't be left flailing for someone to guide and protect me. Kam would not permit a submission that would shelter me from any aspect of reality, nor a lifestyle that would stunt or atrophy any part of me. And, thanks to him, neither would I.

Ask and you shall receive

I asked for a spanking again today – not in the metaphorical sense of misbehaving, but in the literal if somewhat mumbly, ". . . maybe you could spank me . . ." sense. In the immortal phrase, it's "that time of the month" when "I'm not at my best" because "my vagina is bleeding,"* and I thought an ass-smacking might be really cathartic, not to mention a reminder that taking out my hormonal grumpiness on Kam wouldn't be the best idea.

Unfortunately, Kam didn't bring the cane this time. All that was around was my hairbrush.

Damn.

"What kind of spanking do you want?" he asked briskly, scanning my music files for yelp-and-smack-drowning-out ambience music. "Gentle, medium, hard, really hard, or 'holy shit'?"

I nervously contemplated this for a minute.

"Medium . . . please."

He took down my jeans and panties and I lay face down on the bed while he sat beside me, starting out with some sharp, tingling hand spanks. I yelped a bit but tried to relax into it the way I do with the cane, keeping my buttocks unclenched and breathing deeply. I was scared of the hairbrush. I'd just realized I hadn't been spanked with it since we discovered how much I love being caned, and all I remembered was that it HURT.

He started off medium – and yeah, it hurt, but not too badly. The difference was more in quality than intensity – the cane can hurt like holy fuck, but it never has scared me. Something about being paddled just makes me feel afraid. Maybe it's the noise, or the larger area of contact. Anyway, it was a lot harder to relax and I couldn't help tensing up and squirming just a little, although I tried

* *Okay, I ripped that particular euphemism off from The Onion.*

very hard to stay relaxed and still. With the cane, I feel more like staying quiet and I only whimper or make noise to let Kam know what's up with me; with the hairbrush, whimpers are less voluntary and tend to have more of a ring of protest.

After popping me hard and rhythmically, alternating cheeks every five swats or so, and occasionally stopping to stroke my hair and ask how I was doing and if I wanted more, Kam began hitting faster and really hard (not just my perception; he confirmed it afterwards). I got scared again; the hairbrush always makes me feel like I've done something wrong, maybe because it was the implement we used for punishment during our period of "submissive training", and I was having a hard time remembering that Kam wasn't displeased with me. I was crying out and jerking with every stroke . . . and then there was an odd blurring and I realized I wasn't feeling the individual swats so much as I was rolling along on a wave of burning punctuated by sharp popping noises. As soon as I realized this, I started feeling the individual ones again, but then the blurring came back and I could almost relax. It was neat. Still, when Kam finally stopped and asked if I wanted more, I shook my head. I'd had enough.

I realized afterwards that I haven't really had my limits pushed, in terms of pain, for a long time. Not because I'm Wonder Bottom, but because Kam almost never uses spanking as a punishment any more, for a variety of reasons, so most of our spankings for some time have been for pleasure – mine or his. If they're for mine, I can ask him to stop when I feel I've had enough; if they're for his, he's likely to be more interested in taking advantage of the arousal he's produced, long before my limits are reached. Not necessarily a good or bad thing, just an observation.

Another observation: I don't think I'm capable of crying from physical pain, nor from fear, both of which inspire an adrenaline rush that signals my body that this is the very worst time to break down and snivel. I often cry from relief, afterwards, but if Kam ever decided to spank me to tears, I'd have a long spank coming.

> For contemplation he and valor formed;
> For softness she and sweet attractive grace.

That's from Milton's *Paradise Lost*, describing Adam and Eve. We've been discussing the issue of gender in/equality lately in my

Milton class. Coincidentally, I've noticed several blogs taking up the statement, originally asserted by Invidia on The Collar Purple, that "it's not about fair in a D/s relationship. It's about harmony."

I regard Kam's and my D/s relationship as all about fairness. Not only that, but I regard us as equals within it. Yes, our roles are different – among other things, he's the Dom and the boy, while I'm the sub and the girl – but we contribute equally to the relationship in our different ways. Likewise, we benefit equally from the relationship – which is what I consider fair.

Fairness doesn't have to mean sameness. When you buy an apple for fifty cents, you don't consider yourself cheated because the apple doesn't resemble the fifty cents. You would only consider yourself cheated if what you got seemed less valuable than what you gave. D/s is the same way, in my opinion. Yes, the roles are different – one partner plans, gives orders, and wields the implements, while the other submits, obeys and gets the stingy end – but it's only unfair if one partner gets more benefit out of the relationship than the other. And if that's true, I have a hard time understanding why the "cheated" party would stay in such a relationship. Kam assumes the role he feels most comfortable with, and I assume the role I feel most comfortable with. Neither of us would have it any other way.

When I was in elementary school, lunch never began without a ritual trading session – I'll give you one of my Swiss Cake Rolls for six of your Doritos. Four Fig Newtons for your cup of chocolate pudding. Three apple slices for a box of raisins. Whatever the logistics, the gist was that we gave up what we didn't want in exchange for what we did want. That, to me, is fair.

A little while ago, I was leaning across Kam to read a sweet e-mail from Invidia (*wave*), and he took the opportunity to bite my shoulder. Not having expected it and not being in a very sexy frame of mind, I squeaked indignantly and pulled away. Kam followed me, pushed me over, pinned my wrists down and proceeded to kiss and bite me at his leisure and, though I was struggling at first, I soon relaxed, feeling a familiar and comfortable powerlessness, and enjoyed it amazingly. It was a trade; he took away my power over the situation and gave me back pleasure and orgasms.

Seems fair to me. :–)

I'd like to talk about religion. And I will probably use the word "Jesus" multiple times.

So, like, feel free to leave now if you think you will become squirmy.

Hi. So, I'm a Christian. That means, among other things, that I believe in God, as he was made manifest in a Jewish carpenter who lived a couple of thousand years ago. I also love and trust God, and believe that he loves and cares for me, and wants the best for me, and that it is in my best interests to seek to know, and live according to, his will for my life.

Nothing about that is simple, of course – and it isn't easy, either. It is possible to use the idea of God as a crutch to make things seem simpler and easier, but you have to be either really sheltered or really stupid to make that stick.

Anger is the anaesthetic of the mind; it's always nice to have someone to blame, and Christians, of course, are just as prone as anyone else to taking that means of comfort. If you can't blame God (or God's minions on earth), you can easily blame the homos, or the feminists, or the devil, or whoever is most convenient.

It's hard, just getting up again, and going on ahead, and trying to love everyone, and trying to be good. God isn't very good at kissing it all better.

I've heard a lot of talk on blogs lately about total dependence on one's Dom, and the question always hovers around such talk: what would happen if he should leave or (if one assumes he is perfectly trustworthy and, having created or condoned this dependence, will certainly never leave it hanging) die? I've never had the luxury of considering Kam's death as a vague and remote possibility, so perhaps I've been more aware than some of the inherent limitations in even the best, strongest and most loving of human beings. Human beings cannot guarantee anything – except, perhaps, what Jeannette Winterson said she required in a lover: that they will always be on your side.

It's tempting to ask of a Dom that he fulfill the instinctive needs that we all have, but which submissives perhaps naturally feel more than most: a desire for an ordered world, where the rules are always the same and always make sense, and where we know what is right and what will happen to us next. A world where if we are good, we are rewarded, and we always know that we are loved and taken care of.

Heaven cannot thus, Earth cannot ever, give the thing we want. Submission to a loving Dominant is a wonderful thing, and does a lot of good for those whose personalities work that way. It's even possible to create a household where almost everything makes sense. But the household will never be safe. Death and mayhem strike everywhere. That's part of living on earth, as everyone, religious or ir-, can likely agree; everything you treasure is infinitely fragile, and, ultimately, swept away by the tide of destruction and disorder. As Robert Frost once put it, "nothing gold can stay."

I just paused and wondered what, exactly, I'm trying to say here, and to whom I'm trying to say it. I'm not trying to tell anyone who's happy that they are doomed, DOOMED!, because the world SUCKS!, and you should TURN TO JESUS WHO IS THE ONLY THING PERMANENT AND HAPPY-MAKING IN THIS WORLD! Because it's wonderful to be happy, if you are, and anyway, being a Christian is just as miserable as anything else, and maybe more. Like I said, God sucks at kissing it all better.

I think I'm trying to say, to anyone who is sad or unfulfilled or heartbroken or afraid, that being all those things is part of what it means to be human, because it's part of our human nature to long for something more permanent and more fulfilling and less prone to smash your heart into atoms on the kitchen floor than anything we actually know on this earth. And it's also natural to wish that that something could be with us here and now, and not off somewhere in the celestial ether, waiting for us to die so he can explain how it all did make sense after all.

Which is why, though I've explored quite a bit, I can't ultimately understand the love of God through any medium except Christianity – because Christianity is the only religion I've found (that's still extant; Norse mythology, while also quite appealing to me, appears to be extinct, and also unnecessarily complicated, and also to have inspired more rape and pillage than I'm entirely comfortable with, not that Christianity is innocent in that regard either) wherein God also understands what an entirely shitty place this world is to anyone who hungers and thirsts for righteousness.

That's the point of Jesus; God knew it wasn't fair if he didn't take his licks like the rest of us, and so he did, because he wanted us to know that it could be done. We don't have to be happy about it; Jesus wasn't. We don't have to make a "success" of it; Jesus was a homeless street preacher before he was executed as a rabble-rouser. What we do have to do is try our best to love and take care of each other, and drink deep of whatever joy this life has to offer, and try to trust that if God could teach us what we need to learn in any easier way, he would, because he loves us.

Hey. We're subs. We eat tough love for breakfast.

> Behold, we know not anything;
> I can but trust that good shall fall
> At last – far off – at last, to all,
> And every winter change to spring.
>
> So runs my dream; but what am I?
> An infant crying in the night;
> An infant crying for the light,
> And with no language but a cry.
> — Alfred, Lord Tennyson,
> *In Memoriam A. H. H.*

To everyone who said "Thank you" to the last post – Thank you. I can't tell you how much it means to know that my words helped answer or articulate something for you. It's humbling to think. Thank you for that.

M at Sexual Anarchism asked a very interesting question:

> I know that there are submissives out there who are Christian, and there are Christian submissives. Are you submissive because of your religious/spiritual beliefs or for an entirely different reason? Just curious. :)

There are about ten different answers to that question. Let me tackle a couple.

I do NOT submit to Kam because I believe that God ordains that women should submit to men. Jesus never said women should submit to men; in fact, he was one of the earliest feminists, challenging gender inequality and double standards whenever he encountered them, and interacting with women on the same basis of love, compassion and respect on which he interacted with men.

"Women should be silent in church" was cooked up later by insecure male presbyters.

I DO believe that submission is part of who I am – that when God created me, he put that in me on purpose. Therefore, I think one of the things God calls me to is an understanding and practice of the submissive part of my nature. In that sense, yes, I am submissive because of my spiritual beliefs, in the same way that I'm a vegetarian because of my spiritual beliefs, although neither the Bible nor the Christian Church directly advocates vegetarianism; I'm a vegetarian because I believe what Jesus taught: "Verily, verily I say unto you, if you believe something is wrong but are too damn lazy to make any changes in your life or inconvenience yourself the slightest bit in order to live the change you want to see in the world, your complacent lethargy will eventually come back to bite you in the ass."

(I may be paraphrasing a wee bit.)

I also think, though, that one-word labels are not very good at actually describing who people are. I know a lot of people who describe themselves as Christians and whose beliefs are nearly diametrically opposite to mine. I know people who describe themselves as submissives and whose lifestyles are completely repugnant to me. I know people who describe themselves as vegetarians and still eat chicken, and I also know people who are a lot stricter about vegetarianism than me. I know lesbians who are more ambivalent about their attraction to women than I am – and I call myself bisexual. I know blondes whose hair is way lighter than mine, and blondes whose hair is way darker. They're just words. What matters is what they mean to you.

So . . . I don't know whether I'm a "submissive who is Christian" or a "Christian submissive". The only answer I can come up with is that every aspect of who I am informs every other aspect. I'm the kind of submissive I am because I am also a Christian, and a vegetarian, and a feminist, and bisexual, and an academic, and a bookworm, and a Buffy addict – and I'm the kind of Christian I am because I am all those other things, and I'm the kind of Buffyphile I am because of all those other things, and so forth and so on.

One of my basic goals in life is to be the person I wish existed somewhere in the world – be she the smart feminist submissive, the logical activist Christian, or the academic who teases out the implications of the similarity between Ovid's retelling of "Phile-mon and Baucis" and the Genesis account of Isaac's conception. And I believe that desire – to be all those things, to find the needs in the world that I can fill, and to fill them – comes from God, who created me to be what I am, and Jesus, who was what he was created to be, and the Holy Spirit, who guides me in the direction I need to go.

So, yeah. Does that answer your question?

Things I could never live without

Cupid.com asks for "the SIX things you could never live without" as part of your profile. The snarkier answer "Food, water, shelter, oxygen . . ." while the perkier say things like "Lip gloss, Pantene Pro-V for fine hair," and the more sentimental, "Friends, family, my dog . . ."

I was thinking today about what we need (and cannot live without) versus what we want. It seems like it's a lot easier to say you "need" or "couldn't live without" something if you have it and aren't worried about losing it. There's not much I feel that way about.

Take romantic relationships, though. I have always held that it's emotionally unhealthy to crave a romantic relationship in the abstract, when you're single. Relationships are about discovering that someone is such a great fit for you that you want to spend a lot of time with him and express your affection by smooshing your pink bits together and possibly, at some point, merging your DNA. Wanting "a relationship", without even having met the actual person with whom you would be having the relationship in ques-tion, could land and keep you in a bad relationship. In addition, it implies that there is something lacking in you, by yourself – that you need someone else to complete you, instead of having a ful-filling life and soul of your own. Which is wrong. Right?

Except if you think about the theory of D/s, the implication is that we, the kinksters of the world, are all incomplete in that way – we all need someone else, with the opposite set of characteristics, to complete us. A sub has not fulfilled her identity unless s/he has a Dom, and vice versa. Or, if you are some people, a female has not

fulfilled her identity unless she has a Man, and Men need hearth
and whore to come home to after a long day of doing important,
strong, intelligent Man Things. Either way.

I don't always get what I "need", in that sense. I'm a subbier sub
than Kam is a Dommish Dom, and we're frequently completely
vanilla for long stretches. I get in itchy moods where I think the
ideal resolution would be for him to be Dommish and spank or
otherwise Dom me into submission. In a vanilla mood, he wouldn't
think of that, and if I could ask for it, I would already be in the
reasonable frame of mind it would hopefully achieve. So it doesn't
happen.

If it did happen, I could say that when I'm in such a mood, I
"need" him to take control. As it is, he doesn't, and the world keeps
turning, and I deal, or I don't, and get cranky and pissy and ruin a
couple of hours.

The thing is, I consider that my failure, not his. Any situation
where I can't handle my own emotions without help from someone
else is due to a character flaw in me. I couldn't be a slave or 24/7
sub, because that would mean having a 24/7 crutch for my need
instead of having to work on myself so that I can cope gracefully
when I don't get what I "need". And then what if something
happened? Suppose my Dom left me, or died? Suppose he constantly treated me with contempt and emotional carelessness, or
selfishly took advantage of my devotion, and I couldn't leave
because I needed what he gave me? I refuse to let that happen.

For ages I hated going over to other people's places to eat, because
I'm mildly hypoglycemic (means, in practice, that I tend to get
REALLY grumpy when I'm hungry) and I was afraid I wouldn't be
able to eat what they had, or that the servings would be too small to
satisfy me, and I'd end up hungry and miserable. I preferred staying
at home, where I knew I liked the food. Now I have a simple solution:
I eat something before I go to dinner at someone else's. That way I
can eat a small and gracious serving of whatever I'm given and be
properly appreciative and also comfortable. That's sort of my theory
of relationships. If you're satisfied with your life and with who you
are going in, you don't make yourself and your partner miserable by
demanding that he function as your surrogate daddy, shrink, emotional stabilizer and gooey caramel dessert all at once.

I'm not saying that a partner can't be any or all of those things in a healthy relationship. Kam is arguably my gooey caramel dessert, as well as my best friend, confidant, and companion in adventure. Nor am I saying it's easy to be emotionally self-sufficient, because God knows I'm not; I regularly melt into a pile of tearful emotional goo and demand to be mopped up by all my friends in turn, not to mention poor Kam. But I can cope with these bad times by myself, and I don't mind being left to do so; I pull myself together quicker if no one offers to snuggle and comfort me, in fact, because I know it's better when I'm pulled together.

Kam asked me the other day if I was sad that we'd been so vanilla for so long

Here, I think, is the precise, and long, answer.

I don't regret that he's not ordering me around or acting dominant. I've discovered, partly by reading others' blogs, that I am profoundly conflicted about the idea of being bossed around and actually living in submission to someone, in that it makes me hot, but it also makes extremely resentful and uncomfortable. I don't think it enhances our relationship very much when we do it, I don't think it comes naturally to him, and I think it allows me to retreat into a rather immature and unconstructive area of my personality, which makes me uncomfortable both in that I lose other parts of me that I like (better) and in that I'm really not old enough or mature enough yet to trust that such a psychological activity won't "stunt my growth". so to speak. I like being independent. I want to be independent. I'm working on being independent. Taking orders is a step backwards for me right now. (Not saying anything about your lifestyle or personal growth, mind you – just mine.)

I used to think I wanted all that – the whole 24/7 shebang – for two reasons. One is that rough, kinky sex, spanking and scening turn me on to a ridiculous extent, and incorporating kink into everyday life (taking orders on things like chores and daily outfits, etc., and having to report back or risk punishment) made everything in life madly erotic. The most mundane tasks made me wet. Which is all very well, but certainly not enough to counterbalance everything I noted in the previous paragraph. The other reason is that I want to do everything I do "right", and I thought that people who just "played" at BDSM were somehow less "real" or respectable than people for whom it was a genuine lifestyle.

Which leads me to the second part of my answer to the question: Yes, I regret that we're not having more rough sex and erotic pain play, because, as noted, that turns me on to a simply unbelievable extent. I love gentle, tender, loving sex too, but I feel like something is missing from our sex life when we don't have the kink, and anything kinky (hair-pulling, him repositioning me and pushing me about) happening during sex instantly revs my engine.

So, there you go. I don't want a master. I don't want a Dom. I want someone to push me around in the bedroom. Yay!

LETICIA MCKENZIE

http://leticiamckenzie.blogspot.com

Hi! My name is Leticia McKenzie, and welcome to my section of the book!

When I was fourteen or so, I decided that I wanted to be a stripper. Seriously! Nothing would prove my womanhood more than taking my clothes off to the hordes of gasping, horny, lonely men who need somebody to, um, look up to. Somehow, I believed, if I could make some of those lonely men a little bit less lonely, I'd have done good. So I guess it would follow that I would do what all the cool kids are doing these days and start a blog; except, this one would be about, you guessed it, beekeeping. No, seriously, it would be about sex. It would, specifically, be about sex with myself and a few select fantasies.

After a while, at the request of my readers, I stopped being so obsessed with diddling myself and began to branch out into other areas of my life. I'm hoping this section of the book, the Very Best of Leticia McKenzie, will give a good cross-section of who I am, a cross-section that can be peeled and separated and eaten and washed down with pink lemonade. Sound good? Good! Let's get going!

We'll begin with the post that got me on the map as a blogger, my first post regarding the Diddle.

Saturday 3 January 2004

Masturbation. OK, that's what I need to write about. I can't stop. I can't ever stop. For the rest of my life, I'm going to be like this.

Masturbating, masturbating, masturbating, always needing more, never being satisfied with what I have. Shit.

Oh, it wasn't always like this. Back when I started, it was beautiful. Wonderful. I felt affirmed in my womanhood. Then I felt dirty. Defiled. And then . . . well, then I knew I couldn't stop, because I would always be looking for the next hit. I wanted to go back to that first time, the first time I had a fantasy.

Well, since I'm on the subject, perhaps I should share my first masturbation fantasy with all you fine readers. It went something like this: At a sex-ed class, I was an, um, instrument of practice for a room full of horny adolescent boys. A fluffy brunette woman teacher in her thirties (she looked stereotypically Jewish . . . sorry) wanted to demonstrate the proper way to pleasure a woman, so she unbuttoned my shirt and began to play . . .

First, some background material. You should know what I had been reading the previous day before lulling in bed that fine summer morning. For some reason, I was on the People for the Ethical Treatment of Animals website, looking at their nude calendar. Yes, this exists. PETA, having decided that pictures of slaughtered animals was not the best way to win a constituency, went instead for the "naked celebrities posing for animal rights" angle. And, so they say, it went disturbingly well. (For the record, they were beautiful photographs; and the thought of using your [my] sexuality and naked body in support of animal rights just makes me warm and fuzzy inside.) One of the images had a very young model, naked, in front of the class, daintily hiding her fuzzy points and looking determined, having written on the board innumerable times: "I would rather go nude then wear fur." You tell 'em, girl!

So, anyway, also that night, to complete the mental cocktail I was reading "Pornography: Opposing Viewpoints." Opposing Viewpoints is a fairly ridiculous series of books in which they try to give a fair and balanced perspective by reducing issues to a collection of editorials compiled as "Censorship is the Solution to All the World's Problems" or "Censorship Is A Great Big Pain in My Buttocks." In any case, one particularly exasperated blowhard turned to an old issue of *Hustler* [warning: fairly explicit content ahead. No, not really, but it might turn you on, which also means it might disgust you] to indicate why pornography is the root of all evil: the cover had a woman being shoved through a meat grinder, with the caption "More Meat Issue;" the woman was coming out the other end as raw hamburger.

(Isn't that sexy? I mean, really. I would like to be – oops, can't spoil the fantasy . . .)

So I was being – I mean, I was lulling in bed as these images swirled around in my enthusiastic cranium. The teacher unbuttoned my shirt and stripped me naked, passing me around so that the eager students may see how to pleasure a woman. She instructed the students to take note of when I was the happiest; and I was continuously happy, enjoying the attention, mentally and physically. After several rounds of interesting performances – me giving all the boys blow-jobs, them tying me up and whipping me, and branding me – finally, the teacher instructed them to put me through . . . a meat grinder. She said to study my reactions as I was reduced to ground Leticia in a pile on the floor. Truthfully, I enjoyed it; it was like I was being lowered into a warm bath as I excitedly swayed my hips and thrust my arms in the air with a silly grin. Oooh, being reduced to raw meat. I love it.

That's where it got out of control. I had never had thoughts like this. Being reduced to raw meat? Ohhh yes. Oh, it was hot. Hotter than I could imagine. I reached into my pants and . . . oh no, don't reach there . . . yes . . . no . . . yes . . . no . . . ooouuggghhhhh . . . KABOOM! And that's how my room became splattered with blood, come, and Leticia parts.

No, not quite. But still, I was Leticia McKenzie, a virgin no longer. Satisfied with my first fuck, with, er, myself, I went to play Metroid Prime and all was good.

Um, so, anyway, now that I've shared with the entire Internet such an edifying experience, I'm'a go play Halo. Toodles!

(p.s. Strong Bad got me started on the contraction "I'm'a," which apparently means "I'm gonna," which probably means "I'm going to." I use it too often now and I believe my vocabulary is unraveling as a result. C'est la vie.)

After that, my blog was listed on Belle du Jour, and my rather questionable rise to fifteen-minute fame was cemented. And, that, my friends, is how babies are made.

Monday 5 January 2004

I wrote this just now, musing about sex work. Since I think about sex work so much, I decided to write from the perspective of Leticia the Aspiring Prostitute. Here ya go:

I wanna be a prostitute.

Seriously. It's not bad. I want to please a thousand men a day and hear their simultaneous cries of joy and agony with relief and satisfaction. I have done my job. I have turned men on.

I want to walk down the street in day-glo short shorts and go-go boots and give men the knowing glance that I'm for sale, that the space between my legs is for rent and that I can cheer up any sullen mood.

I want to eat men, I want them inside me, inside my vagina's clamp, sucking them in to my world. I want to trap men in my arms, never to come back. One taste of Leticia and you will be begging for more.

I want to melt, I want to be consumed. I want to be a commodity. I want to be licked off the floor by eager men wanting more of the tantalizing Leticia taste. I want to be eaten, in full, without clothes, so that somebody can know what I taste like. I want to be part of the world.

(If you haven't guessed, I'm lonely.)

Dante is a boy that is very important to me, so, to summarize all my feelings about him, I wrote this quite recently. This is the place that it would go most logically, as it is never been posted to my blog and is thus exclusive material. Keep in mind, though, unlike the other posts regarding Dante it is written with somewhat clearer hindsight.

NEVER POSTED

I met Dante on a park bench outside the school. I had just moved to Poseidontown, and I hadn't made many friends and I was something of a nerd, so when I saw this group of boys playing Pokémon on a park bench, I was instantly intrigued. I went home on the bus with Dante. My mother didn't like that I had brought a boy home without telling her, which made me really sad because she usually welcomes guests. I invited Dante into my room and showed him my worldly possessions. Most importantly, though, as I bonded with him, I learned that he was the only person I had ever met who knew the Sonic level designs as deeply as I do.

I started to find a crush on him. He is very attractive. He's like nothing you've ever seen, and it's a shame I can't describe him (for the sake of his anonymity) because he's the most precious, precious man I've ever laid eyes upon. Something in me wants to know about every nook and cranny of that boy's body, and won't stop until I know it intimately, as intimately as we know the levels of Sonic.

So, back to that subject, Dante and I were really good friends until I finally told him that I loved him. I was an ickle fifteen and hadn't yet found my voice, but I still had to tell him or else I would die. We kissed after a long night of drinking soda and playing Sonic 3, and my life was never again the same.

Well, I'm overdramatizing, but you get the idea. Suddenly, it reversed. He told me something that I'll never forget, that he liked me back, that he had always liked me back, and that all he wanted was to be with me. I ran out of breath. I didn't know what to do. I slept in another room and thought about what should happen next.

Why don't I want to be with him? I thought. I've been chasing this man for months now. But . . . it felt to me that I had gone too far with what had simply been a girly-crush, and now I was trapped.

Moreover, Dante really needed me, and this breaks my heart. He has had a verifiably awful past, including a rotating cast of fathers, and I had to be there for him or else, as he warned, "the darkness will overcome me." We became "us", not exactly soulmates, more that I would be the one to motivate him to do good in this world, or at the very least, stay alive. I couldn't handle being one half of us. I freaked out and I stopped talking to him. I must have hurt the poor guy's feelings.

After all, before I finally kissed him, every time I saw him I wanted to. Under the tree, on our porch before saying goodnight, just walking home late in a serene evening in the summer . . . but, you gotta understand, it was a crush. Calf love.

Oh, but it was more than that. Dante's an enigma. I pride myself in being able to figure people out, and to see far inside their souls.

Dante, I couldn't. It was like he was blocking me, and that made it all the better. If Dante doesn't know how he will react to each day when he gets up in the morning, how will he react when we have long, hot sex in the shower? How far could I get into this Dante enigma? He was like my personal project. If his emotions are constantly in conflict, would it completely unravel him to have me as a girlfriend? Will I finally get to see the wonderful person beneath all those layers of darkness?

After a while, we both forgot about it, and it was hard to tell him how I really felt. Finally, I came clean; it wasn't a fluke, Dante, I really am attracted to you. The problem is, I can't figure you out. You're a mystery, Dante, and no matter how much I enjoy it it scares me. I'm afraid of what I don't understand, and I hope you can understand this. Goodbye, Dante, I hope we meet again.

Except, it didn't go like that, we kept being friends and I finally had the feelings off of my chest. I felt that I had a reliable backdoor into his heart, for the time when I'm mature enough to face the people I love and not judge them by what I perceive as their motivations, but that was shattered when he met Another Girl.

Another Girl shares Dante's dark past and rotating cast of fathers. It's a tragic story that's finally been put to rest with these two people coming together. She wants to be a teacher and he wants to be a doctor, and soon they plan to marry and set out into the real world in search of fame and fortune, or at least a steady living. They both live out of Dante's mother's house and are embarrassingly happy together, embarrassing in that not even I, the great Leticia McKenzie, could please Dante as much as that wench. (Jealousy talking. Jealousy talking.) But, truth be told, I had my chance, and it's up to Dante, and I ought to find my own man.

It kills me to say this, because in my private fantasy world, I really was going to be Dante's savior. It hurt me that Dante put so much energy into regretting his dark past, because he could have put that energy into moving beyond it. His childhood isn't who he is, he is who he is now. But, alas, the job is not for me. The job belongs to Another Girl, and she's doing quite a good job as it is. I'd better bow out while I can.

Moreover, my mother complex tells me to fix everything I can, to make everything perfect for everybody. Those who know me know that I am constantly trying to fix every situation I'm in, and always telling everyone to play nice and be polite. Nobody knows that, between my ears, a fiery war of me against me rages on every time I have to make a decision. I calm the world around me in hopes of calming the world within me.

So I take things one day at a time. Not really, but it's an ideal to which I aspire. When I'm angry or confused, I try to look at what I can do and what I can't do, and what I can do is limited to what's inside my own body. I can be there for Dante and be his friend. I cannot force myself upon him and be his savior, no matter how nervous I was about that role at first, or how much I feel I deserve it. Only Dante can do that, and not me nor Another Girl should attempt it. We can show him the water. The rest is up to him.

It pleases me to see that Dante has become a family man, providing food for his darling fiancée and planning the family finances. I hope he can do better than my condescending image of him that I've projected onto him ever since I met him. For now, inside my own head, this is Leticia McKenzie, saying goodnight.

Saturday 24 January 2004

Hey, yo, one and all. This is Leticia McKenzie, reporting from Poseidontown's Sad Sorry Sluts Division. *(I say things like that a lot. Don't do it. It's bad for your health.)*

I can't say what's gotten me down so much. Maybe it's my tears, and how I can never get them to come at the right moment. I can't get myself to feel – but yeah, I cried once during Pokémon when Ash left Charizard and it was SO SAD . . . but I can't get myself to cry over things that are important.

Like Dante. Yeah, if I had more emotional fortitude, I could be his mistress. But no, I need the person I'm having sex with to have a relationship with me *(that might be good . . .)*; I'm too fragile and insecure for anything else. I couldn't handle the thought of my sex making somebody happy, who will then forget about me when the lights are dimmed and the candles are lit and he goes to have real love. *(Yeah, that might make present-day me not so happy either.)*

So I had a dream. I had friends over at this family vacation home, but I promptly forgot about my friends anyway. I looked at my room; wow, there were three beds in it. I could call my other friends right now and have that girly sleepover that I always wanted to have. I needed intimacy, I needed bonding, I needed to sit in the middle of the bedroom floor in my pajamas and giggle and talk about boys for hours like all the other girls did in, oh, elementary school. I needed friends.

So anyway, there was this raft in the backyard. Er, the backyard was a great big lake; it was the evening, and the sun was setting beautifully. I sat on a raft a step away from the back door, admiring the sunset and writing in my diary. For some reason, I was naked (this happens at least once a dream) and I yearned to swim out to the sunset, to touch it, to taste it, to feel its warmth. It was late, but the water was not yet cold, and I wanted it to envelop my naked body.

But, no, I put my clothes on and went inside instead. I accidentally dropped my diary in the water, so I needed to dry it off. Besides, I had to go do my homework. What would I have done if my parents had seen me naked? I would have died. And so on and so forth. End of dream.

So, if anyone has Beautiful Sunset real estate out there, make me an offer . . .

Most of my dreams have that sort of anticlimax. I'm sure yours do, too. In fact, I'm sure you've been in all my dreams, and you've told me all your dirty secrets. In fact, you also think about boys when you masturbate. Don't lie, I know you too well.

I'm going to get on my high horse and say that my fifteen-year-old enthusiasm for being a stripper someday was something every teenage girl goes through, and if they do not learn to deal with it, they manifest it in some negative fashion like forming an identity around being a sexpot, and I know full well by the things that twelve-year-olds wear these days in America that I am not alone in that regard. The problem is that teenage girls are not equipped to deal with their emerging sexuality in America, when it ought to be something that their parents and family guide them through; instead, we keep quiet about sex and our teenage girls, like me, head to their bedrooms and listen to Britney Spears to learn about sex. No good.

Here's another one of my silly fantasies. You will notice that I get off on capitalism. I do kind of like economics. Maybe I will become an economist, and then write economic porn on the side. I think my first book will be called, "Double-Dip Recession . . .

Wednesday 11 February 2004

Last night I really enjoyed the following fantasy, in which Leticia the Popstar was told by her agent that, unfortunately, she over-looked a clause in her contract that said she would have to be run, naked, vertically, through the Song Machine that, while she sang, would turn her into pure audio for recording on a smash-hit album. I get off on corporate fantasies. Weird. (Yes, I had been reading too much Jennifer Government.)

Oh, but before that, my naked popstar trio was kidnapped by space bandits who placed us in a giant . . . clamp thing (you know . . . the WinZip logo!) at the back of their ship and turned the crank. (The space bandits were teenagers, with scruffy hair and impeccable hygiene. I think they rebelled and stole their rich dad's space shuttle to go around picking up naked popstars. But anyway . . .) We moaned and giggled and forced weak smiles as the ceiling lowered and eventually we were crushed into . . . something. I think a Game Boy Advance cartridge. I seem to fantasize about those too. What?

(oh, the cruel and yet pleasurable entrapment of plastic . . .)

Indeed. You should all try it sometime. Anything that makes me imagine being turned into a merchandizable object makes me happy. In this case, it's the fact that I'm being flattened into information. Maybe I should write cyberpunk porn, instead of economic porn. So many choices ahead of me! I should have stuck with saying "I wanna be a nurse" like all the other girls.

Saturday 13 March 2004

All the girls in Leticia's home ec class were happy to learn they were making human muffins that day, so they ganged up on Leticia, ripped off her clothes, and threw her in the bread machine, which kneaded and prodded and baked her into a fine, warm

Leticiaberry Muffin. The teacher was delighted; she always wanted to know what that awkward girl tasted like. The class ate her up and licked her from their fingers; indeed, she got more attention as a muffin than she ever would have as a human.

I fantasized that I was with my broad-shouldered husband, relaxing in a big black boiling pot, to be eaten by cannibals. I, being an airhead, was completely oblivious to this predicament, and I looked up at my husband, lovingly telling him "Isn't this great? We're getting a warm bath." Being the wonderful imaginary husband that he is, he just lay there, holding me tenderly, appreciating the time we had together. We kept that same sappy expression as we were laid, naked, on a platter surrounded decoratively by fruits and vegetables, and as we watched our limbs being carved off ("oooh, I have some nice fat over here, cut this off") and swallowed, toes and all. Our only nervous moment was when our heads, the final course, were seperated to be eaten like apples, but we didn't seem to mind. We enjoyed the time we spent together. We were a happy marriage.

"Dearest? They seem to be eating us up."

"Don't worry, honey, everything's going to be all right. . . . Hey, that's my leg!"

"Oooh, my thigh's gone too . . ."

"Honey, I don't think these are nice people . . ."

"Don't worry. They say true giving is the giving of yourself."

"But wait! Honey!" (chomp! his head gets eaten.)

"Oooh, I like you best like this . . ." (licks his nipple and then takes a great big bite out of his chest.) "Oooh . . ."

Thursday 18 March 2004

Well, I leave for England today (yahoo!), so I won't be writing much today, probably. Most of my day will be spent playing Mario & Luigi on the plane. I'll miss you all, my darlings.

(But stay tuned for updates from Leticia's Fantastic England Adventure.)

Friday 19 March 2004

Hey, ho, lovely Leticiaites! We're kicking it liiiive from somewhere in England (my undisclosed location), which I have now declared the People's Republic of Brielleistan, which shall be the sister nation of Leticiastan. From here, we shall conquer the world! A dildo in every home, I say!

So anyway, it took a plane, my mom's car, three trains, and a bus to get home, and I was up for a good twenty-six hours before finally crashing at my dad's Quaker National Headquarters. Seriously; this place (my undisclosed location) is Quaker City, a mansion complex in which I keep looking around to find George Fox's preserved brain, or perhaps the Quaker Central Hivemind. In any case, this place is lovely; everything is white and clean and boring, just the way I like it. Ah, Quakerness, religion of peeling paint and folding chairs.

Okay! So about the flight. I, Leticia Jeanette McKenzie, have seen my personal hell. My personal hell is as follows: I am on a plane. There are people on each side of me, attractive women that I will have to spend nine hours within breathing distance of and yet never getting to know their names. I will not be able to get out without making one of them pack up her nine-hour livelihood and stand in the aisle while I re-inflate myself and discover the joys of standing. The lights are broken, and despite the fact that I bought two Game Boy Advance games for the flight I will never get a chance to play them. And, I cannot go to sleep, because there is not enough space for me to put my head down because the kid in front is leaning back in his chair, playing HIS Game Boy Advance SP, WHICH HAS A LIGHT. It took all of my pacifist leanings not to beat his head in with a shovel. Oh, but it would have been fun. Then I would've just switched our Game Boys and hoped he wouldn't know the difference, accept his boyhood probably wouldn't have allowed him to play a pink Game Boy with sparkly star stickers all over it. I think his existence would've been negated. Poof.

(That is, a puff of smoke, not, you know, a poof.)

Aaaaanyway, so the kind flight attendant with a goatee (and I deserve credit for not using my feminine charms to drag him into the bathroom to have sex with me, which would have been kind of

sexy in a not-sexy kind of way. Airplane bathrooms are thrilling, in
that you are peeing at 7000m in the air and could be jettisoned at
any moment) let me play my Game Boy for a few hours while
sitting in the coffee-making area, which is right next to the
emergency exit, which gave me the thrill of playing Mario & Luigi
when I could be sucked into deep space at any moment. (It also
gave me the thrilling WHIRRRRRR of the world rushing past me,
which drowned out any catchy music Sonic Advance 2 might have
had. Sonic Advance 2, by the way, really kicks the llama's ass.) This
was absolute bliss; I was given so much space that it was compar-
able to a bench on a bus (which might as well have been the
Construct from The Matrix in comparison to the gerbil cages we
were normally kept in), meaning I could actually extend my
muscles and stretch for approximately half a meter without trip-
ping the sexy flight attendants who were constantly passing me (oh
yes). But it had to come to an end; one non-sexy flight attendant
made me sit back in my gerbil cage and so I watched the Matrix
Revolutions in Headrest-O-Vision for the rest of the flight.

To be continued with my impressions of London, based entirely
on the train station, the heaping wads of advertisements taking over
civilization, and the naked women. Dear Lordy, the naked women.
My masturbation fantasies are so tame by comparison. If you ran
each and every one of my friends through the Magazine Machine
you would NEVER have as many naked women as . . . okay, this is
a dumb simile. But you get the point! Good night!

(Or, good morning, for me . . .)

Saturday 20 March 2004

Things I have noticed about London:

1) Pretty

Everything is arranged in nice, polygonal corridors, albeit with
advertisements spewed in every conceivable corner (Mike Myers
scares me enough without being 6 feet high). The airport, however,
despite its clearly marked paths was incredibly labyrinthine, and
together with all the stone pillars I had a feeling a gun was about to

materialize in front of my viewpoint and hideous aliens were going to jump out at me. But in any case, everywhere where Americans design someplace to be confoundingly hard to navigate, the British just seem to put everything in a circle. This is HEAVEN for somebody like me with no sense of direction.

The London Underground turns me on. Without all those advertisements (seriously; they stretch down long hallways, and adspace is bought in bulk), it might be the coolest thing in the universe. However, given that they are constantly trying to beam thoughts of insecurity into your brain with every wall, it is not quite as cool as Jet Grind Radio and a muffin.

Naked women. Good GOD the naked women. I had a feeling that, when I first saw a newsstand and its legions of barely clothed nymphs, that they were all going to jump out at me and assimilate me into one of their kind, which wouldn't be so bad if we got to have pajama parties and cake-baking contests. But no, these girls were there to show you that YOU aren't good enough, you need to be sexier like me and so you should buy ten thousand billion things that nobody needs; but more importantly (and more honestly; this makes me more partial to men's magazines than women's), they more often said "Oooh, stare at me all you want, but you'll never have me. Ha!" I honestly saw – this is going to shock Americans and bore Britons – a naked woman orgy on the cover of a men's magazine with the caption "Blonde Sex Party." (Hell yeah! I'm there, but my hair may or may not require bleaching – my secret identity requires you not to know.) All these girls were assisting each other in covering up their naughty bits; how touching. I wanna join!

. . . But anyway, all in all, just from that one newsstand there were more naked women than a busload of, er, naked women. Dammit! I cannot think of a good simile for this. More naked women than a baseball team of . . . naked women. Hey! That's cool! I'm going to direct a drama anime about a baseball team of naked women. It'll be called "Dirty Nymph Diaries" and it is coming your way next season on the All Leticia's Female Nudity Empowerment Channel. (Call for rates. Just call the number on your screen and say "Naked, my whole pie plus!")

Oh, but my point was, anybody who says that America is awash in sex should get their head clubbed by a British newsstand.

Britons are awash in sex, and I reckon they're happier for it; we're just awash in sexual anxiety and dishonesty. This is how we can play all sorts of radio songs about sexual coercion, but oh no, if it's performance involves showing part of a nipple, we can't take it! This is America, you know, not Britoninishitstan!

That said, every guy who signs my "Yes, All I Really Want is Sex With Hot Blondes" online petition (lesbians too) (I'll think of an alternative for gay guys and straight women) will get a kiss from me and a "I Tell It Like It Is!" button. We will be on our way to sexual honesty.

Where the hell was I? Oh yes! Double-decker buses are quite thrilling, especially because, from the viewpoint on the front of the bus, it looks like you are flying a great big hoverbike, narrowly threading your way through tunnels and coming very close to beheading random pedestrians and stop signs. Fun fun. I considered drawing crosshairs on the windshield just to authenticate my experience, but I'm sure I would be arrested and forced to give the twenty grovels. (Is that the misdemeanor punishment in Britain? It should be.)

Aaaaanyway, something about sex and blondes. No! Wait! Jet Set Radio: England would kick the llama's ass. Especially because I saw lots of graffiti on the train tunnels, and it was actually quite good. I think the best way to wipe out graffiti would be to commission wayward youths to do murals for the train tunnels, and the city could find a way to distribute territory evenly between the gangs. They could get professional branding companies to give each gang a sexy logo. See? Diplomacy at work! We would be getting kids off the streets with style.

Wasn't this supposed to be a numbered list? Oops. In any case, the next thing I noticed was that:

2) British accents are sexier than I thought

And everybody has them. You know, I kind of thought they were a novelty. Gosh, Americans are so silly. We must have the silliest accent of them all. I cringe at the thought of what my accent sounds like to a foreigner. "Hi! I like to slouch and eat Cheese Doodles while watching Fox News! How about you?" But in any case, I think every accent is sexy (just British in particular; and everybody knows everything Japanese is hot), so my question is, are American accents particularly sexy? Or are they just weird? Answers on a postcard, please.

So, after taking my plane, three trains, a bus, a hamster, and a rocking horse back to Quaker Central Command, I collapsed into bed. Ohhh that felt good. I could've melted right there. In fact, I think I did, as I woke up (here it comes . . .) with all my clothes off, imagining myself traversing through the giant blank land of the Internet and falling into one of the many small, rectangular pits, reaching away for dear life as I was ground into pure information applesauce. Oh, yes, baby. Ohh . . . Ohh . . . I trudged all the way to the shower and came into it. This is the best room ever.

You may have noticed I have a habit of being self-conscious and of second-guessing myself, but during this little episode, not once. I was in a beautiful dream, but it was real, where I was butt-naked in a small, personal land where nobody would notice if I trudged off to the bathroom to please myself. I was high, I was dreaming, I was . . . pure. I was 100 per cent pure Leticia energy. I was a nymph. I was glorious. I was who I was. For one moment, I was floating on pure eroticism.

. . . Then I had to clean everything up, find my clothes, and hope my dad never, ever finds out. Then I went back to bed and had a dream where I accepted myself as a lesbian. Beautiful.

(Actual self acceptance was delayed until May 2005. Eventual acceptance may face additional delays depending on outside forces, such as really hot guys. We'll see.)

(And the alternative petition is "All I Really Want Is to Have Sex With Leticia's Imaginary Asian Boyfriend Who Delicately Spreads Whipped Cream and Honey on Her Naked Body while She Relaxes and Plays Sonic Advance 2." Ha!)

(*You may think to yourself, "is she really a lesbian?" I think to myself, "am I really a straight woman?" Someday, we'll figure it out.*)

Y'know, right now, in particular, I really really really wanna be run through the Magazine Machine.

Something about London . . .

Monday 22 March 2004

By the way, if you've never read *Bellow* *(http://kathrynjane.blog-spot.com)*, do so now. Really. Stop reading my blog. Now. What?! You're still reading?! Cut that out! Okay here's an E-mail she sent me a long time ago:

Ms McK –

Thank you for calling my blog "really freaking good" in bold letters. I was originally going to write that it made me want to kiss you, but then I remembered that that's not really up your alley. So instead: It made me want to stand you in the middle of a room naked and have hundreds of people write on you with feather quill pens. Each person would only get to write one word on exactly one square inch of your skin. Then they'd lay Leticia The Living Novel down on a paper cutter and dice you into one-inch cubes and Fedex you in boxes filled with packing peanuts to Book of the Month Clubs around the country, where people would open you and devour their square-inch Leticia Leaflets with their eyes. After that, they'd shelve you in their homes next to Tolstoy and Sade, and you'd have to wait there, forever, shattered by the ecstasy of always hoping that another person was just . . . about . . . to read you.

Please don't tell your mom I wrote that.

Kathryn

My reply:

That . . . is the best . . . thing . . . ever.

– Leticia

(Ten thousand Leticia points plus stock options. At least.)

Now *go*.

Wednesday 24 March 2004

I'm sad.

In downtown Undisclosed Location I found a photo book called "Hippie." Yes, I knew the only reason I wanted to look at it for the naked women I would invariably find between its covers – not for titillation (entirely; you all know my lesbian tendencies) but because . . . I wanna – be – a naked woman. It's not fair. I want to be that one girl who was clutching her boyfriend as they strolled naked through their beautiful garden, perfectly in-keeping with the hippie philosophy of celebrating life and contemplation. I . . . I . . .

Where's Poseidontown's hippie-land? We're such a liberal city and I have yet to find such a place where I fit in. Someday, dammit, someday . . .

(On the positive side, we have the nicest punk kids you'll ever see; the kids downtown smoking pot and begging for change are at least ten times nicer than the well-dressed businessmen who would sooner spit in their hats than give them pity as forgotten children.)

Back to the previous topic: "I wanna be naked" appears many many times in my diary, from about three years ago to one year ago, ending entirely when I read Promiscuities and realized that I, in fact, am not alone. In fact, every teenage girl wants to be looked at. Well, I mean, duh. But it doesn't really sink in when the adults in your life effectively tell you you're a whore.

But more importantly, I . . . wanna be loose of my material trappings. You know? When I was a kid . . . (embarrassing story ahead) I saw the cover of the Demi Moore movie, *Striptease*, on one of those junk mailings. On it was Demi Moore, naked, elegantly covering up her naughty bits. I . . . I . . . it was intense. I had never seen a naked body before, being from small-town Hicksburg (name changed to protect the innocent), and . . . OK, here goes. Before I took a bath, I would take off all my clothes and look in the mirror and . . . pose myself as Demi Moore. I wanted to have that command of my body. And . . . I loved to have that time, that excuse, while the tub was filling up with water, to spend time with myself au naturel, and to pretend I was some glamorous striptease star. There. I was, I mean, I intend to say, that is, I . . .

I wanna be naked.

Saturday 27 March 2004

Well, hello! It's 3 a.m., and I can't get to sleep, because of jet lag. So, you're stuck with me!

I got a whole bunch of responses from the "hippie" post. Thanks, I had no idea so many people felt the same way . . . (sob) Adolescence sucks! It's just an experiment in thinking you're the – only-one – in-the – world. Moving on . . .

(THANK YOU to the kid who E-mailed me saying she did the Demi Moore thing too. We are going to make plans to hang out sometime, only to do Demi Moore impressions in the mirror and eat cookies while our obedient male servants [who are kind enough only to wear loincloths and battle scars] lavish our naked bodies in cherry sauce and whipped cream. Really.)

(. . . And some artsy French photographer will have a field day with us.)

(. . . And a giant piston will mash me into a cake but I'm not sure how that fits in.)

No, there wasn't a kid playing a Nintendo Ultra Nitro 37px D20 on the plane, but the woman in front of me did seem to enjoy mashing my head in with the back of her chair when I was trying to nap. I believe my head is now lightly tenderized. And finally I'm really hungry for some of that vegetable curry I had in London, which is the best thing in the universe. G'bye.

The following post is probably the most popular one I've written so far. It's a sad one, though, so don't read it expecting me to talk about being turned into jello or something. Even the president of teenage sex blogging has a private life, and like it or not, people die and insurance agents swindle their customers and TV companies churn out terrible sitcoms year after year, and there are even sad things at Leticialand. So take a deep breath and come back when you're done masturbating; tragedy can be quite a buzzkill.

Sunday 28 March 2004

My friend slashed his arms.

These days, the hip thing to do when you're contemplating suicide is to run a blade into the undersides of your arms, calling on the courage to press down on your wrists. This leads to permanent scarring and a permanent seat in the House of Cool.

My friend is into emo – the songs written for teenage boys to rhapsodize on how the girl never took him to prom and therefore civilization is ending. You know, the teenage feeling that everything you do could make or break the rest of your life, that your worth in society for the next seventy years is determined by your actions in middle school. (*If you are into emo, stick with me for just a little bit before you throw the book across the room. You won't stay mad at me. Promise.*)

This is a load of hooey, but I felt it too, when I was in middle school. I contemplated suicide because I felt that society should no longer have to deal with Leticia the outcast, Leticia the dysfunctional cog in the otherwise perfect machine of Hicksburg, Leticia the orange splotch on the otherwise neat street. It took the strength of my two best friends – and the knowledge of how sad they would be if I were to kill myself – to keep myself from doing the deed.

So I can't help but feel anything but disdain for Linkin Park when I hear them articulate that feeling – "Crawling in my skin, these wounds they will not heal" – as if somehow, the insignificant mistakes and mishaps of high school will scar you for the rest of your life. The skinny girl didn't ask you to prom? Your girlfriend got drunk and fucked the football captain? Or, for us girls, your first foray into non-virginhood wasn't all it was cracked up to be? "Fear is how I burn, confusing what is real!"

(To be fair, many people do have right scarring experiences in teenagehood – having abusive parents or being marked the neighboorhood slut ranking among them – but people can and do recover, and you need to empower yourself to move beyond them rather than wallow in your own misery. Don't let your shortcomings become your identity.)

So I went to the bookstore and found a book on emo culture and tried to discern why my friend wanted to slash his wrists. It was trendy, I figured; my friend was obviously contemplating suicide (and this is a popular friend of mine; I continuously heard him talked about by my peers as the most thoughtful and mature preteen they know of. That is, until he started smoking pot. I hate pot. Drugs are not cool. That stupid animated mascot from fifth grade was right. But I'm getting ahead of myself), but could he also have been motivated to make these scars because all his friends were doing it?

But, you know, I was looking in the wrong place. I realized, about a chapter in, that I was only reading the book so that I could find a way to justify the "I Hate Linkin Park Because It Made My Friend Slash His Wrists" rant that was making its way to my fingers. Of course Linkin Park didn't make him slash his wrists. Teenage angst, and contemplation of suicide, are both perfectly normal (if bizarre and shocking) aspects of growing up. I just wish he didn't have to damage his beautiful body for life in order to express his emotions. So I grieve, and I try to shove the blame as quickly as possible at the most convenient target, which is Bands Who Make Wallowing In Your Own Emotional Despair Cool Again.

My dad listens to the blues. Throughout my childhood, I always wondered what he got out of it. If you can listen to any commercially available music in the world, why would you want to listen to a guy bitch and moan about how he shot somebody in Memphis and his girlfriend left him but she weighed 300 pounds anyway and MWAH WAH WAAAAAAAAAAAAAAAAH (boom boom boom boom boom boom) . . . and there's no money left in his bank account and John Q. Mobster is coming to bust his kneecaps. Why the hell does my good Christian father wash dishes to this?

But one day he watched a documentary on blues ("Bluesland," for those who are following me), and the well-dressed, somber, heavyset black man (with his deep sexy voice . . . oooh) told us, "I want to eat applesauce-covered Leticia in one mighty slurp." No! No! How did that get in there?! (rewind . . .) He said, "We all get the blues sometimes – and nothing gets rid of the blues like blues music." He went on to describe the "two blues devils, fightin' " and how listening to the blues can sometimes provide an articulation and a release for the blues inside of all of us, even if we never shot nobody in Memphis. I found that charming; I play videogames, and I can often find humorous release of my inner passions on the flashing box.

So, it's not all Linkin Park's fault, just like it's not all Doom's fault, or Mortal Kombat's fault, or jazz music's fault, or swing music's fault, or Shakespeare's fault. We have our own ways of articulating our inner passions. I just don't know what to do about my friend's arms.

(I did what I supposed I should do: I hugged him and said "We love you!" I hope it helped, you know . . . I didn't get that in Hicksburg . . .)

(wah wah . . . crawling in my skin . . .)

I got a lot of responses for writing about suicide. I just don't know what to say. Part of it is that I recommended that every teenager who likes manga should read Confidential Confessions vol. 1, by Reiko Momochi, because it articulates the teenage feelings of loneliness and desperation with honesty and depth, and doesn't hold back on showing where that attitude leads. Other than that . . . what can I say? You only get one life, make the most of it.

Tuesday 30 March 2004

After I said this:

> These days, the hip thing to do when you're contemplating suicide is to run a blade into the undersides of your arms, calling on the courage to press down on your wrists. This leads to permanent scarring and a permanent seat in the House of Cool.

someone (*actually a good friend and regular writer*) E-mailed me and said this:

> Sweetie, dont make light of it. We do it because we have issues, not because it makes us cool.

Sorry, sorry, sorry! I said that only because I was really really angry and not because I actually thought it was true. Okay, I did actually think it was true, because I was really really angry at this person for slashing his arms. I was quick to blame it on something. Mea culpa.

(If I were mature, I wouldn't have a blog . . .)

So I'm sorry if I made it sound like people cut their arms only to be cool . . . I was only frustrated with the people who DO make it cool.

He E-mailed me back, saying "thanks," which I am very grateful for as mine was a pretty weak apology. It's a problem that cutting is sweeping the nation, and it's an even bigger problem that cutting has become cool in certain circles; that bothers me, but not as much as when people cut themselves in earnest.

Tuesday 25 May 2004

After reading this post at Kitten Blue (*http://kittenblue.blogspot.-com/*), I felt motivated enough to comment:

> Today I bought my first thong. It's another milestone for me, I've always been a avid lover of big pants, but there's always been something very naughty about thongs to me, and the fact you need confidence (and a half-decent butt) to wear one says a lot. Well, finally, I feel good enough about my butt to wear one. Go me.

Girls, boys are the most easily amused creatures on Earth. They DO NOT GIVE A FLYING FUCK whether or not one boob is bigger than the other or if your butt cheeks do not meet ISO 9000 standards. There are the horniest creatures God ever made, and it's a wonder that they don't go for lamp-posts if you put them in tank-tops. It doesn't sound like it's true, but it is: a winning personality is what keeps a boy coming back for more, and sex-wise, being confident in your body matters a lot more than what your body actually looks like. Boys think EVERY female-looking body is the most beautiful thing in the world. I could fluff some bread-dough and pour flour on it, and then give it frosting for lips and stick a bikini on it (as well as some dime-store googly eyes) and set it out in the street and pretty soon, there will be a horde of Boy-os Sapiens asking for her phone number. It's that simple.

It's not your body, it's your confidence in your body.

(Trust me. Leticia knows EVERYTHING about boys.)

In response, she wrote, on her blog, which you ought to go read: "In reply to Leticia's post, in my case, my butt-confidence (or lack of) stems from how I feel inside, not from how I think guys see me. If the boyfriend doesn't like my butt, he can go elsewhere, simple as that. Feel good outside, feel good inside. That's just how I work, I guess."

A fantasy:

I did kind of enjoy imagining myself and my women friends relaxing in a serene hot spring, taking in the sights and the smells when suddenly, a gurgling sound alerts us to that there is something wrong. Suddenly all the water begins to swirl into the bottom of the pond, and we grab onto a ledge for dear life but it is no use as we are haplessly sucked in. A tough, bulky guy with a bandanna and a leather jacket (particularly Bass Armstrong from Dead or Alive, but don't tell anybody) grins to himself and chuckles as he swings around the plug he has liberated, while in the background, me and my lady friends are swept down the drain. Perfect.

Whatever happens to us after that is up to you.

Thursday 3 June 2004

I get to see a woman I haven't seen in a long time in a few days, a woman who was my mother figure for the better part of my teenage-hood and without whom I do not know where I would be. She loved me enough to take me to coffee periodically and listen to me bitch just because she knew how much I needed it. She would always listen and she would ask before she talked and she always meant the best for me.

So now I should be really happy to see her again, but I'm not, and this is the only reason why: I'm terrified I'm not going to impress her enough. I need to show her how much more mature I am. I need to have a conversation with energy levels in the high nineties. I feel this so much that I was writing down – in the middle of writing class – what I was going to say to her, under the heading "talking points".

And what I never realized (and still don't) is that this woman doesn't love the Leticia who pines after her own success and draws up complicated charts and graphs out of her own insecurity, but the Leticia who asks for love and nothing more, the Leticia who knows she isn't perfect and yet still strives to be the best woman she can be. More than that, though, I think the Leticia she loves best is the one she barely ever sees, the one who lets her guard down just for a brief moment when she's with a friend.

I could learn a lot from her.

Thursday 10 June 2004

I dreamt about an adorable young girl with white powdery make-up and a bright red kimono who was actually a con artist and you should stay away from her at all costs.

. . . Weird.

A friend of mine, over the Internet, told me he fantasizes of turning me into a gingerbread cookie.

No . . . boy . . . has . . . ever . . . told . . . me . . . that.

And it's gross.

But no boy has ever told me that.

Wah!

Saturday 17 July 2004

I always thought it was stupid how all my friends would complain that the only boys they like are gay, that the only ones with sensitivity and/or fashion sense seem to bat for the other team. I mean, what does that mean for heterosexuality? I, for one, want a boy who is inclined to spread whipped cream on my pussy. So here is where my story begins . . .

We'll call him Sephiroth. Sephy is the definition of the pretty-boy. He has long hair. He has a cute body. He is the only boy whose clothes I want to see in tatters on the floor of my room between a stack of comic books and a GameCube controller. He is gentle. He is eloquent. He is my type.

And he is gay.

Phooey! Curse you, God, and your unfathomable reasons for making straight women attracted to gay men and straight men attracted to lesbians. Wait a minute . . . (pauses and flexes her muscles inward with intense fury) Quiet! I'm growing out my armpit hair! After this, all I'll need to do is get a mohawk and plaid shorts in order to get a train of guys to watch my every move.

This, by the way, is the biggest lesson against homophobia: guys, you really ought to listen to gay men more. They know where it's at. Let some of that gay-ness rub off on you. We dig that. Trust me.

Also, wear a kilt, because we (I) dig that.

Leticia

(Sephiroth once said, "You know, gender doesn't really matter to me so as long as you have the equipment. I'm no good with vaginas." Har har! Fuck you.)

(And I mean that in the kindest, gentlest manner, by which I mean that you need to rip my clothes off, right now, in the car, and play that one song from Jet Set Radio Future while you do it. Get down on the floor! [Say what?] I say get down on the floor? [Say what?] I say get down! I wanna see something I've never seen before . . .)

Tuesday 20 July 2004

Hi! I'm sorry that things have been a bit empty in the House of Leticia as of late. I've been very busy with homework. Do not fear, soon I will have my papers in and I can do important things again.

In other news, Sephiroth encouraged me to "walk around topless sometime." Dear, you have no idea . . .

(didn't he say he was gay? I'm starting to wonder about that kid . . .)

(pleasebestraightpleasebestraightpleasebestraight)

By the way, I fiddled with his chain wallet as a means of expressing affection. His chain wallet. Strange. I wonder if one might get any sensual pleasure out of that. I suppose it is attached to you . . . and comes out of your midsection . . . and represents masculine power . . . and could conceivably be stroked in a girly and adorable fashion . . .

And yet, it is cold and lifeless. Nothing like its parallel that I hope I have made painfully obvious.

Let me think . . . I've spoken many a time on the subject of the female body, but not on the penis. How do I feel about the penis? Well . . . I find it kind of amusing, almost as though men cannot contain all their masculinity so it sort of slips downward into their safekeeping pouch, where they can use it to pleasure women and have pissing contests. (. . .) It is . . . kind of creepy, in that it's like the one body part that doesn't seem to have any compositional value, other than as kind of a center point for the rest of the anatomy to revolve around. And . . . its ability to, um, transform is actually kind of beautiful. Like those chronically overused time-lapse photos of flowers blooming, it's like . . . the physical expression of eroticism. It's the chemical reaction to a man being aroused, so it . . . makes me happy.

A lot of feminist authors write about phallic symbolism . . . and they're onto something, as "gladiator" literally means penetrator and men have always have had aggressive social classes and women have always been relegated to kitchen duty. Well, I say . . . attack the problem, not the person, or the penis, for that matter, because it isn't, you know, it's fault! It's just hanging there, innocently, because every guy has one, and every guy is entitled to the responsibility of one. A penis has a lot of power right there . . . it can make babies, it can please women, it can hurt women, it can allure women, it can be (unfortunately) the focus of a relationship . . . so much symbolism right there, and sometimes I feel sorry for the boys for having to carry all that emotional baggage between their legs. Oh well . . . all you tough men can handle it, right?

The reason I'm babbling on the subject is because I've been recently thinking about the penis, Sephiroth's, in particular, and I realized that I've never given them all that much thought before. They're . . . there. Only recently have I realized . . . they're actually quite beautiful, with all that masculine stature and snake-like allure . . . the way it winds down between the testicles, like something out of Gothic arcitecture. Just think, all the secrets to life are held right in there, and someday, I just . . . might . . . get my tongue on one . . .

And that scares me. Where did all this come from? Wait, don't I like girls? Well, I thought I did, until now . . .

Crikey.

Leticia

(By the way . . . if Sephiroth says one more time that he is no good with vaginas, then I am sending out a personal vagina trainer, paying her expenses, and not quitting until he is the best vagina maestro in all of Poseidontown. And then . . . he'll have nowhere to run. Bwa ha ha!)

(He's said before that I'm very pretty, and he's very affectionate toward his gal pals . . . yet I am beyond his reach, since he really does want to be with a man. See? He's like me, only male. Crikey.)

NEVER POSTED – written on Saturday 14 August 2004

I was listening to a song from Jet Set Radio Future. A very pretty song, it was by Russell Simmons (no relation to Richard . . .), and it was about, well . . . having sex with his wife. Getting bored one day and having finished all my homework, I began to consort with myself, gently, when I had the brilliant idea of sexing myself to Russell Simmons song, "I'm Not a Model."

("Get down on the floor! Say what? I said get down on the floor! Say what? I say get down! I wanna see something I've never seen before")

I just about cycled through every fantasy I like to imagine a boy doing to me until finally, I laid back.

("Gonna get down! Gonna get down!")

I came precisely in time with the song; being a song representing sex, I orgasmed exactly where the musician has his orgasm, and I looked to my ceiling expecting for rays of light to burst through the roof and carry me off to Orgasm-Land, where pretty pink fairies play in rivers of lemonade and palmtrees reach up into the heavens and emit a protective barrier from all who would steal their precious fruit without obtaining permission first. And I loved it. And I slept well.

Until . . . I got the shivers. I realized . . . where the hell's this Russell Simmons person? I mean . . . I don't know him . . . you don't know him . . . he's kind of a strange person if he writes songs about having sex with his wife, and then they get licensed for a video game about graffiti (he got lucky; he had the right label at the right time). But I fucking NEED HIM. I JUST HAD SEX WITH RUSSELL SIMMONS AND IT CAME WITH NO CUD-DLING WHATSOEVER.

Goddamn, I was FURIOUS! The shortcomings of this song are

IMMENSE! What's the point of masturbating to it if the music will not envelop me in loveliness and project the image of its singer giving me a back massage while little pink fairies paint my skin with occult images that kind of tickle? What's the point if the music will not flow through every one of my pores until it eats me from the inside out and my existence is negated? What's the point if I am not lifted through my clothes into the heavens in which I hot-tub with Angelina Jolie? WHAT'S THE FUCKING POINT!!

Then I forgot about it and probably went to play Jet Set Radio Future. But still, you all know the moral of the story . . . do not masturbate to a song without having the singer there, in person, naked, showered, with dreadlocks, and maybe a little bit of chest hair to accentuate his, um, patterns, and a really deep voice and smooth motions, and give him a glass of endless pink lemonade that you can either drink or have it poured all over you, and then fuck him until the night turns to morning, and then the sky turns pink and it starts raining babies. Good night.

(By the way, my patent on music that will actually cuddle you is in the sorting process. The patent office is rubber-stamping things like crazy, so with any luck, you will soon be able to project the essence of any musical number into your bedroom. This thing could sell millions! If you had such a machine, what song would you like to have sex with? I'm going to go with "Pokémon Johto," the theme song from *Pokémon 3 The Movie*, for now. Bye bye!)

Afterword

If you're my age, I hope you can identify with these entries. They're silly, yes, but they represent a lot of my sexual development that I wouldn't have been able to share without my anonymity. I'm glad to have it as an archive, a record of what made me the woman I am now.

Growing up is tough, and as I've learned, figuring out what to do with your middle spot is probably the easiest lesson learned. But looking at boys and realizing you see something besides their clothes, figuring out who you want to ask to the prom, wondering what you're going to do aout the boys who tease you in the hallway

. . . it's what makes high school nerve-rackingly difficult, and trigonometry easy by comparison.

If there's one thing I've learned from this blog, it's that I am worth it, and I hope that in my next life it won't take eight months of blogging to realize it. I hope you all know that too; and wherever you go, the spirit of Leticia McKenzie – not me, but Leticia – will always be inside of you, cheering you on as you go through life's troubles. Have no fear!

– Leticia McKenzie, 20 August 2004

NAKED LOFT PARTY

Lex Konrad

http://www.nakedloftparty.com

After Hours Orgy

7 July 2003

> *"Don't you know what it means to become an orgy guy? It changes everything. I'd have to dress different. I'd have to act different. I'd have to grow a mustache and get all kinds of robes and lotions and I'd need a new bedspread and new curtains. I'd have to get thick carpeting and weird lighting. I'd have to get new friends. I'd have to get orgy friends."*
>
> – Jerry Seinfeld

Are we swingers now? I hope not. Swingers have a bit of a bad reputation. You know, fake-wood paneled romper rooms full of mirrors, desperate middle-aged couples revealing their cottage cheese thighs to other middle-aged couples, fat hairy balding white guys licking their lips at the prospect of seeing their saggy wives get plowed up the ass by strange men, buffet tables piled high with steaming pigflesh. I mean, would you really want to "swing" with these people? Not that there's anything inherently wrong with all this. It's just not my thing. Call me an elitist but we're still young and hot. If we're gonna do this then we're gonna do it right.

Now, to clarify, Leslie and I have been actively meeting, fucking and dating women together for about two and a half years. It started innocently enough with us dating people separately during a lame open-relationship phase. Then one day she happened to stop by my apartment while I was going down on my date, a sweet young strawberry blonde from Texas with perfect C cups. Thus began a long period of increasingly outrageous sexual hijinks. Picking up and seducing hot young things became second nature to us. We had threesomes, foursomes and private sex parties. We had girlfriends and mistresses. Not once, however, did I think of myself as a true swinger or an "orgy guy", nor were we involved in anything larger than our own private debauchery. We were also leery of being in an environment where there might be other sausage around, or at least I was. People used to ask me why I did it and I would say it was because I wanted to have something to smile to myself about as I sat rotting away in my old age.

Recently I had the dubious pleasure of finding out that we're part of an emerging trend. Apparently there's a whole new generation of Americans who are discovering the varied pleasures of fucking in groups of three or more. This new post-swinger generation attends velvet rope orgies and rents private suites at swank hotels. They drink champagne. They don't do buffets. It's not called swinging anymore, it's called play. This is the new new thing. The nauseating hyperbole that surrounds the new hedonism makes me almost want to get out of the erotic lifestyle altogether. Almost.

Last Saturday we attended SKIN, our second off-premises "play" party. In swinger lingo, off-premises means you can flirt, dance, tease and even remove some clothing, but orgiastic sex has to be taken to apartments and hotel suites. We did a full on-premises orgy a couple of weeks ago, but as shy newcomers we didn't do much more than watch. Ironic that we were more comfortable picking up women in regular nightclubs than at parties specifically designed for such activity, but so be it.

After we tumbled out of the cab onto Bowery Street, directly in front of the lounge, we stood around for a couple minutes, unsure of whether we were at the right spot. Fortunately the bouncer took one look at Leslie and waved us over. I was relieved that we looked the part. Or was I? It was still a challenge to embrace that orgy-guy image. Inside, it would have been easy to imagine we were at a regular nightclub except that everyone was unusually well dressed and the women were unusually attractive. On the whole these were the kind of people who commute in from Connecticut and not the usual hipsters who haunt the urban canyons of downtown Manhattan on a typical Saturday night.

We paid the cover and stood around for the better part of an hour, feeling if not necessarily looking out of place. People eyed one another hungrily yet warily, probably unsure as to whether they were to become predators or prey. Things finally began to flow when we went out for a smoke and met a busty blonde whose husband was hanging out somewhere inside. As most people seemed to be that night, she was relatively new to group play and really hadn't seen or done much at all. It was a relief actually, as I suddenly felt wise and experienced in these matters. Eventually the night took on a kind of whirlwind quality as women doffed their tops to have their breasts spray-painted and people headed downstairs to flirt on the dance floor. I can't remember what music was playing. Always the center of attention somehow, Leslie ended up in nothing but a G-string and blue-and-silver body paint, her breasts and ass writhing against the lithe frames of other young women. She had handprints on her delicious ass from someone who had placed his hand there and let the artist spray over them. The tantalizing silhouettes of breasts, nipples and asses undulated behind a backlit screen as Leslie gently teased and played with other women, partners changing fluidly. I forgot myself, standing around dumbstruck with the other men, lost in a tide of bodies, colors and shapes.

The night accelerated at a queasy pace. People began to discuss after-parties, boundaries, hotel suites, cellular numbers. Gina, a thin, sharp-faced blonde, and her husband Jacques, a handsome Egyptian man, wanted to bring us back to their room. They were also relatively new to this. Anxious young swingers with a ten-month-old at home. Gina and I had talked for a while about how to pick up single bisexual females, and then about the vicissitudes of playing with other couples. She wanted to go further than Jacques though, who told me (quite understandably) that he didn't want anyone else fucking his wife. "I'd just like to feel another man's arms around me," she confided. Oddly I didn't feel sexual at all but I didn't want the party to end either. I was *intrigued* by these people.

The after-party brought us to the Soho Grand. Five or six couples and an alluring woman in a black leather skirt crammed into a tiny air-conditioned room with what must have been a queen-sized bed at most. Jim and Kathy, a hipsterish couple with whom I hadn't interacted much at all, had come through at the last minute and provided our little crew of couples with a place to play. Leslie and I stood there dumbstruck as couples began to array themselves around the bed and Kathy began to eat Susan, a curvaceous brunette with stupendously large knockers. Knockers is really the only word to describe breasts that large. "They're real," she told me as I squeezed them a few minutes later. Her man looked a little bit like the porn star TT Boy, something we all joked about. Eventually Kayla, a gorgeous, sweet brown-haired girl from Bermuda, went to work on my girlfriend, hungry lapping at Leslie's tight cunt as Leslie sat on the floor with her back against the bed, legs splayed. Kayla's husband and I looked on appreciatively. He looked like a young version of the black guy on that TV series *Everwood*. As Kayla came up for air I pulled the fabric of her blue dress inward and a pair of beautiful tits popped out. I kept telling her husband how beautiful she looked.

I dropped my pants and Leslie began tugging on my cock, to no avail. Somehow in the midst of all this sex I just wasn't feeling aroused. It was all too overwhelming. Too close. It's interactive porn, I kept telling myself, but there's a world of difference between sitting on your couch with your cock in one hand and actually being on *stage*. We conferenced in the bathroom as the girls blew their men on and around the bed, which was the only thing everyone seemed comfortable with at the time. Leslie told me she couldn't come with Kayla, but not for lack of desire. I was semi-hard at best. Round one was soon over as a few couples finished up and left. I squeezed Kayla's tits one last time in lieu of a goodbye kiss. I'd love to fuck that girl. It was time for a smoke. On the way out Kathy was sitting on the floor with her legs spread, blocking our point of egress. Leslie and I each put one of her plump tits in our mouths as I ran an index finger along her pussy.

Outside, as the sun came up, we debated leaving. Maybe I wasn't cut out for this. But we had left some shit upstairs anyway. We had to go back in. As we entered the room we were greeted by a very different sight. Kathy, who was a saucy, pale Irish girl, was on the floor bent over the bed. Nancy, the intriguing short-haired brunette who had come by herself, was perched atop Kathy, her hands spreading Kathy's ass-cheeks as Jim violated Kathy's pussy with a golden vibrator. Kathy was sucking Susan's pussy as Susan lay in the center of the bed with her legs spread. The red flames of body paint that had streaked up Susan's chest had already been licked clean around her nipples. Jim spat on Kathy's ass and inserted his thumb for good measure. Leslie pulled off her dress and went to cradle Susan's head in her lap. TT Boy watched attentively as both Kathy and Susan let out cries of pure ecstasy. Faced with this vignette framed by the morning sunlight streaming in through the blinds, I became aroused. In the immortal words of Dirk Diggler, I thought to myself, I wanna fuck.

And fuck I did. Susan detached herself from Kathy's mouth and let TT Boy put his cock in her missionary style. I let Leslie suck on my turgid penis for a minute and then followed suit. I entered Leslie from behind and made her suck Susan's ample breasts as I pumped away. Nancy positioned herself on a chair by the TV, legs slightly spread, and watched the scene unfold. Leslie and Susan were propelled into each other by the cocks that were pounding into them. Susan had a clit ring. I made eye contact with Nancy and licked my lips. She smiled seductively. Being watched was suddenly important to me. I wanted everyone to see my flesh going into Leslie's tight little hole. I wanted to be seen. I wanted to be heard. I wanted them to appreciate my newly shaved balls. I wanted to be filmed.

BDSM was something I had very little experience with, never having been involved in it nor ever having the slightest interest in watching it. It turned out that both Nancy and Kathy were subs, which I would have known by the collars if I weren't among the uninitiated. Kathy had this habit of saying "thank you" every time her ass was smacked by Jim, sometimes even crying out multiple times "thankyouthankyouthankyou." He put a black hood over her head, handcuffed her, applied a bar to her ankles to keep her legs spread apart, brutally tortured her ass with various whips, and fucked her hard from behind. But it was soft somehow. Respectful. Loving even. And all the stimuli that had overwhelmed me before now fed an outrageous sexual appetite. This is how Rocco Siffredi must feel when he's lining up seven virgin asses and fucking them all in a row, I thought. I came. Leslie came. TT Boy and Susan left after lounging around on the couch and making pleasant chitchat with us.

Soon everyone was watching as I fucked Leslie again. We had

become the show. I played with Kathy's ass as she kissed and
fondled Leslie, occasionally dipping my finger into Kathy's cunt.
Kathy's ass was black and blue and though I liked squeezing it I
couldn't bring myself to slap it hard. An Andrew Blake video was
playing on the television and some entirely inappropriate music
was blaring from the radio. But it hardly mattered. I fucked Leslie
from behind, admiring her puckered little asshole as Kathy moved
behind me to lick and suck on my balls. I stood up as Kathy
positioned herself under us in a sixty-nine position with Leslie.
"Aren't you going to fuck her?" she asked sweetly. I obliged and
was then pleasantly surprised when my cock slid out of Leslie and
found its way into Kathy's mouth. I alternated between mouth and
cunt. Mouth and cunt. For ever, it seemed. Kathy helped get it
back in Leslie's wet hole when required. A good assistant she was.
Nancy sat next to us for a closer look, captivated by the scene that
unfolded before her. Jim eyed us from the foot of the bed. After
what seemed like a blissful eternity I came inside Leslie, erupting
into a coughing fit as I forgot to swallow and instead inhaled my
saliva. My penis popped out and the last of my ejaculate dribbled
onto Kathy's chin. "Don't worry," said Jim. "She won't mind." It
was *that* good.

This after-party changed everything. I have to dress different. I
have to act different. I have to grow a mustache and get all kinds of
robes and lotions and I need a new bedspread and new curtains. I
have to get thick carpeting and weird lighting. I have to get new
friends. Orgy friends. I've become an orgy guy.

The Why of it All

3 September 2003

I was at the naked loft party last Saturday pondering the terrain
inside people's heads, trying to understand the why of it all.
Perhaps group sex isn't quite as strange as mainstream culture
would have us believe. Sex is social, after all. Even for the chronic
masturbator, fist pumping away furiously as he sits hunched in his
easy chair, sexual gratification is still essentially about the *other*.
And if a person can be expected to fit at least one other into his
erotic scenarios, what's so unnatural about bringing along a few

more? Yet the sex party takes this social urge to the extreme, and I get the sense that some people would explode in a mist of jizz if they didn't have this outlet.

Particularly interesting to me are the people who need to see and be seen. Sure, many of us have our exhibitionistic or voyeuristic tendencies, but some people have elevated this to an art form. There was one couple who spent the better part of the night screwing in the center of the giant play room. Apparently not sated by the long session, the male half pranced over to a curtain and parted it to leer at the action in a side room, stroking himself furiously like a coke-addled mouse taps at its pellet-dispenser. I watched this unfold as I lay on a saggy mattress in a post-blow-job haze, stroking a cat. Later on we spoke with this couple as we all shared a cab back into Manhattan and it was still tough to uncover the "why". What is it that makes some steal off into a corner while others proudly put themselves up for display? For me, desiring a certain amount of privacy is probably less a matter of inhibition than of connection. I like being watched, but for the most part I like to know who's doing the watching. Similarly, I enjoy watching but usually only get off on seeing people I have an interest in fondling at some point. I gotta have some skin in the game.

To be sure, there were some tasty vignettes though. Two brown-skinned girls lay side by side uttering salacious moans as their dates lapped them up. A cute couple walked around most of the night, unsure of what to do with themselves, until finally the big-titted lass hiked her skirt and mounted her man as he sat on a couch. A threesome was going on in the little room where we had fucked The Cock and Schoolgirl at a previous party; one girl ground her hips into a young man as he pounded another girl in the missionary position. At first it looked as if the girl behind him might have been fucking him in the ass with a strap-on, and Leslie and I looked at each other as if to say "that's different". As it turned out the girl was just grabbing him. That night Les and I enjoyed our share of exhibitionist play, but we had the most fun tucked away together in one of the little loft spaces. I fucked her from behind while sort of suspending myself from a pipe. Only my upper body was visible from the room below.

And so, too, looking at the bodies arrayed around me, I was contemplating the nature of attraction, a subject that's been very much on my mind since the Cindy debacle. These parties have opened my mind. I've met women who wouldn't have earned a second glance from me on the street yet turned out to be gifted lovers and very pretty girls who offered little beyond the purely mechanical aspects of sex. The stuff that happens between my ears is a big part of the "why" for me. I can't help but think that people who are overly rigid in their physical requirements are missing out on something significant.

Things to do in New York when you're dead

7 November 2003

Wake up in the grip of a hangover. Medicate yourself with a swig of cough medicine, a liter of water, two generic ibuprofens, a glass of wine and a ciggy. Watch a movie you missed when it was out in the theaters. Your girlfriend's pretty eyes well up with tears. Decide her face looks silly when it cries. Soon enough it will be dark. Throw on last night's costume and make a mad dash for the L train. "I hate Halloween," a woman says as you walk by, but you ignore her.

Pick up the pace after you exit the station in some dilapidated Brooklyn neighborhood, broken glass everywhere, grass poking out through cracks in the sidewalk, and sodium streetlamps painting everything a sickly yellow. Down that street? No, this one. "C'mon," you say, grabbing your girlfriend's hand, "let's hurry." Try not to give into the feeling that you are dead tired. Flinch when a man walking behind you calls out. It's OK though. It's just Jimmy, also on his way to the party.

Hand your money to the bouncer. Tell the girl with the swastika on her arm that she has balls dressing up like that in New York. Talk to some people. Talk talk talk. Say hello to Daniella, who seems in a hurry to start fucking. See some girls you recognize – those you fucked, those you fooled around with, those you used to want to fuck, those you might fuck under the right conditions, those you would fuck right now, and those you would never fuck.

You need to sit down for a minute. Just fucking relax. Compose yourself. The couch comforts you; gets you out of the way of the guests streaming in and the people walking around with video cameras, cold lens-eyes staring back at you. A reporter approaches and asks for an interview, so you oblige. You do your best to explain why people like to get naked in groups and fuck. Don't flinch when he asks you how many people you've hooked up with. You don't want to think about this. Just smile and tell him it's not about keeping score.

Make pleasant conversation with a girl who's being chased around by the video cameras. A hot young photographer with bursting cleavage wants to do a photo shoot. Let her take you into the back. The girl being followed by the cameras balks at the last minute, so it's just you and your girlfriend. The photographer is bossy but careful to keep your faces out of the pictures. *Click click click.* She orders your girlfriend to put her hand on you. You wink and tell the photographer she can put her hands on you too. Get a little aroused as your girlfriend grabs your cock through your slacks. You are suddenly aware you possess a dick.

Realize you want to be in control. You want to go further than anyone else. You want to be the alpha. This is a tall order at an orgy. It is easier to be free when those around you are in chains.

Head back to the kitchen for another drink and watch your girlfriend frolic with two semi-nude women. *Click click click.* More photos. "No, put your hand there," the photographer says.

Coin a new term: *swingersploitation.*

The party is half over now and it's time to take a piss. Note the traces of vomit on the toilet seat. Why is it that people drink themselves sick so quickly? Probably nerves. You are dead tired and you are pissing into the toilet and it has a little vomit on it. You step out of the bathroom and directly into the path of a ghost from the past. She looks unremarkable and throws you a half-smile. Shrug your shoulders and go somewhere else.

Talk to some people for a while. Touch some girls. Eventually you'll find your girlfriend in a little blue room conversing with a little black fairy who has heaving breasts. Across from you a black woman fishes out her boyfriend's big black cock and sucks on it. Miguel and Leandra enter the room, followed by another black couple. Everyone is sexy. Cup your hand now and spank Leandra's ass properly, feeling her wetness when your finger slips a bit and finds its way to her pussy lips. Watch the black fairy slip out of her costume. The orgy is now growing around you. Play with the girls but don't forget to pay attention to your girlfriend.

The room is now a cramped sauna. Take your girlfriend's hand and flee to the back, to a cool, dark little room with an empty bed. This is where you fuck her the way she deserves to be fucked. She screams, but it's not like you are putting on a show. For an orgy person, having sex in a dark corner of a crowded party feels as intimate as having sex at home. Ghostly figures sometimes walk through the room on their way to find new cocks and cunts but you do not flinch, nor do you take extra pleasure in their presence, their furtive glances. When you are about to come all you can think is "blue, blue, blue". Your orgasm sits down with you for a while to have a chat over tea. You are Ivan Karamazov and it is the Devil.

Afterwards you find Schoolgirl wandering the halls wearing nothing but a corset. Suck her tiny pink nipples. Spank her tiny white ass. Be mindful of your technique. Remember to cup your hand – it's only good for her when your palm stings and your ears ring. Watch her and your girlfriend for a while. Compliment them both on the excellent show. Say it with feeling. Even better, let them see that your cock is hard.

The party is winding down now. Go sit on the couches by the dance floor and stare at the ceiling, the reflected lights of the disco ball swirling around like hundreds of restless ghosts. Watch The Cock and Schoolgirl slip into a side room and make fucking noises. Strange noises. Laugh when a girl sitting nearby asks "Was that a duck?" Tell the wisecracking girl you have only recently overcome your spanking inhibitions, having been conditioned in college to believe taking such liberties with a woman is wrong. Look up to realize she is towering over you and bending over to see what you can do. Her breasts hang heavily. Lift her tiny skirt and give it a go, pausing between smacks to inspect the bruises on her rear end.

Grab your girlfriend on the way out. Don't be jealous that she's French-kissing another man. On the way home in a hired car, note the tiny colored lights dotting the support columns between the doors. Watch the Empire State gleaming in the distance through the tired metal skeleton of the Williamsburg Bridge. You cannot understand why the white lights are still on. Safely back in your neighborhood again, pay the driver and stumble out. When you see a marathoner on the street wish her luck. You've just run your own marathon of sorts, which is all the more impressive since you are dead.

A Real Education

12 January 2004

> "*Suddenly, I was public property in a small way. It was an odd sensation. In a certain sense, you do write to seduce the world, but then when it happens, you begin to feel like a whore.*"
>
> Erica Jong, *Fear of Flying*

Blogging, I've read, is a good way to meet people. There are certainly plenty of examples of guys whose online musings have inspired meetings out there in what we call the real world. Some writers even make such encounters their explicit intent. I hadn't given the idea of meeting someone much thought until a couple of months ago when I began to receive correspondence from female readers. Men generally want to know where the party is, or else seem to think I need more dick in my life. Women are masters of the subtle hint – their notes are unassuming.

When a female reader was bold enough to invite me out to "chat sometime, fully clothed, maybe over coffee," I was curious to see how she'd respond to the real me. I rolled into the cavernous Freight 410 on Thursday night, scanning the post-work crowd for a woman named Natalia. Not seeing her on my first run through, I strode up to the bar and ordered a beer. I left a message on her cell, thinking about returning home in a while and snuggling up on the couch next to Les. Just a drink or two, I thought. Gotta see this through.

Natalia called. "I'm walking up to you," she said. I spied movement in my peripheral vision and turned to face a pretty, fresh-faced black girl with straight, shoulder-length hair and a tight body. She wore snug lavender pants and a black tee that strained against her ample breasts. I smiled. I couldn't help myself.

"You look great," I said. I told her I'd never met anyone through the NLP. She said she'd never met anyone online; it had taken her a month-and-a-half to get up the nerve to write to me. She's young, a recent NYU grad. We talked about books and I was happy to discover she's an avid reader – so few of the girls I meet have any patience for literature. As we talked, she opened her body to me, breasts grazing my arm. "These are double dees," she said, flashing two fingers in a vee formation. Natalia asked what I want out of life. "I want to have sex with beautiful women," I said, "make a decent living, and completely change the way people think. In any order you like."

"I'm not really sure what I'm supposed to do now that I've met you," she said.

"Well, why did you ask me out?"

"I told you; we go to a lot of the same places. I was fascinated by the idea that I might have run into you somewhere before. And I've always had these fantasies about group sex. I want to know more."

"No, why *really* did you ask me out?"

She smiled coyly, "I don't know. I recently broke up with my boyfriend."

"That's not good enough," I chided. "I know why you came here, I know why you read me, and I know what you want. Look at these people around you. Underneath this veneer of civility there's an unspoken erotic tension. You want to lift that veil. You aren't satisfied with idle fantasies. You're ready to begin your real education."

I fixed my eyes upon hers, feeling the eroticism of her innocence, her expression a mixture of curiosity, desire and trepidation. "Are you afraid of me?"

She nodded slowly, her big eyes mirroring my gaze. I looked away, fearing I might fall in.

"Good," I responded casually. "I'm afraid you won't be as excited by me when the fear wears off."

"I'm going to the bathroom. Watch my drink . . . and don't put any powder in it." She rubbed her index finger and thumb together over the highball glass.

I smiled. "You've got to be kidding me. Where would the fun be in that? Now turn around and run along. I want to check out your ass." My eyes followed her firm peach of a rump up the stairs and watched it disappear behind the bathroom door.

When Natalia emerged from the loo I walked back to have a turn. I met her at the bottom of the stairs and tried impulsively to impose my lips upon her. She pulled back a bit so I grabbed her narrow waist and drew her to me. She smiled and threw back her head. My lips grazed her neck. Finally she stopped squirming and allowed me a chaste kiss. I released her and went to take a piss ("Don't put any powder in *my* drink," I said). When I returned an Asian guy was hovering over her, a colleague of hers. For a moment I feared Natalia might be a female player, not quite as guileless as she came across. I excused myself for a smoke. When I came back he was still there, sitting in my seat now. She looked into my eyes and turned to face me, blowing off her colleague as politely as possible.

"You might be too young for me," I said.

A doleful expression transformed the map of her face. Her eyes grew even larger, if such a thing were possible. I almost regretted what I had said. "Really?"

"You and your puppy dog eyes. You have to stop – a man has no defense against that. Look, this summer I almost swore off girls under twenty-five."

"And why is that?"

"On the whole they're conniving, selfish, overly dramatic and have no idea what they want."

"I don't know what I want."

"Oh, but you do. You do."

We took a cab to the East Village to meet a friend of Natalia's. In the back seat we studied each other's faces. "What?" one of us would ask, smiling. "Nothing," the other would respond.

Natalia's friend was tall, black, with short hair. She was at the Black Star with a German guy who had an inch on me. Not that I paid much attention. Natalia and I stood there, face-to-face, dancing but not dancing, both of us delirious. I pressed her to me and felt her knockers rub against my chest. I grabbed her firm peach of an ass. We sat down against the wall and kissed wantonly. Every time I pulled back she would take my lower lip between her soft, full lips and suck. I squeezed her breasts and placed my hand down the back of her pants. I placed her hand over the bulge of my cock.

"You need to go to a sex party," I was saying, rattling off sections of my sexual syllabus, "you need to try threesomes, foursomes. Maybe guys at either end, too. You, of course, have to fuck me and Les. In the orgy scene there are a lot of people looking to fuck any hole, as long as it's new – still, you need to see it. Our private parties are more intimate. I want to fuck a person, not just a hole. I want there to be some aftermath. I want to change someone."

I asked her if she'd had any experiences with women. "Yes, one time," she said.

"What? First base? Second base?"

"I don't know. We kissed and I touched her."

"Down *there*?"

"Down *there*," she laughed. "That's funny. Yes, I touched her down *there*."

We decided to leave the bar and I spent ten minutes looking for Natalia's errant coat. She was oddly serene throughout all this. I finally found it in a corner far away from where we had been sitting. Outside we kissed and talked about what to do next. Imposing on Leslie this late wasn't an option; Natalia's place in Brooklyn seemed far far away in the sharp cold. "I want to stay with you," she said. Her friend suggested a party over at Lotus. I bummed a Gauloise from the German before he left us.

Lotus was packed, so we headed downstairs to a cozy back room. Natalia and I danced in earnest this time, her tight body writhing against me expertly. She mouthed the words to every song. We went to get a drink and when we returned our coats had disappeared. We just looked at each other, shrugged, and sat down. Soon she was on top of me, giving me a lap dance that quickly degenerated into dry humping. I placed one hand on her D-cups while straining to reach her clitoris with the other. I pulled my middle finger out and stuck it in her mouth, making her taste herself, and she went to work on it as if it were a cock. *Heyyyy yaaaaaah*, the music said.

The night took on a surreal, druggy quality. This isn't real, I thought. This ain't happening. After the back-and-forth of recent months, her willingness almost seemed suspect. "You're going to be my sex slave," I whispered in her ear, "and I'm going to be yours."

She smiled and gazed upon me more confidently now. "You smell like baby powder."

Natalia's friend came back leading another gentleman friend by the hand. "Damn, you two need to go into the back if you're going to be doing this," she scolded, gesturing at an empty lounge. We made our way back there and I pushed Natalia onto the couch, lifting her shirt and taking her chocolate nipples between my lips. A flashlight shone in our direction. I pulled Natalia's shirt down and looked over to see some guy standing a few feet away, giving us a stern look. "Aye, what are you lookin at?" I said. He informed us we'd have to stop. Can't risk anyone having too much fun. Oh how I longed for the good old days of Centro Fly, of after-hours orgies in the VIP room when the cleaning crew kept their heads down and swept around us, of late nights at Chelsea Grill when the girls' tops came off and anything could happen.

Soon we were on our way out. The wandering coats had miraculously checked themselves, so at least we wouldn't be clinging together coatless in the extreme cold. I considered returning home but was determined to see Natalia naked. Her friend invited us over for drinks but Natalia shook her head. "No, he's coming home with me," she said confidently. Brooklyn, I thought, egads. The gentleman friend vanished into the cold and the three of us piled into a cab. I'm committed now, I remember thinking as we left the safe confines of Manhattan, skyscrapers receding into the void.

"So, you're cheating on your girlfriend?" the friend asked.

I laughed, "No, not at all. She knows what I'm up to tonight."

"Well, I'm not going to argue with you, but it sure sounds like cheating to me."

I wasn't about to go into a long-winded explanation. People believe whatever it is they want to believe; whatever keeps them sane. Natalia squeezed my hand and nuzzled her cheek against my chest. "You don't have to justify your life to anyone," she said softly.

A few minutes later Natalia and I were bracing against the cold, fiddling with the frozen lock to her apartment – I imagined being trapped on the desolate streets among sleepy row houses. We both worked at the lock for a while until finally it gave way. We made our way up the darkened stairs and into her room, where she packed a bowl and handed the colorful glass pipe to me. She stripped down to a red thong and a matching bra. Her ass was everything it had promised to be – tight, round, just waiting to cushion my thrusts.

"Are you still afraid of me?" I asked as I was unhooking her bra, watching her massive tits tumble out.

"A little . . . but I'm glad you're here. I don't have much experience with guys; I've never taken someone home like this."

"I prefer it that way. You aren't jaded. You'll be all the more excited because everything's so new to you. Consider this part of your education. You don't have anything to worry about around me. I'm gonna push you, but in a good way." I gave her breasts a firm squeeze, pausing to admire them. "Funny how our date turned out."

"If this had been a regular date I wouldn't have brought you home."

"So, you're like my groupie now."

She laughed. "Quit it."

I let my hands cruise over her body, feeling the smoothness of her dark skin. My cock was nagging me so I brought it into the open. I began to remove her thong and she brought her hand down in token resistance. I pinned her arms behind her head and pulled the panties down, revealing a tight little cunt decorated with a thin welcome mat of pubic hair. She was giving me that shy expression I had first seen at Freight, trepidation and desire mingling in her innocent eyes. "Don't worry; I wouldn't fuck you tonight even if you were ready. I try not to fuck on the first date."

"You *try* not to?"

"Yeah, well, sometimes it can't be avoided."

I teased her clitoris and then pushed a couple of fingers deep inside her. She gasped. I pounded her with my fingers, working my thumb against her labia. I talked to her, said the dirty things that begged to be said. I told her I would fuck both of her holes, that I'd pound her from behind while she buried her face in Leslie's cunt. Soon she was shuddering, quaking. She pushed my hand away. We repeated this cycle several times, sometimes bringing my tongue into play.

"I bet you're a good fuck," she said.

"I'd like to think so." I placed her hand on my cock and guided it up and down my shaft. I straddled her and placed my tool between her tits, occasionally pushing forward to tease her lips with it. I made her stick her tongue out and lick me. I was anxious to sully her in some way, to mark myself upon her. She lay on her stomach with her head at my feet while I toyed with her ass and stroked my cock. God thought highly enough of the female asshole to place it less than an inch away from the cunt. How can the anus not be eroticized? I told her I was going to come on her and pointed my cock at her left buttock, greeting the wave of release that washed over me. I watched as that trembling thing between my legs painted the left side of her ass in thick, syrupy, unhurried spurts. Immediately I felt exhausted.

"Did you like that?" I asked, admiring my copious output as I lazily traced wet circles in her soft skin.

"It felt warm," she purred. I toweled her off and collapsed next to her with a sigh.

In the morning I watched Natalia go about her ritual, gazing intently at her ass and breasts every time she bent over to retrieve something from the floor. The television droned on quietly in the background, calling all Americans to morning prayers in praise of work, money, celebrity.

"Do you know what you're going to write about me yet?"

"I need to sleep on it," I said as I stood up, blinking in the light. "I'm trying to figure out what happened last night." It was as if I'd started here and had yet to experience the beginning.

On the train into Manhattan a comfortable silence settled over us as we slouched on graffiti-repellent plastic seats. I fantasized about tall glasses of orange juice. Natalia eyed me intently as I studied the advertising copy directly across from us. I turned to look at her. "You still smell like baby powder," she said.

Spill

23 January 2004

It's gonna spill, that's for damn sure; you just don't know where. The organ performs a basic task. Sometimes it shoots, rather impressively, onto, say, the bedroom wall or a waiting pair of breasts or the back of a toilet. Not like the other organ, with its blood and acidic lubricant; with its capacity for entry and egress. Seepage supplanting spillage. How did you come to revere this other thing, this mess, this quim?

The mouth is a filthy hole, of course: an asshole in reverse; a slightly different collection of microbial flora – split a lip and you need a shot to protect you from yourself. May as well tongue an anus. But mouths are everywhere; the other organs are not.

"Are you surprised I'm the one who peed on her?" the enigmatic girl asks.

You choke on your smoke. Urine is sterile though: less dangerous than blood and saliva and semen and shit. Piss on a wound if there's no clean water available. Peepee girls. Pissy pussies. You wonder, is it an evolutionary category-error that we piss, more or less, through our genitals?

"Well, yes, I suppose. A little. You seem so . . . reserved."

And she is. Laconic. Indifferent. Still waters. Running waters. The stream interrupted slightly by her labia, little rivulets running down her legs perhaps, the main flow splattering the recipient's breasts. That unmistakable *psssssssssss*. Must smell like piss, but then again most pussies smell a little pissy sometimes. Not unpleasant really, pissy pussies are.

"I'm like that around people I don't know well."

"And this is a regular thing for you?"

"A boyfriend introduced it to me and now it's part of my repertoire."

You wonder what else is.

Nova introduces you to another friend. "These are my lovers, Leslie and Aleks," she says brightly. She places her hands on you, on Leslie, sometimes grabbing your ass or grazing the twitch in your pants. Refreshingly, she has nothing to hide. The friend plays a set. You laugh. You smile. You bid all farewell and take your girls home.

It's gonna spill, that's for damn sure; you just don't know where. The girls had their turns. You delight in the merger of the everyday mouth with an organ that is mostly forced to hide in shame. The tongue writhes, dances. There's a factory in there – noisily churning, slurping, producing pleasure – but she's just toying with you. You know she can finish you if she wants.

"Do you want me to keep going?" Nova asks.

Ohgodyes. Now she's serious, mouth chasing the tight seal of her wet hand, heavy breasts grazing your thighs. Try to kiss Leslie but lose motor control as everything goes out of focus. In her mouth? No. Couldn't be. You breathlessly announce the event, giving her one last chance to get out of harm's way, but Nova's lips clamp on with firm resolve as you spill into her mouth, pumping in enough calories to power her body for a couple of minutes. You writhe as she milks you until your pleasure centers are overtaxed.

She swallows your spill. You find this delightfully intimate.

Babylon

16 March 2004

It's nine o'clock in the p.m. and I'm doing the dishes, lost in some internal monologue. I haven't slept much but I tell myself I'll catch up tonight. There's a monster in me and I'm trying to put it to rest. It lives in my head or up my ass or perched atop my cock or wherever it is that personal demons live. A quick glance in the bathroom mirror reveals the toll of a late night spent hunched over my desk. I need some air. I need to fill my sunken eyes with life again.

Leslie's out on a date. She calls again, asking me if I want to come out.

"Is she hot?" I ask out of reflex.

"Yeah, she's hot," Les answers brightly, alcohol dragging out her syllables.

"Did you give her the memo?"

"She understands our situation."

"Is Nova coming out?"

"She's in Brooklyn."

Just a drink or two. Socialize a bit. I tell myself it will be a quiet night this time, that I'm most definitely probably possibly not going to fuck this girl. I shower but I don't shave my nuts, thinking this will serve as a final line of defense. Who am I kidding? It's the Maginot Line of virtue. As I lace up my shoes a surge of lust hits me like sudden indigestion. Where'd that come from? It's not so bad out so I opt to traverse the north end of the park on foot. The lake reminds me of the dead guy. Speed-walking now. My heart thumps.

And it drops when I see her. Susan the willowy brunette – pretty face, pert breasts teasing me from behind the frame of her plunging neckline. Hot all right. A little fragile and sweet. It'll be like filling her up. Wonder how she looks with that top off? I say hello to the ladies and walk over to the bar to buy a round.

The bartender smiles at me. "You always show up with beautiful women," she says.

"We make a great team," I say, nodding in Leslie's direction.

I return to the table bearing drinks. The girls talk about dicks.

"It has to be a certain size otherwise it just doesn't do it for me," Susan says.

"Good grief!" I interject. "We're already talking about *cock*?"

"Don't worry," admonishes Leslie. "I told her you have a really nice one."

Susan looks down. I nearly blush. Leslie removes a sticker from its backing and places it over the creamy skin of Susan's right tit. "I'M A BIG DOG," the sticker reads. Les heads for the bathroom. I study Susan's face and practice holding eye contact. Her features are sharp, small, a tad doll-like. She tells me she's part Irish, Italian and Cherokee. I can almost see it.

She broke up with her boyfriend a few months back and now wants to meet girls for fun. Strictly no strings attached, as they say. One could say this is crass but Susan comes across as charming and intelligent. I sometimes wonder about this kind of bravado though: isn't there middle ground between the zipless fuck and the all-consuming quest for the One? I think of Nova and feel a little guilty. It's been two months and we haven't yet established any rules. At least we're honest with each other.

"The girls my ex and I were with seemed more interested in him than me," Susan's telling me. "I got tired of that."

"Well, Les is most definitely bi."

Susan goes all dreamy. "Oh God, she's so hot. I want to feel her hands all over me." She casts her eyes downward again, straight hair framing her delicate lines. "Do you think Leslie's into me?"

"No. She told me earlier she thinks of you as a friend."

"Are you serious?"

I chuckle. "No, I'm *fucking* with you."

"So you don't mind if I have a purely sexual relationship with your girlfriend?"

I wonder whether her scenario includes me. I don't ask.

Leslie and I stand outside smoking. I tell her about my conversation with Susan. "I'm not sure about her, though," I conclude.

"You don't like her?"

"No, no, it's not that. She's nice and everything. I'm just not sure she's into me."

"We'll find out soon enough."

"And there's our girlfriend."

"I know. I've been talking about her all night. I'd like to introduce the two of them."

"Well, this is different, I suppose. We don't need another girlfriend but variety is nice, just mixing it up every once in a while. Maybe the four of us can play together."

"That would be quite a party. Who knows? Susan seems up for anything."

We leave our table behind and hang out by the bar so as to really have at the sauce. Les introduces me to a winsome blonde but I'm not really following the conversation. I glance over my shoulder and see that Susan's being chatted up by an older gentleman in a suit. He has his arm around her. This, I decide, is a capital offense.

"Guess I'll go over and shut him down," I say, smiling wickedly.

Susan turns to me. She wants to be rescued . . . I can read the subtle pleading in her eyes. She spills a tiny amount of the drink the Fool bought for her.

"We need to get you out of those wet clothes," I say, and stroke her back lightly.

"That line works for you?" the Fool asks.

"Oh yes – all the time," I say, adopting a facetious tone. "I usually deliver it a bit differently, however."

"Show me," coos Susan.

"Well, first I place a drop of my drink on her, like this." I dip my index finger into a glass of ice water and press a drop into Susan's blouse.

"Then I lean in *real* close, like this." I invade Susan's personal space, my lips centimeters from her ear. I exhale slowly and slip my arm around her waist. "See? She's showing me the nape of her neck. That means she trusts me. Now let's get you out of those wet clothes, baby."

Susan grins. "Mmm . . . you're smooth."

"I'm too old for all that nonsense," the Fool responds indignantly. "I'd rather be direct."

"I simply enjoy making women feel sexy. You, my friend, are way too octopus-like and obvious. You either can't read her body language or else you don't care (and that's even worse). Hell, I've *forgotten* more about picking up women than guys like you will ever know."

The Fool has a smile plastered on his face. He doesn't yet realize he's done my work for me, driven Susan into my own octopus embrace. "I should be taking notes," he says.

"I'll keep my arm around you," I whisper to Susan. "That'll do the trick. Your hair smells wonderful, by the way."

Soon the nymphs are leaning over me and kissing, forming an arch as I sit between them. I grasp an ass firmly in each palm. There is no urgency in their lips, their tongues. It's not exactly lust I feel but warmth, like I'm sitting on the beach in Tulum and sipping a cocktail.

Back at the apartment the women don't waste any time. The panties fly off and Susan's flicking her tongue across Leslie's muff. Susan bends over the couch now, a tiny tattoo visible on her right ass cheek. I pound her inviting cunt with a couple fingers. I smack a tight buttock and it jiggles. Susan moans.

"I want to taste you," I say to Susan. She smiles. She lies back on the couch and I lose myself in the folds of her hairless pussy. I sneak a peek at her face, now twisted in pleasure. Her hip bones protrude. She grabs my head and grinds against me. She mumbles incoherently and it dawns on me that she's coming.

We're in the bedroom and I'm fucking Leslie from behind as Susan grabs at Leslie's gorgeous rump. I slip out of Leslie and Susan takes me into her mouth, jerking my shaft as she licks me clean. "Is this thing big enough for you?" I ask, smiling and gently tugging at her hair.

I push into Susan as she lies on her back, filling her up, fulfilling the evening's prophecy. It's a slippery slope up there – I'm committed now. I gently brush the hair from Susan's sweaty brow. I flip her over and push a thumb against her asshole as my pelvis smacks against her. She's breathless. I order her to bury her face in Leslie's pussy. "God you're going to make me come again," Susan purrs. And then she's lying there, spent, a little air escaping her cunt.

I clamber atop Leslie and brush my lips against hers as I thrust into her. The heat inside her is simply too much and soon we're both gasping, releasing into our tight embrace.

Susan's already sleeping. Leslie's drifting off. I stumble into the living room to smoke a cigarette. I pop in a Steely Dan album.

I stand by the bed for a minute and watch the girls sleep. I crawl under the covers and close my eyes.

Automagic Pilot

21 May 2004

Wolf down a plate of mac-n-cheese. Finish your beer. Throw on those pants with the frayed edges and a few small holes in them. You bought them that way. Grab a shirt off the hanger – the one Nova calls your "dirty shirt".

Beware of the woman who lies in wait behind a parked van. Too late: she's sprung her trap and nabbed your cab. Another taxi comes along in a minute, cutting across three lanes and nearly sideswiping an ice cream truck. Your girlfriend shoos the lumbering beast off. Outta the way! *Doo dee dum dee doo*, the truck drones on.

Navigate the city grid to Jack-n-Jill's, down past sleepy doorman buildings where money comes home to roost. Be prepared for that look Jack always gives you because you're always late. The two girls are gussied up and appear not at all the way you remember them. Make an exaggerated formal gesture of kissing the German girl's hand – something she'll remember – and then chill on the couch. Laconic tonight, aren't you? Nothing a few drinks won't fix.

Natalia's spent the past two hours preening and prepping. You call her and she's still holed up at home, walking around topless and fretting over her assortment of dresses. Tell her you'll meet her in 20 minutes. Your girlfriend rides with Jack-n-Jill and you, lucky you, get to escort the girls. It's starting to rain now and the cab scoots down the Franklin D. Roosevelt like a hydrofoil.

Stake out a space downstairs by the bar, buy a drink and watch 'em all roll in, first your girlfriend & company, then Ms. C (of the vicious circle) and her curious, rebounding friend, then Film Boy and Cherry Girl. A brunette in a red dress struts by and runs a soothing hand down the small of your back. Flash a sidelong glance and smile – there'll be time to deal with this later. Someone's calling your name and when you see her your eyes bug out. She used to work for you. "What are *you* doing here?" she asks. Ask her the same question.

Wander out for a smoke just in time to meet Natalia on her way in. "I hope you're wearing something sexy under that jacket," you say. Yes she is. Head back down and dance for awhile. Interact. Spy the woman in red. Your girlfriend lifts her skirt and sticks her ass in front of a camera, a woman spanks it, and a dozen monitors moon the room. Your girlfriend's kissing everyone now, including the cocktail waitress who keeps trying to get you to buy a vial of mystery liquor.

You're upstairs chatting with Jamie. It's been two years since you last saw this girl but she acts like it's only been a week. She's pretty . . . and witheringly vapid. Go ahead and see if you can push her buttons. "I still have those naked pictures of you . . . you and those big tits and that sexy ass," you tell her. She laughs. Natalia appears at your side. Make the necessary introductions.

Leave with the German girl when she tugs at your arm, concern etched in the furrows of her brow. She pulls you outside into the downpour, around the corner, and you see your girlfriend huddled on the curb, soaking wet, head hanging heavily. What a mess. You're both hauling her up, getting her to stand, scolding her for overdoing it. Try to find a cab but give up after 20 minutes in the rain, after some yuppie steals your ride and you're *this* close to hauling him out by the neck.

Take your girlfriend inside and tell Jamie to get her a glass of water. Run downstairs and let everyone know what's going on. When you come back up Jack-n-Jill are outside helping your girlfriend into a cab. Hand the driver 20 bucks and then stare in bewilderment – the driver's saying something but it's coming across as white noise. Before you can react Jill throws in another 20 and the beast is satisfied. Broken meter . . . goddamned crook from Crapistan. Make a note of the number and tell the cabbie he'd better get your mate home safe and sound. Tell her you'll call in five minutes. Slam the door.

And, of course, once she's at home she calls you to say she feels fine.

Go to the bodega with Natalia and grab some ciggies. On the way back you see Film Boy and Cherry Girl hailing a taxi. They invite you to an absinthe party. Turn down their invite – later on you'll be glad you did. You find the German girl, meaning to thank her for taking care of your girlfriend, and the two of you sit upstairs drinking water. The way she's staring at you . . . you know it's coming. "I'm going to do something *mad*," she says. Don't flinch when she grabs you and presses her lips to yours, when all you can think is that *impulsive* is the word you would have used, or *crazy* even . . . but not *mad*. Stick your hand up her skirt and feel her cunt over her panties. She's cute, actually. "Shall we go, uh, downstairs?" you ask, feeling a tad awkward. When you stand she puts her arms around your neck and kisses you again.

The night's winding down. You find the cocktail waitress by the dance floor and she's hounding you again, asking you to do a body shot with her. "Look, how much commission do you make off this crap?" you ask. She tells you. "Well, why don't I just give you the money and lick you wherever I want." When you say this, place your hand on her ass for emphasis. She won't mind.

It's a wrap. Natalia's right here, in her underwear, lying next to you as your girlfriend's pretty mouth clamps onto your member. Everyone's split, run off to after hours, gone home to sleep, fuck, masturbate, watch television. Everyone's on automagic pilot.

Echoes

7 August 2004

We sat hunched over the kitchen counter as Leslie made drinks and Layla fiddled with her one-hitter. Only now, under the lights, did I really notice Layla's eyes – bright and blue and unsettling. The words flowed easily among us but we didn't speak of what we were so obviously ready to do. It was Leslie who broke the tension, pressing her body into Layla's. Soon the women held each other, swaying to the music.

"I'm hot," said Leslie.

"Then we have to get you out of that top," Layla replied, pulling Leslie's blouse over her head. The girls gave each other tender kisses while I took pictures. "You're so beautiful," Leslie kept telling Layla. The rest of their clothes soon melted to the floor, revealing wonderfully taut young bodies. A tattoo of a butterfly trapped in a spider's web adorned Layla's pubic area, forming a neat triangle over Layla's shorn cunt. The spider lurked in a corner.

Layla leaned against me as I sat on a stool, her naked ass pressed into my clothed lap. Leslie knelt before her and stuck her tongue into Layla's pussy, causing Layla to gasp and throw her head back. My cock ached to be free but I dared not release it. I raised my hands to Layla's breasts, kissing her neck and teasing her earlobe with the tip of my tongue, losing myself in her scent. After a dreamy eternity they switched positions and now it was Layla sprawled at Leslie's feet. I stood and Leslie fished my cock out, letting it twitch before our playmate's face. Layla, being a well-mannered guest, promptly wrapped her lips around me.

The two women retired to the couch, where Layla buried her face between Leslie's thighs, Layla's spine curving gently upward, her soft, voluptuous ass seeming to levitate. This is how I captured them, holding the camera and trying to concentrate on something other than my own lust, and when the shutter clicked the moment was already lost to memory. They wanted me to join them. I wanted to torture myself a little while longer . . .

"I want to see how you do it," Layla beckoned. I obediently curled up between Leslie's legs and lapped at the center of my universe, Layla's saliva mingling with Leslie's own juices, Layla's hand grasping at my erection. Hungry for me, Leslie crawled onto the coffee table and bent over to service me as I reclined on the couch, her beautiful ass jutting proudly skyward. Layla brought up the rear, winking at me across the expanse of Leslie's curves. My girlfriend's silky tongue slithered over me and I counted my blessings.

I was doubly blessed: Leslie insisted that Layla have a turn upon the table and Layla eagerly complied. The way a woman uses her mouth says everything, I think, that needs to be said – Layla swallowed me whole, cupped my balls, wrapped her tongue around me, and Leslie's machinations at the other end were making Layla breathless, causing her to utter loud, lusty moans that can only be described as pornographic. I grabbed a fistful of Layla's hair and babbled encouraging words.

Flush now, with a pulsing ache between my legs, I penetrated Leslie as Layla cradled her. I wondered whether we might just break the table but I doubt I would have stopped if we had. I dismounted, finally, to give Leslie a rest and watched for a moment as Leslie took Layla again. Unable to contain myself, I cried out: "I want some of that!" I flipped off my slippers and rested my knees upon them, brought my open mouth to rest against Layla's pretty pussy, became the butterfly trapped in her spider's web. I closed my eyes . . .

"Daisy chain," I said, working my fingers into Layla as she settled down to the business of making Leslie come. We had finally left the coffee table behind for the softness of the bed. And Les did come. Beautifully. I arranged the women in a 69 position and slipped into Leslie from behind. Ever the faithful assistant, Layla licked me clean whenever I popped out and then helped inch me back in again. With Layla's tongue against my balls, I bent over and snuck fingers into both of her wet holes, all the while grinding into Leslie, watching her tongue dart across Layla's clitoris.

The poor girl had waited long enough for her orgasm, so Leslie and I uncoupled and dove in, taking turns, lapping away relentlessly, sucking at Layla's labia as her moans grew louder. And then we divided the labor, Leslie concentrating on Layla's clitoris as my fingers pistoned in Layla's pink. This could have gone on all night and I wouldn't have minded. Soon Layla was a quivering mess, drawing her legs together. Leslie and I were both panting as if the orgasm had been ours. I rose and stood at the foot of the bed, the two women watching me as I rolled on a condom.

Propped above Layla, I gently tapped her butterfly with the head of my cock. "Careful . . . you'll be trapped in my web," she said as I eased into her.

I smiled. "Funny, I was just thinking that." She gave way, warm and wet around me. Leslie suckled at her pert breasts. "How's this?" I asked as I shook the bed with my thrusts.

"*Ohhh*," Layla gasped.

I slowed down, pulling most of the way out and then sliding forward. "How about this?"

"*Mmmm*," she moaned.

I pushed Layla's legs up against her chest and went deeper, feeling every inch of her. I lost track of time. Had it been minutes or hours? "God, I'm going to come so hard," I said. And I did come. And my mind was empty.

Later on we rested on the couch in our post-sex haze, listening to a Pink Floyd album. Layla sang along. "I'm the king," I heard myself say, "Leslie's my queen . . . and you're our princess." Growing by infinitesimal increments, fueled by the gentle friction of skin upon skin, arousal took hold again. Layla's hands found Leslie and Leslie's hands found Layla. Leaning up against the cushions, I fucked Layla under Leslie's rapidly circling fingers, my eyes fixed upon Layla's pretty pussy, the living room filled with the echoes of our coupling. And then I came full circle, making love to my girlfriend as Layla cradled her. I kissed Layla, then Leslie, and awaited the night's final revelation. When it finally arrived I slumped forward, my head nestled in Layla's arms . . .

Outside, the palest blue light crept across the landscape, a veil over memories of night, coming to rouse the city from erotic dreams. Leslie and I settled into bed with our princess between us.

"Goodnight, my king and queen," she said.

"Goodnight, princess," said Leslie and I.

And the night, already lost to memory, echoed in my mind.

LAURA'S WINDOW OR MY LIFE
AS A FORMER PROSTITUTE

http://happyhooking.blogspot.com

Monday 9 February

Wow. My very first post as a blogger. How momentous a moment.

Here I intend to keep a diary for myself of what's going on in my life, so at some point I can look back and remember things I may forget that I probably shouldn't. I think it will be interesting to be able to see the evolution of my thought processes, mostly.

Lately I've been thinking a lot about an activity I began doing a bit over a month ago, and that's having sex with men for money. When a friend of mine initially told me a few years ago that she'd done it one time to pay her rent, I recall being shocked. I could never ever do that, I thought, no matter how desperate for cash I was. After all, I thought, it's just wrong. How your perspective on right and wrong can change considerably when you actually think about vs. just accepting something as wrong because you've been told forever that it just "is".

And now it's late, and I've got heartburn and don't want to be sitting in front of this machine any longer. Note to self: purchase more Mylanta and don't eat cookies at midnight.

Wednesday 11 February

On Tuesday I met a very nice gentleman for coffee, whereupon we sized each other up a bit, made some idle chit chat, and then retired to a local motel for adult activities. He was short, funny, and Italian. We talked a lot about smokers being persecuted and ostracized, and golf. The sex itself was actually pretty good, and then the hour was up and he asked if he could see me again. Walked away with a 30 per cent tip, even. I felt rather amused with myself on the drive home . . . I'm still rather amazed that I can get paid for doing something so fun.

Friday 13 February

Had my first somewhat icky experience this morning.

Had an appointment with a man today. He insisted that it be early. I'm not a morning person by any stretch, but I decided it would be OK this time. So I arrived at his place at 8.45 a.m. Big messy house – evidence of kids everywhere, but that's OK. What wasn't OK was that when scheduling the appointment I'd asked for some coffee upon my arrival, so we could sit and chat and get to know each other a little bit before the "event". However, when I got there he informed me that he'd forgotten to get my coffee and tried to kiss me before I'd even taken my coat off. Jeez Louise. It seemed as if he also forgot to use deodorant that morning, because his pits were ripe. My God. I was not even the slightest bit turned on, and was very relieved when it only took him about a minute of fucking me to come. He was disappointed, and I didn't care. I just wanted this relatively harmless but unpleasant for me hour to end. Fortunately he didn't say anything when I didn't attempt to fill out the hour with anything else besides chit-chat, and finally, after 45 minutes, I was able to escape.

When I got home from this, I heard from my "quick" client via email. He's totally no nonsense. Just likes a less than two-minute blow-job, pays me, and I'm out of there. And his office is only seven minutes away, so the whole experience is well worth the hundred bucks it nets me. I have to wonder though, why he wouldn't just jerk off for a quick release? But it's his money, so I'm not going to ask him lest he not call me the next time he feels the need for some "relief", as he puts it.

Monday 16 February

My boyfriend (with whom I have an "open relationship") went
away for last night, so I had an unprecedented opportunity to do
some "night work". I posted an ad in the morning, and by noon
had received the usual gazillion responses. This ad was very non-
specific about me and what I'd be available for, so the responses
were particularly strange. One man wanted me to show up at his
shoe store after hours wearing nothing underneath my long coat
and get fitted for shoes, another wished for a blow-job in the public
toilet in front of the city's library, and another wanted lingerie and
toe-sucking. I'm sure there's someone out there that would be
willing to comply with these requests, but it's not me.

I wound up chatting in IM with the sweetest 21-year old boy – a
senior in college in the city. He was smart, polite, and absolutely
adorable in his photos he sent me to preview. I felt very comfortable chatting with him, and so we made an appointment to get
together late. I didn't realize I'd be visiting him in his dorm room!
(The furniture in his room gave me déjà vu from my own college
years.)

We talked for a long time before anything happened. I told him
before I even got there that I didn't want to be in any kind of rush,
and so we'd just pretend I was only with him for an hour. He liked
that idea, of course.

I really enjoyed his company. He was so sweet and it was a total
pleasure for me. I almost told him to just keep his money, but alas,
there are bills to pay.

Saturday 21 February

Wednesday I was blown off by a man I'd corresponded with for
weeks. That's one of the real irritating things about doing this
independently. You spend all sorts of time marketing – creating
enticing ads, responding and trying to weed out the creeps, making
appointments – and then, when they fall through at the last minute,
cursing because you could have scheduled some other actual willing person who wasn't just wasting your time.

Friday 27 February

Just got an instant message from the gentleman I saw earlier in the day yesterday, telling me what a good time he had with me. I had a really good time with him as well, so it's certainly nice to hear. He gave me a Minneola orange on my way out the door, and giggled a lot before, during and after.

Monday 1 March

I thought receiving the gift of a Minneola was odd the other day, but yesterday I was given Loganberry Preserves by a man I'd spent the afternoon with. Yes, preserves! I think it was kind of a big deal that he'd given them to me, since he had to go all the way to Seattle to get it. It's odd the things you talk about when you're lying naked with a stranger.

I'm surprised at how busy I've been with this. I wasn't expecting to be seeing men almost daily. I thought it would just be a now and again thing, to help make ends meet. A fun way to make ends meet. But the money is so easy, and for the most part I've met only nice guys that I actually enjoyed spending time with.

I find it interesting how much some of the men I've met like to talk. Sometimes I think they've hired me just as much for having someone to listen to their stories, as a warm willing body to fuck.

Friday 5 March

I saw a rather unusual older man in his luxurious five-story condo downtown yesterday. When I arrived, he immediately ushered me up all these flights of stairs, past impeccably decorated rooms into this gorgeous bedroom, replete with a bed with more pillows on it than any man or woman should ever possess. "What should I do? Should I take off my clothes?" he asks. So I said, "Sure." And so he did – down to his actual tighty whities, and I removed a bunch of mine, but left on my lingerie. Then he proceeded to lie face down on the bed, with a very stiff posture. He didn't look particularly comfortable. I figured perhaps he wanted a back rub, so I tried to do that for a couple of minutes but that's not really my specialty, so I asked him if he'd like to roll over. So he did, and I gave him a blow-job – and it took several minutes of blowing for him to actually get hard. He didn't really look at me, just lay there with this kind of scrunched expression on his face. Finally he asks me if I'll take off my bra, and then he proceeded to kind of pinch one of my nipples while I finished up with the head. After he came, we talked about his job, and traveling. He loosened up finally, thank goodness. Before I left, he asked me if he could contact me again. I had an email waiting when I came home. He told me I was extremely nice and it was a pleasure to have had me in his home. And today another one from him wanting to reserve two hours of my time tomorrow. Go figure!

Wednesday 10 March

Had lunch with a charming Englishman on Monday. Tall, thin, attractive, great accent. I followed him back to his place and spent a couple hours in bed with him. We discussed books and work and so on. He was very sweet. "Oh, that feels so lovely," sounds fabulous in a British accent, I must say. It made me want to keep doing what I was doing so he'd say it again. At the end of our time together, he actually said, "Since you had a good time too, how about if I pay you half?" And I said, "No, how about you pay me what we originally discussed?" with a smile. He looked a little bashful and paid up. I think he'll probably call me again when he can afford it.

Thursday 11 March

I've been thinking about what to say when my clients inevitably ask me "So, why do you do this?" I need to come up with some snappy but sufficient response, because it's not something I really want to discuss at great length with them. Most of them don't want to hear that I'm doing it for the money, which is only partly true anyway. If I tell them I do it because I really enjoy no-strings sex, then I fear they'll argue with me about why should they have to pay for it then? This topic needs much further explanation, and perhaps writing about it will allow me to sort it out a bit better in my mind. More on it later, I suppose.

Sunday 14 March

This is a repeat customer weekend. Yesterday afternoon I went to see once again the gentleman referenced on 5 March, with the incredibly well-appointed and luxurious five-story condo. He was much more relaxed this time, thank goodness. We took our clothes off and got in bed, and indicating my breasts, he asked, "What do these like?" (as if they were separate entities with their own wishes). The other amusing thing was, after he played with my boobs for a while, I asked him what he would like, and he said, "Make me scream. Make me scream 'Mother.'" I just looked at him and laughed and said, "Now, I think that would be kind of weird!" I ended up sucking on his cock like a champ again. It took forever! And again, hardly any reaction the entire time from him, until the end. That's when he reported it was the best he'd ever had. He said after that, "God, I don't know what to say." I said, "You don't have to say anything." He said he was kind of embarrassed that it was the best he'd had, to which I informed him that if it makes him feel any better, I get that from most everyone whose cock ends up in my mouth so he's in good company.

Tuesday 16 March

I was thinking yesterday about how when I first started doing this, I'd have butterflies while getting ready for my "date" and I'd be nervous about whether or not I'd be well received when I arrived or if there's something I forgot to do before running out of the house. Would he like me? Would he be disappointed with my looks or personality? Could I carry this off? I barely even think about that stuff now. I just go through what has become a routine for getting ready for an appointment. Lay out outfit and lingerie. Shower with Dove soap and shampoo that smells yummy. Shave legs, armpits and pussy (I wish I could work up the courage to wax!) and exfoliate skin, apply Nivea Q10 lotion all over, get dressed, dry hair and put on makeup. Check manicure and pedicure. Make sure

I have directions and the date's phone number in case I get lost. Check purse to make sure I've got enough condoms and mints or breath spray. Tada, I'm done and I'm off.

I'm going to compose a new ad now. Those years working in marketing have paid off, since my ads always net numerous replies that I carefully weed through and have been able to turn into new clients. My angle has so far been basically what's known in the trade as a "girlfriend experience". Apparently a girlfriend experience includes kissing and generally more affectionate treatment than an ordinary experience with a whore. I position myself as a sexy, smart, funny, "normal" woman with a dirty mind, who isn't a seasoned professional (which I suppose I am really not, yet), and so far it's worked like a charm. Many of the men that answer my ad tell me they did so because I don't sound like all of the other girls that are advertising and they felt compelled to get in touch. (And maybe they say that to all the girls they try to hire. Who knows?) Perhaps eventually I won't have to advertise anymore and will have a bevy of regulars to fill up my schedule.

Wednesday 17 March

More on the "why I do this" topic:

I've been thinking, and I have to admit that a large part of it is an ego thing. It amazes me still that there are perfectly attractive; even dare I say – hot! men that are willing to fork out big bucks to play with me. I'm just an ordinary early thirty-something woman, not some supermodel. In a previous part of my life, I'd have been hesitant to even smile at some of these men, for fear that they wouldn't smile back, much less actually chat one up. And now I'm sitting around picking and choosing from a virtual plethora of "applicants". Who will I let pay me for my company next – when I feel like it, not because I have to. It's amusing to no end.

Thursday 18 March

I was asked a question by a reader about what it says about human nature that the purchasing of sex is so prevalent. While I've never sat down with a client and specifically asked the question, "So, why exactly did you decide to rent me today?" I have gathered from the conversations I've had with them that there seems to be a common thread or two.

One common thread is the men I've seen so far have been more often than not either married or involved in a long-term relationship, rather than single. It isn't they're not getting sex at all, so they have to buy some in order to satisfy some basic need. Nope. Prior to doing this that is what I would have assumed. Renting a whore for an hour or two seems to be satisfying the need for *variety in sex vs. the need for sex itself*. From what I can tell, these men are happy in their relationships and prefer to not risk these relationships by having an affair to get some "strange". An affair might become an emotional entanglement, but they don't have to worry about that with a prostitute. They're paying to have a cut and dried experience. Sex and conversation. It's the ultimate easy no-strings attached situation.

I think also the purchase of sex is prevalent because most people fear rejection and a sure thing is a good thing. Why wine and dine a woman and wonder if she's going to give it up for you at the end of the date, when you can spend virtually the same amount of money (and much less time!) on a prostitute without all the pretense? You're definitely going to get your blow-job, or get laid, or whatever it is you've negotiated. Some people might disagree, but most men pay for sex in one way or another – and hiring a call girl is just a more efficient way of doing it for some.

Wednesday 24 March

The accordion player was an odd duck indeed. He wasn't unpleasant, just definitely unusual. He was very interested in the whole "professional" aspect of what I do, and wound up giving me a book called *Turning Pro* from his bookshelf. "You could make a LOT of money doing this," he said. I got the impression that he thought I'd never done this before him. I decided that perhaps that was part of the fantasy for him – the whole breaking in a "new girl" thing – and I didn't want to burst his bubble so I just let him think what he wanted to think. He didn't want to kiss or fuck. Just massage and oral.

I watched this HBO on Demand special with my boyfriend called *Hookers and Pimps*. It was basically about streetwalkers. Afterwards I was teasing him and asked him if he had any money. We negotiated – he started off by offering 15 cents! I ended up giving him a blow-job and letting him fuck me from behind on the couch for $5. Ha!

Thursday 25 March

Many folks have written to ask me what a typical appointment with a client is like. How does it work? What happens? How do you get from the initial contact to the sex?

Obviously I can speak only for how I do it, since I have no idea how it works with other escorts.

When a potential client answers one of my ads via email, if I find his response compelling enough, I'll send him more information about me. I have a standard reply which includes information such as my availability, physical description, hourly rate for companionship, and a couple of photos. I explain that since I want the experience to be fun for both of us, physical chemistry is important to me and therefore I need to see a photo of him as well before I'll consider meeting. This puts some potential clients off, but I don't really care. I'd rather lose that business than have to reject the man face to face later on.

Once it's been established that he'd like to see me and I'd be happy to see him, there is generally an email exchange or chat via IM to determine the when and where. I do not have appointments in my home, but I do make both hotel and house calls. I like to arrange to have a cup of coffee in a public place (since I meet during the day) so we can talk and make sure that we'd both be comfortable and would like to go through with the experience. The talking is hardly ever about what is about to happen. It's usually about his job or my "real job". "Tell me about what you do," is a sure winner. Usually this part only takes ten minutes or so and I don't include it in the "hour". Generally what happens is eventually there will be a silence and it's time for him to decide. I'll say,

"So . . ." and smile with an inquisitive look on my face. That's worked every time.

I'll then follow the gentleman to his hotel or home. Men that have seen escorts before will then generally offer a beverage (even though we just had one). There's usually a couple more minutes of chit chat at this point. If he doesn't take the lead to get the ball rolling once we're in a private place, I've found that all it takes is for me to give him a kiss. If we're not in a bedroom and he's nervous and seems to need direction, I'll suggest we move somewhere comfortable.

It's at that point that I'll ask what he'd like. Some men just come right out and are very specific and others are will say something like, "Well, whatever you want to do." (I find that kind of funny, since theoretically I'm providing the service.)

And then the fun really begins . . .

Wednesday 31 March

It's been a few days, I know.

I've had three appointments since I last wrote. All painless. Whee!

One was with a local shop owner who wanted a hot oil massage and a hand-job. Easy as pie. He lit candles in his bedroom and heated up his oil in the microwave. He was just so delighted with the experience. It was kind of sweet. He mentioned my nails being great as I was lightly scratching his back. I said, "Yeah, and they're real too. I don't understand the whole fake nails thing. Actually, I don't understand fake anything." And as the words were leaving my lips, I noticed that the gentleman was wearing a toupee. I don't know how I didn't notice it before, but I didn't. Whoops. Fortunately he was all blissed out and didn't seem to notice my remark. He had a spare bottle of that massage oil which he wound up giving to me after I said I liked the way it smelled.

Another was a British academic. All he wanted to do was play with my boobs extensively and masturbate while I tickled his balls. Oh, and of course he wished to come on my tits and of course I let him.

And the last was someone I didn't really want to see, but I'm glad

I did. He was suggesting all kinds of activities to me via chat that I didn't want to participate in and I just wasn't looking forward to it, but decided to go anyway. He was surprisingly normal in person. Amusing, even. I said to him that I assumed this wasn't the first time he'd done this and he said that yes, he had experience with escorts. I asked him what his other experiences were like. He told me that they ranged from awful to today – and that I was an "exceptional GFE." Awww. Flattery will get you everywhere. It got me into the shower with him which I think was what netted me the 100 per cent tip I received.

Monday 5 April

I had what had to be the most effortless appointment ever today.

I arrived at the gentleman's hotel, and he greeted me politely and offered me a glass of wine. He'd brought along a CD player and had some new agey music playing which, albeit a tad cheesy, was a nice change from the usual hotel room silence. After talking with me for about 20 minutes, we finally got down to business. And what was that business, you wonder? Yours truly got to lie there and have her feet rubbed, her toes sucked, and then some pretty fabulous oral sex for an hour. No reciprocation on my part was required whatsoever. And that was it! Hot damn.

Sometimes a prospective client will have a huge laundry list of questions for me about what I'll do and what he can do.

- Can I take photos of you with my cock in your mouth? (No way.)
- Can I lick your ass? (Sure.)
- Will you lick my ass? (No.)
- Can I fuck your ass? (Nope.)
- Is it OK if I come on you? (Yes.)
- Can I kiss you? (I sure hope you do.)
- How about coming on your face or your tits? (Just avoid my eyes, please.)
- Can I fuck you from behind? (Of course.)
- Is it OK if I call you names? (Sure.)
- Can I slap your ass? (As long as you don't bruise me.)

- Pull your hair? (As long as you don't pull it out.)
- Will you talk dirty? (I certainly can but usually don't unless really inspired.)

The list is endless and I try to be both frank and patient about discussing my boundaries, since I don't want to have to deal with uncomfortable situations in person when it can be avoided with advance conversation. What I find quite interesting, however, is that those with the most detailed and specific questions about what can actually happen during the course of a session with me, seem to be perfectly happy with the same basic stuff as those with hardly any questions at all.

The young guy I saw yesterday was one with tons of advance questions. I think what happened was he'd scripted out this whole porno movie situation in his head so much before I showed up and was so excited about the ideas he had about what we could do that I hardly even had to touch him before he came. I assured him it was OK and that perhaps it was good to get the first one out of the way so quickly. His second orgasm took longer, but getting there didn't involve much of anything he seemed so concerned about when he had all the questions. And then we lounged around some talking about his job, and then he got up and got dressed. He said he had a fantastic time. I wondered if he was disappointed that there was no ass-slapping or dirty talking or hair-pulling or even fucking, for that matter.

This isn't the first time this sort of thing has happened.

I wonder if it's got something to do with men overestimating what it's going to take for them to be satisfied? Perhaps they think they're going to need way more stimulation than they actually do in reality?

I find it interesting to read other people's perspectives on what I do. I found this opinion online: "I have a really hard time with the indignity of prostitution. I can't help but feel that prostitution is not just about selling sex, but about selling the whole woman, and commanding her, having her at one's (sexual) whim. I also feel pretty sure that prostitutes are often subjected to far worse treatment and degradation than any other laborer except maybe plantation slaves, and that this degradation and abuse is part and parcel of the sex that they sell."

Indignity.

Hmm. I have to say that when I was waiting tables at night to supplement my income I felt far more exploited and undignified than I have ever felt doing this. Having a shift manager who was seven years younger than myself and about half as intelligent ordering me about and questioning my every move just because he thoroughly enjoyed his little power trip was quite possibly the most degrading experience I've ever had. Having to crawl around on the floor wiping crumbs off the bottoms of chair rails after being on my feet for six hours, smiling at rude people who snapped their fingers at me and frequently would shout "Hey you, waitress," – these things were far more soul-crushing to me than anything that's ever happened to me during an appointment with a client.

Tuesday 6 April

With a couple of exceptions that I've blogged about, I've liked all my clients. I find it very difficult to be intimate with someone whose company I do not enjoy. I think as an independent escort in the unique position to be able to pick and choose who I spend my time with, the likelihood of having to endure the company of someone I do not like is much lower than that of a girl working for an agency. If I get a bad vibe from someone during the initial stages of contact, I can opt not to meet them. (I actually only wish to meet a small percentage of those who contact me.) Granted, being independent has its cons as well – for I have to spend time writing ads, managing the replies, and setting up appointments. It's a lot of work and can be quite time-consuming.

I do find similarities between my clients. They've been attractive, intelligent, interesting nice guys with some disposable income. It could just be that I've gotten good at weeding out the unattractive morons during the initial contact process, or it could be that the ads I create tend to appeal to the sort of client I seek. I think it's a combination of the two.

About 80 percent of my clients have been either married or involved in a long-term relationship. I do not judge them for coming to see me and I think no less of them than I do the unattached clients. In fact, I think they're smarter to see me than to have an affair with their secretary or their next door neighbor in order to get some sexual fulfillment. They don't have to worry that I'm going to fall in love and start calling up their wives or girlfriends or boiling bunnies on their stoves.

Thursday 15 April

Finally, another appointment to report on. Unfortunately, however, it was pretty dull as far as these things go. Another lawyer. (What is it with lawyers and hookers? High-stress job/disposable income/limited time?) Met for coffee, had a fairly boring conversation about my real job (or maybe it's just boring to me since I feel like I'm always answering the same exact questions) and then I followed him home. Very obviously married with children. We retired to his home office. We sat on his couch. I asked him what he had in mind, and what he had in mind was oral – and could he come twice? I must say this was the very first time I've ever given a blowjob right next to a child's Playskool desk, something I noted at the time and found kind of oddly amusing. He was pretty chill about the whole experience. I could tell he's hired working girls before. I think he enjoyed the experience more than I did. Most of the time (unless the guy turns out to be an ass) I have fun. I mean, I really actually enjoy myself. But today – well, it felt more like work than fun. I'm not even sure exactly why. The gentleman was perfectly nice and polite and attractive. Maybe it was the Bruce Springsteen CD that was on in the background. Ha.

And, on another note, a reader wrote and asked how I cope with my period and appointments. Well, I simply don't make appointments when Aunt Flo is in town. And no, I've never had anyone specifically ask me if I'd see him during my period. However, I have seen women posting ads specifically saying that they have their periods right now, so there must be a market for that sort of thing. I guess there's a market for most everything, really.

Thursday 22 April

Several ladies have written asking how one goes about getting started doing this sort of thing. Anyway . . . I'm by no means an expert at this, and I certainly don't advise leaping into something like this lightly. I urge you to do your research. There's plenty of information online about sex work and I implore you to do a whole lot of reading before rushing out and setting up shop.

OK, so . . .

First off, think. How's your self-esteem? Are you assertive and confident? Patient? Do you genuinely like people? Can you talk to anyone? Are you well versed on safe sex practices? Do you have any guilt issues about casual sex? Are you happy being a "giver" when it comes to sex? Are you good at saying no? Just some stuff to consider.:)

I have no idea how most independent escorts go about getting involved, I only know how my friend and I did it and it was as simple as writing an ad and posting it online. There are numerous web sites where you can place adult ads for free and, before I'd invest any money in advertising one's services, I'd go the free route just to make sure it's something you're actually comfortable doing. You have to be careful how you word your ad, because it's illegal to offer sex for money, so basically you have to imply that's what you're doing, vs. coming right out and saying it. Read a bunch of ads and see what others say and then craft yours to be a bit different. What makes you desirable? Why would a man want to spend his hard-earned cash to spend time with you? Think about what makes you special and talk about it in your ad. Also, one thing you can do is do a search on escort web sites and see how they phrase what they're offering. You can also get an idea of what the going rates are for various services in your geographic area that way, too. When I posted my first ad, I was unprepared for the response. I had no idea I'd get so many replies. It became evident rather quickly that, no matter what you write, a lot of the men responding to your ad have paid absolutely no attention whatsoever to anything you've said. For instance, you might say in your ad that you're only available during the day and you can't host (that means you're not going to be having them over at your place), and you'll get an inbox full of mail from guys saying, "I'm interested. Where are you located and can I come see you tonight?" It's plenty frustrating. You start to wonder if all men are idiots. However, just keep in mind the old 80/20 rule. Basically, 80 percent of all your responses will be crap, and 20 percent will be worth further investigation. Speaking of email, it's a good idea to set up an email account with yahoo or hotmail or one of the other free email services to separate your "real" email address from your "working girl" address. Obviously, it's safest not to put your last name on the account.

Be prepared to send a recent photo or two of yourself. Fuzz out your features if you want. I don't, but lots of escorts that advertise online do. I'm sure it's a less effective way to get clients if they can't see what they're getting, but obviously it must work to some degree if people are actually doing it. I have a standard reply that I send to the interesting responses I get (and frankly, like I said, only about two out of ten are worth even sending your standard reply to). Basically I give a physical description, a general outline of my personality, my "fee for companionship" and when I'm available. I ask for a photo if they haven't already sent me one, and ask when they think they might like to see me. I don't like going into too much detail about specific sexual stuff in these emails because one never knows if you're corresponding with a real prospective client or some kind of law enforcement official, so you have to be very careful. If you're getting a weird vibe from someone it's best to just move on. Better safe than sorry.

Sometimes you play email tag for weeks trying to set something up with someone, and sometimes you advertise in the morning and by noon time you've got your afternoon client scheduled. It can be hit or miss. You have to expect you're going to be blown off sometimes, and that's pretty sucky.

I'm not sure how other girls do it, and maybe I'm unusual, but I generally always make them meet me somewhere public first. A cup of coffee is a good idea, or a drink if it's in the evening. That way, if I get a bad vibe I can excuse myself. I didn't meet first in public once and what a disaster that turned out to be. I've certainly learned my lesson since then and I've become a lot more confident about saying the word "no". It's much easier once you've said no a bunch of times and found out people generally accept it without too much hassle. Also, tell someone where you are going to be and who you are going to be with. Tell your client you're going to do that and if he's not willing to tell you his real name and show you his ID, then you shouldn't be willing to go through with the rest. I've never had a single man refuse to give me this information when I've asked for it.

So that's pretty much it, in a nutshell. I'm sure I've probably forgotten something important, so feel free to comment with questions and I'll do my best to answer them.

Friday 23 April

And speaking of penis size, Jay asked if working girls tell their clients how huge their cocks are, like as part of some Whore Script or something. If there is such a script, no one has sent it to me yet. The only time I ever mention anything about a guy's largeness is if his manhood actually is exemplary. And so far, only one has been noteworthy enough for me to comment on it regarding its grand scale.

For all I know, though, it could be part of some escorts' repertoires to stroke not only the client's body, but his ego too. I just don't see the point, myself. I mean, if a guy is average and you're telling him he's gigantic, he's going to know you're being flattering and not honest, so why say anything at all? I prefer to comment on his pretty green eyes, or his manly shoulders or his cute ass – something true and real.

Eric wanted to know how I went from being shocked at my friend's admission that she'd been escorting to doing it myself. Excellent question. It wasn't as if one second I went from shock to participating myself or anything like that. My shock wasn't really revulsion – I thought, I could never do that, it's just wrong! But that thought lasted for only a short time. As soon as I could evaluate the concept, I changed my mind. Logical thought instead of just accepting a perceived moral truth. And then, once I'd gotten through that, it was more like I'd never considered the idea that a normal person could do such a thing. I'd had this concept in my head that you had to be either extraordinarily attractive in order to be one of the more highly paid call girl types, or you were a $20 crack whore. It never occurred to me that there is a market for a more or less normal woman like myself. Also, I had no idea how to actually go about it. So, over time, I pumped my friend for information and decided, hell, if she can do it, why can't I?

Also, he wanted to know if size matters.

Ha!

I certainly can't speak for all women when I say that why yes, it does. But it does matter to me. But it's probably not how you think. Believe it or not, every sized penis has its advantages and disadvantages. (And that's one of the reasons variety is the spice of life.) If I'm in the mood to fuck (vaginally), then there's nothing better than a nice thick cock. But if I'm going to be giving oral sex, give me an average to smaller cock and I'm a happy camper. Once in a while I like to engage in a little backdoor action, and that's when I most prefer a more wee friend. (Although that's not an activity I ever do with clients, regardless of size.) So yes, for me, size does matter – but it matters only in what activities are the most pleasurable, though. I can find something entertaining to do with any sized cock!

Monday 26 April

I had an appointment this morning with a new client – a very pleasant, polite and handsome Scandinavian IT guy. The only remarkable thing about our meeting was that he was married with a young baby. I've started to notice a trend. I've had my share of new fathers at this point. I guess for brand new moms sex is probably the last thing on their minds, so it's no wonder.

I've been asked by a number of readers what I'd do if a wife ever came home while I was there. I think I would probably just let the husband handle the wife and I would leave as quickly as possible and hope she doesn't shoot me before I can go. I'm not sure how else you could handle something like that, really. I'm pretty non-conflict oriented in general, so I don't think I'd want to stick around for any drama that would be sure to ensue.

Tuesday 27 April

BUSTED

Imagine my surprise this morning when I got an IM that says "Have you seen this?" And there was a link to this blog, my blog, right there in the little chat window.

I was chatting with my best friend, Y.

Oh my.

My initial reaction was to pretend I hadn't seen it, much less wrote it, but I knew he didn't believe me. He let me pretend, just as I'd have let him. However, he's not even remotely stupid. He knows me so very well. The way I write and the things I say and how I think. We arranged to have lunch today and I decided I'd just tell him in person. I wanted it to be a face to face discussion with eye contact and all.

So we have lunch and I keep thinking, OK, I'm going to just bring it up. But I didn't. I don't know why. I was there, sitting across from this person who I feel the most comfortable being totally me with, who doesn't ever judge me, who totally just gets me (and vice versa) AND with whom I've shared some of the best ever sexual experiences of my life – and I didn't know how to just bust out with the truth! There were quite a few pregnant pauses. It was a little surreal, since I knew he knew I knew he knew. One of the things I love so much about Y is that he didn't pressure me about it at all. He just cooly pointed out to me that's he'd read it and that was that. He knew that when I was ready I'd spill. Exactly the way I'd have handled it, if the tables were turned.

So after lunch, we're sitting in my car and I'm still not spilling. And all this time elapses. We're yakking at each other, as we're wont to do, but he's got to get back to work and I know this and I know I have to SAY SOMETHING. But there is no one on earth I like kissing more than Y, and I wanted a kiss first before I came out with it, in case when I did tell him he was so horrified at me that he never wanted another kiss. I'm so silly sometimes.

So I get my lovely kiss and then take a deep breath and I look right at him and say, "So you're quite the Sherlock Holmes." And he starts to laugh. And so then I told him about how I knew he didn't believe me earlier, and how I knew that if anyone was going to find the blog and recognize it was me it would have been him. So I talked and talked and he sat and listened and smiled, and finally I stopped and said, "Are you judging me? Um . . ." And he said something to the effect of "God no, of course not. I think it's . . . hot." And then he grinned at me like he does and smooched me some more.

I'm really so very pleased and totally relieved to have had that conversation. If I planned to continue the charade with him I would have had to have taken great pains to never reveal anything even remotely personal ever again, just to make sure he definitely didn't really think it was me. I would have felt like I had to censor myself. Also, I've always been totally honest with him about everything, and I have felt pretty strange about keeping this secret from him anyway. I should have known it would have been OK to discuss with him.

Life can be so weird and good sometimes.

Thursday 29 April

Heather wrote and wanted to know if for the benefit of the ladies, I'd care to share some of my more popular blow-job techniques.

Sure, I thought. However, when I contemplated it, I realized that the Mechanical Guide to Good Head didn't need to be re-written by me. Anyone can find dozens of really great tips for what to do with your tongue and lips and hands by just doing a Google search on "fellatio".

I've asked numerous lovers to try to give me some insight on what it is that I do that makes it good. A blow-job doesn't seem like rocket science to me, so the idea that I have some kind of mechanical skill that lots of other women don't have just seemed kind of preposterous. So, I've asked and been met with a lot of "I don't know. It's just . . ., you're just . . . uh, I really don't know what it is." I've suggested that perhaps it's enthusiasm for the task? "Yeah, it's that, sure, but there's something else, too." The smartest and best of those lovers told me it was empathy.

I had a boyfriend in high school, and like most teenagers that are sexually active, we were like bunny rabbits. We spent a great deal of time having sex which I greatly enjoyed, but I never orgasmed. I realized after a year of this almost constant sex what the issue was — why I wasn't coming. It was because I wasn't ever fully in the moment. If we were fooling around in a parked car, I'd be thinking about getting caught by the police. If we were fooling around in my bedroom, I'd be thinking about the fact that my Mom was down-stairs or my sister might just burst in at any moment or that I really should be doing my Calculus homework. So, for the most part, I was having fun but it was distracted fun. I wasn't "in the moment".

When I had this little epiphany and started focusing on exactly what was going on, vs. thinking about other things, I started having orgasms. Something extra came along with figuring out how important focus was during sex – I started becoming very aware of my partner. Once I learned to pay attention to the way my own body was feeling, I think I just naturally started paying very close attention to the reactions I was able to provoke in my partner. I know this seems like common sense and everyone thinks, yeah, yeah, I pay attention during sex. But do you really? Now think about the best sex you've had, and I'd be willing to bet that a good part of the reason it was the best then is because you were both totally in the moment with one another.

When a client is paying me for my attentions, hopefully that's what he's getting – my full attention. Ideally, I'm able to not think about anything else besides how I'm making him feel. Obviously there are situations that occur where I'm not able or don't want to put myself into that mindset, but more often than not that's what I'm doing. I'm listening to what he has to say, thinking about it, watching him, looking in his eyes . . . just being fully present. What I do next with my lips or my hands or my tongue just happens based on how I imagine what I am doing actually feels to him. I don't have any sort of set Blow-job Technique. There's no step by step. I just focus on his eyes and the rest just happens.

Tuesday 8 June

A curious reader wanted to know what are the differences between having sex with my boyfriend and having sex with clients.

The sex I have with my boyfriend is rarely surprising. When you've been sleeping with someone for more than a decade, you tend to know all their moves, and vice versa. You know what they do, how they do it, how long they'll do it for, and in what order the things they do will happen. If you're me, you also know that there's not a whole lot of animal lust going on, either, but you accept that as perfectly normal. I know that the pleasuring that is going on is done out of love, not passion, and that's OK.

When I'm with a client, I don't know anything for sure. Every client is like a new puzzle to figure out and therefore it is a challenge for me. I have to pay much closer attention to whatever it is that I'm doing, since it's not a tried and true method as it is with my boyfriend. My clients aren't motivated by love to have sex with me, they're motivated by more base feelings – like lust, for instance. They want to have sex with me because they're horny and they find me attractive, not because I cook them dinner and snuggle with them during *The Sopranos*.

I'm not even sure if that is the information the curious reader was looking for, but it was a stab.

Wednesday 9 June

Math was never my best subject in school. One of the best teachers I've ever had encouraged me to tutor Algebra, even though I felt I was struggling myself. She told me that by trying to teach others, I'd begin to understand it better myself. She was absolutely right. I think perhaps this blog is a lot like that for me. I'm gaining a greater understanding of myself by constantly being questioned. I think that's a good thing. It's like free therapy.

Pistachio asked me, since I've obviously slept with a number of people over the course of escorting (and thus sampled a whole lotta merchandise, I suppose), what do I think makes a good lover? I think it mostly boils down to a few particular qualities. I'm all for the type of person who doesn't have a whole lot of inhibitions about themselves, their bodies, and what turns them on. I think if you're ashamed of yourself, you can't be fully present in the moment because you're too busy with your self-consciousness. The best kinds of lovers aren't afraid to say what's on their mind, to try something just because they think it might feel really good, or to simply just lose themselves in pleasure. Good lovers want to communicate and experiment and play. I could go on and on, but it's late, and I need my beauty sleep.

I don't wish to go into too much detail discussing the myriad of ways over the course of my very, very long relationship with my boyfriend that I have attempted to make him a more sexual person. I spent the first couple of years anguishing over his low sex drive – Is it me? Does he not find me attractive? Am I lousy in bed? After deciding that no, it couldn't possibly be me, I proactively tried to get him to try new things with me to find something that would interest him – everything from new positions to role playing, BDSM stuff, bringing home girlfriends for him to play with, etc. This wasn't something that went on for a couple of months, this was YEARS of trying to be as creative as humanly possible with little result. His libido was still as low as ever. I finally gave up trying.

Anyway, I'm not going to go into the whole history of my relationship and exactly how it ended up being open, but it did, and where things were not fine for a very long time, now they are. If you feel bad for my boyfriend, or want to judge me, that's fine. I can't and don't care. I don't wish to justify my relationship and it's intricacies any more and I won't. How we're dealing with our relationship is not an issue I care to discuss anymore.

Tuesday 22 June

I admit it. I have a predilection for men in their twenties when it comes to sex.

Until the question was asked about how does sex with a man in his forties compare to sex with a younger man, I'd never really thought about why I find myself gravitating towards young whippersnappers. It was just a something I noticed about myself but not something I'd ever analyzed. But it's fun to ponder one's own motivations, and this is what I've come up with as an explanation.

I think the main reason is I'm not a huge fan of quickies. What I mean by that is I prefer the kind of sex that takes all afternoon or all evening. (Or all weekend.) I've found that younger men tend to be better suited towards that than older men, simply because it doesn't take very long for their batteries to recharge. When a younger guy comes, it doesn't mean the entire event is finished, it just means it's time to relax and talk for a few minutes before he's ready to play again. And again. And maybe again after that. I can't say that every young guy I've ever been with has been the Energizer Bunny, but it's been my experience that more young men are then older men. It's just physiology.

Older men, in my experience, are also a bit more set in their ways than younger men. While I'm sure there are exceptions to the rule, I've found it's much more difficult to teach an old dog new tricks than a young dog. The older men I've been with have also tended to be less experimental, perhaps because they're comfortable with their own "formula" or because they're carrying around more societal baggage about what's sexually acceptable behavior.

However, if it weren't for the older men I've been with, I'd probably know about half as much about what makes my body feel good, how to make someone else's feel lovely too, and the sorts of things that do turn me on. There's definitely something to be said about learning the ropes from an expert.

Thursday 24 June

I've been asked if I'd post one of my ads here, so readers could see what I have to say about myself. I'd rather not. I don't really want this blog to be that closely associated with my advertising.

Speaking of advertising, I haven't in quite a while now, and I have no particular plans to do so any time in the near future.

I've been thinking about it quite a bit, and I feel as though I might be at the point where I've satisfied my curiosity about the world of sex for hire. I'm not making any promises about that, for I know I may just change my mind. Obviously, I'll post about it if I do decide to place another ad or spend some time with a "regular". But I've been turning down appointments left and right though, and while I don't particularly enjoy disappointing people, I'm just not into it right now and I don't think it would be fair to a client to see him when I'm not feeling enthusiastic.

I guess I'll have to change the name of this blog if I actually commit to retiring, eh?

Friday 25 June

John asked:

Are you sure you aren't losing interest in being a whore just because someone you know found out about it? There was another blog that is indirectly linked to this one, with a similar situation. She wasn't having sex for money, just a lot of it, and for free. I guess that made her a slut and not a whore. Not sure if it matters. Anyway, she was outed by her husband and promptly announced that she didn't feel like writing about it anymore and deleted her blog. I wonder if that is happening here.

Your blog is interesting and I wonder if you just like having sex AND getting money for it. You seem to carefully pick and choose the customers, like you are picking a date. Maybe all women do that to some extent anyway. It sounds like this type of dating game is getting dull now for you. No more excitement from the "big secret".

It was an interesting read. Maybe you'll come up with another good game soon.

Yes, I'm quite positive that I'm not "losing interest in being a whore" (as you put it) because someone I know found out. That happened almost two months ago and didn't dampen my enthusiasm in the slightest. In fact, it was fun to have someone whose opinion I value just as much as my own to talk about it with. I'm pretty sure my boredom is due to my curiosity about what it's like to be a sex worker being sated. I've had plenty of experiences, most of them good, and most very similar to each other in lots of ways. I'm sure the similarity has a lot to do with the fact that I tend to find myself choosing to spend time with the same sort of men over and over. I'm sure if I just decided to be indiscriminate in my appointment setting, I'd wind up having a wider variety of types of experiences, but I'm just not willing to do that. I rather like being alive and healthy and don't get any kind of rush out of the idea of meeting with possible weirdoes just because it might be more interesting to do so than to spend time with the "normal" ones I've been seeing.

Perhaps I just have a short attention span for hobbies. I've always been the kind of person that gets intensely interested in something, does it with great gusto for a while and then, when it starts feeling old hat and like there's not much more to learn from it, my enthusiasm wanes.

I don't have any intention of "promptly deleting" my blog. I'm not even sure if I've turned my last trick, so to speak. (I like to keep my options open.) I plan on sticking around as long as folks are still interested in my musings.

Wednesday 7 July

I guess I must have done a really inadequate job of explaining that my gig as an escort is over since lots of people keep asking me about the addition of the word "former" in my banner.

Nothing bad happened. There was no "event" that precipitated the decision. I just stopped feeling enthusiastic about doing it. I got tired of the small talk (answering the same questions over and over, basically), not to mention the work involved in creating ads, screening clients, and arranging my schedule to suit others. It's a lot of effort, and while it was fun for a time, it became less amusing over time and started feeling a lot more like work than play.

So that's it. Nothing more complicated than that. I'm sorry there's not a more thrilling explanation to the big mystery.

Tuesday 20 July

Regret is an interesting topic for me. I might be a bit unusual in the respect that I rarely ever look upon things I've done with regret, but I do regret things I have not done. Even if a choice I've made has turned out to be a bad decision, I just look upon that as a lesson I've learned, rather than something to beat myself up for forever. One grows from their mistakes and, if you never allow yourself to make any, how can you learn anything?

I feel a little bit sad for people who decide on a particular path, and then refuse to deviate because they have committed themselves to it even when they've found that perhaps the path isn't as interesting or fulfilling as they originally thought it would be. I feel very strongly that one should constantly evaluate their path. Take risks. Allow one's self to be imperfect. Experience everything you can, don't worry so much about making mistakes, and grow and grow and grow.

Sunday 25 July

Sometimes I wonder if it's because I spent the first twenty-two years of my life being so very good and doing what was expected of me, that I've enjoyed so much being spectacularly bad and relished doing the absolute unexpected for the last twelve or so. (And, by bad, I do not mean ever purposely causing anyone harm. I haven't stopped trying to be a kind person.)

Perhaps I just didn't have the courage when I was younger to do anything but the expected. I recall spending an awful lot of time and energy worrying and being afraid of what people would think if I didn't do what I was supposed to do. Somewhere along the line I realized that people can't think anything if they don't know anything. If you plan well and don't get caught, you can fly under the radar.

"Why did you hook?" people ask. I think part of the answer lies in the above. Getting away with the unexpected while maintaining my good girl image was what hooked me.

GEEKSLUT

Stephen Cox

http://geekslut.org

Saturday 19 April 2003

Cops, damn. I've had my share, Sergeant Biff.

Biff was an MP (Military Police). After Pacunus, he was my second serious relationship. He was a hard motherfucker, tough and serious. To this day I think it was because of that name, Biff. He hated it. I'd harass him about it just to set him off. And set him off I did. I was his little officer bitch and he was my big daddy sergeant.

Biff had a broken-down trailer outside of post. With a Grand Am sitting on concrete blocks in front and an empty freezer in the back, it was a classic poor-white-trash trailer.

Three things were important to Biff: beer, getting his dick sucked, and guns. He had a huge gun collection. Shit, some were classics that were handed down to him from his father and his father's father. He tried to intimidate me with them. I played along cause I dug sucking his dick. His dick was long, fleshy, fat and stretched toward the floor when hard. A cocksucker's dream.

He'd sit back in his lazy-boy like the King of fucking Siam; his hairy legs spread, beer in one hand, a gun in the other, watching me work on his cock. Occasionally he'd put down the gun and light up a cigarette, that's when the games would begin.

Games like kicking me around the trailer, standing on my hard cock, making me sit beside the toilet while he pissed (yeah he'd miss the bowl), or sucking his ass while he cocked a gun outside my view.

Biff never really hurt me. He got into my head and made me his for a while. It ended cause of beer. Biff was a mean drunk. One night he got crackbrained and while I was jamming to the Bad Brains (wearing headphones and watching TV) he put his cigarette out on me. He thought it was funny. It hurt like fuck and pissed me the fuck off so I kicked the shit out of him. That ended it. We still saw each other around post and Atlanta but I never got to suck his dick again.

Sunday 27 April 2003

Oh, here's what I wrote Friday while waiting in the hospital for the heart cath – I was high, so high.

The motherfuckers are making me wait till 3 p.m. No food, water or shit until after the procedure. But I'm starving? Their answer, DRUGS . . . yeah, baby. I'm not one to pass up a cheap high.

I'm so fucking horny. Been playing with myself, and playing a little game with the nurses. Of course they notice but no one has said anything, yet. Hey, it's their fault for giving me this high.

While stroking my hard-on Johnny comes into focus, I get harder. Johnny was this hot redheaded surfer boy I used to fuck with back when I was sick as a dog. Johnny was also in town to die in his mother's arms but, like me, he had good timing. Six one, covered with KS, skinny as a rail – we were both kind-of at the same place, and horny as shit. He had a nice dick too, a perfect pipe, not too big, not too small. And those damn IV antibiotics would get us so fucking hard. We dug playing toilet games, screwing in the shower with his hose, pissing on each other, fucking and sucking on the toilet, shit like that.

The usual MO with us was to get high on our pain, mood, and sleeping pills. We'd mix them up, share them and usually smoke some weed to ease the wired feeling. Then hook our IVs to our ports, our cocks would soon rise like flag poles and we'd fuck all night. It was sleazy and fun, kind of hot in a morbid way. It was good therapy; sex is always good unless, of course, you use it as a weapon. We were fighting death and sex and the drugs were our way of blowing off steam and our charged come.

Johnny also introduced me to Ma Jaya Sati Bhagavati, a crazy cool guru lady from Brooklyn who saw Jesus in her basement and had an epiphany. She's the spiritual leader of the Kashi Ashram in Central Florida. I spent many weekends on the Ashram with Johnny. It doubled as a hospice, so we were well cared for. We didn't fuck on the grounds out of respect for Ma, but we sure did in Johnny's truck right outside the gate. Ma's a great lady and she taught me a lot.

This has a sad ending though. After recovering we kind of parted. I moved to Ft Lauderdale and Johnny got hooked into a horrible meth addiction. He abandoned the Ashram, Ma, his friends and even me. But I heard from him a year or so later.

He called me out of the blue and asked me to pick him up at Imperial Point Hospital emergency room. I did. He was thin and cracked out of his mind. He had passed out on the road and the FHP (Florida Highway Police) picked him up and hauled his ass in. He was arguing with two local police officers when I arrived. Not a smart thing to do but, like I said, he was orbiting Saturn. They were about to arrest him. I manage to convince the cops to release Johnny into my custody. Much to my surprise they did, but not Johnny's truck. I still don't know if Johnny got his truck back. Anyway, the cops *ordered* me to take Johnny home. I did.

There are two types of drug dealers in the world: those that deal for profit, and those that deal to support a habit. Johnny was supporting a habit. And he was in deep shit cause he consumed his own product and owed the wrong people. So I dropped him off and we fucked. I fucked him hard. I was pissed and took it out on his ass.

Tuesday 29 April 2003

So it looks like the heart crisis is over, for now. Good. Let's get back to sex. Actually, let's get back to cops. Robby, a cop in NYC I used to fuck with.

It was late. I was riding the subway on my way home from a big party held at Columbia University. A gay student club used to throw them monthly on Fridays. They were fun parties and I always scored twink butt and dick (which I LOVE, LOVE, LOVE).

I wasn't really cruising the subway car . . . well, OK, I AM

ALWAYS CRUISING but, you know what I mean, I wasn't REALLY looking to score. I had already gotten a few numbers and screwed my brains out with some twink. I was tired.

The subway car was almost empty. But the people that were in it I studied. You do that late at night. Not much else to do except sleep, which was risky in those days. In walks in a young cop, tight uniform, about 5'10", twirling his nightstick in his hand and chewing gum. OK, I couldn't help myself, I studied him. Yeah, I know, cops get nervous when you watch them.

He sat down across from me. Now I got nervous. "OK," I thought, "I'm fucked". I began counting the bottles I had in my pocket – one K. "Good," I thought. "Not that much." He just stared at me.

Finally he asked, "I know you, Sir?"

"No, Officer," I replied. Or something like that. I can't remember the exact words. Let's just say I studied him enough to beat off later fantasizing that he slammed me on the floor and fucked me silly with his nightstick.

Skip a month or so, I'm sitting at a monthly GLCC meeting. I went with Ed. I was his date, sort of. Ed liked taking me cause I was muscular, bubbly, pretty and hung on his arm. The room went silent and the meeting got started. I scanned the room looking for potential dick (it's a reflex) and guess who I spot spotting me, the cop from the subway.

He nodded and my mouth went dry. He discreetly got up and walked to the toilet. I jumped up loudly and the room watched me as I ran to the toilet. LOL, God.

I walked in and scanned the toilet quickly (I can scan any toilet in two seconds flat). Blue and white tiled floor, one window, a row of sinks and mirrors and four stalls. There was one person in one stall. Of course it was him. I slid in front of the sinks and made like I was doing my hair in the mirror. I was such a girl!

The stall door opened and he grabbed me from behind, pushing his body against me, slamming me into the sinks, breathing heavily into my ear. I could smell his breath, and feel his hands on my ass and squeezing my dick and balls. He was drunk, very drunk. I took advantage of it. I'm not stupid.

He then freaked out or something. He got nervous that someone might walk in and see him with me. I reminded him that he WAS at a GLCC meeting. Didn't matter, he threw me (yes, he threw me) across the room. I landed against the door, slamming it shut. He pressed against me and madly started kissing me. He was stronger than I thought. I took the opportunity to feel him up, an incredible compact muscular body. He was really a beauty. I realized he was whacked but I didn't care . . . stupid, well sort of stupid.

I invited him back to my place. He took my number instead. Well, I was surprised . . . but cool. I went back to the meeting. I'm not sure where he went. I then realized that I had not gotten his name. Shit. (I got it later.)

The meeting ended. No sight of him. Ed and I said our goodbyes and I went home and logged onto MaleStop, a local gay BBS (Bulletin Board System. BBSs were what us geeks used before AOL and Instant Messenger), searching for geek dick. I found it and it was named Jonah.

Jonah. He was infamous in NYC. He might still be around. Jonah had the biggest dick. Thirteen and half inches (and I'm not kidding), long and thick as my wrist, it was incredible. But, Jonah had one problem . . . he was a nut job. I don't know what it is but, the bigger the dick, the crazier the man. Maybe it's because we, as a society, put so much importance on dick size. I mean, there have been plenty of times I've overlooked obvious, twisted problems with a guy just because he had a ten-inch dick. Only to get slammed, hurt or jailed later on. Anyway, back to Jonah.

We hooked up at my apartment. Jonah was a geek, like me. Unlike me, though, his black hair was never combed and he had big thick glasses. He arrived wearing tight light blue Spandex shorts and a white T-shirt. "Oh, dear," I thought. I could only imagine what the doorman thought.

We talked a while about D&D and other shit. I could hardly think. All I could think about was the outline of that baseball bat in his shorts. He knew it. In fact, he encouraged it. Jonah lived for his dick. His whole life was wrapped around his dick. Every conversation somehow got back to his dick. Don't get me wrong, Jonah was smart. But he was the type of guy that complained that no one liked him for him. It was all about his dick he complained, and it probably was. Thing was, Jonah wanted it that way.

"They all want my dick, that's all!" he said.

"Well, no shit, your point?" I thought. I said, "What do you expect? Look how you are dressed."

He then proceeded to describe what he did to boys with his dick. I was already hot; now I was sliding off the sofa. He went on with his description and my head spun. Finally he flipped it out.

"Shit. When was the last time you washed it?" I asked/choked.

He cracked a wide smile. Jonah had big fat lips too. Something else we had in common.

"It doesn't really matter, does it?" he stated. He was cocky, too. Also like me but, for different reasons.

He flopped it around, signaling me to chow down. I prayed to the Gods for protection and dived on it.

Thursday 1 May 2003

I liked Jonah. And not just for his dick. He had trouble getting hard so I knew he'd never fuck me. He'd try and try but usually I'd end up frustrated. He'd tease my ass and get me hot by telling me how good his cock would feel balls deep inside me. I'd squirm and have visions of being impaled on his dick, rotating like his little school-girl bitch. I'd suck the head of his cock clean; slide my fat tongue under his foreskin, softly sucking the skin, making sure I'd get it all. And his nasty ass, I'd take care of that too. That's what he wanted, someone to worship him and his dick. I did, for a while, a short while.

But I couldn't include Jonah in my life. I could've brought him along to the parties with me. I knew the only thing that trumped a hot body on the circuit was dick. And he had dick for days, BUT he embarrassed me. He didn't act *right*. He didn't dress *right*. He didn't do anything *right*. So Jonah and his dick were hidden from the friends that I thought mattered so much. I was over his dick – Ok, maybe not, but I WAS over him. I didn't want a relationship with Jonah. So I avoided it by concentrating on his dick, which suited him fine. I think he thought THAT was a relationship.

Jonah and his dick would soon take a backdoor to other diversions. I was fucking with so many men at this time that juggling them became a problem. I had to keep a calendar just to keep the guys straight, you know, who was who and shit like that. There was

Trevor, a beautiful black man married with kids. We'd meet at my
place twice a week for a lunchtime fuck. I'd spit on his ass and slam
him down, fuck him hard while yelling how much of a faggot he
was. Condoms . . . please . . . what condoms? He didn't ask, I
didn't ask. There was Claude, an actor with a really fat dick and
BIG low-hanging bouncy balls. He'd bump Tina (meth), shove K
up my ass and fuck me for hours in front of a mirror. I'd watch us,
him on top of me, behind me, his balls swinging slapping my ass.
He'd watch himself smile and ask, "Am I fucking you good, boy?"
Claude would ask me that several times a night. Like he needed to
HEAR me tell him he was the best. He'd wait for my answer,
"Yeah, sure . . . fuck, man. Fuck me, fuck me," I'd usually reply.

I was SO bored. That would change though; I was about to take a
dark and violent turn, again.

One night, 4am:

Ring. Ring. Ring. Ring.

"Fuck, yeah?" I asked into the phone. I was hung over and my
ass was hurting. Claude had left a few hours ago.

"Yo, man, it's Robby"

"Who? Man, what the fuck? You know what time it is? Who is
this?" I asked quickly.

"Fuck the time, man, it's Robby. I'm calling you, dude."

I was wide awake now and pissed. "Who the fuck is fucking
Robby?"

"Robby, man! We were kissing and shit – the GLCC meeting!!!"
he yelled.

It clicked. A good month had gone by but it clicked. It would
have clicked faster if he didn't sound like he was from Long Island.
"Oh, yeah, man. What the fuck you calling me so early? Shit, I just
got to sleep."

"I wanna see you, dude."

With that I got up, got his number (now I knew his name) and we
made a date for that evening. There was something about that cop
that got to me. Giving me THAT feeling I'm addicted to. The
feeling you feel in your balls or on the edge of your nipples – like
you're about to get it good, real neat and fine. My instincts were
telling me to walk no, RUN fast . . . But THAT feeling, THAT
addiction won out.

I've attracted a lot of violent men (and women – but more on that later). I'm not sure why. Maybe it's because fighting turns my crank. I loved fighting when I was a kid, in the Army and in New York. Got the scars to prove it, too. Something like a Fight Club would've made my world real rosy and kept me with a walking hard-on. The idea of making out with fat busted lips, blood flowing, is SO fucking hot. I've outgrown this kink, I think; but, back then I was in the middle of it.

I've always been a secretive person, a typical double Scorpio. Only telling what needed to be told. Half truths and half lies. None of my lovers ever knew the whole story. I make this statement because going forward some of my revelations may be difficult to swallow. I certainly wasn't violent with most of my lovers, just a few. I'll try to describe the reasons for the violence, but, for those few who know me and are reading this now – know that time and AIDS have changed things.

Monday 18 August 2003

Working at the gym. Just the usual smoking through the weights and joking with the fellas. No "bitches" this time, just us men popping and grinding, checking each other out and talking about the "bitches" . . . and cars. I spot this guy spot me. He kind of booms over, smiling. I'm thinking, "Wow, new meat."

Nahh. I hear, "Hey man, been a while."

Damn. Damn. Damn.

"Yeah? Who are you?"

He does look familiar. He's about my height, not as big but very cut-up, both arms covered with tattoos, head shaved close. Real close. A skinhead. A hot fucker that I would make a point not to forget to soon . . .

Anyway, turned out I did know him. Years ago. Used to fuck around with him. Back then he was a just another poz skinny big-dicked boy that I threw around, bouncing off the walls.

Used to make him sit naked on the floor in front of me while I sat and watched TV. Pressing his dick into the floor with my right 13-inch Army-issue steel-tipped jump boot. Man, he'd howl when I'd stand, crushing his dick into the floor and announce, "I need a brew." Something I did EVERY fucking commercial. I'd watch him watch the TV, waiting for the commercials. Waiting for the pay off. He got it. He loved it. He'd be like, "No, no, no, no. I'll get it. I'll get it." He'd cry, tears swelling in his eyes.

I'd grind and twist my boot harder on his dick till his tears got bigger and he'd grab my leg, whining . . . and then I'd let mister nice guy pop out. "Sure, man, go get it, dog-boy."

He'd fetch the beer and we'd start the process all over again. Then we'd fuck HARD and we'd sleep HARD with him wrapped in my arms, his head resting on my bicep, nose stuck in my armpit (using my bicep as a pillow). I'd listen to him breathe and sleep and then drift off myself. Funny I remember that. The sleeping part, I mean.

I used to do a lot of rough shit with this kid. Man, he was fun. And he took it all, too. I wanted to keep him as mine. Protect him. Teach him. Keep him healthy. I'd failed in something like this before, but this time I was smarter.

But one day he just disappeared. Happens a lot with young gay men. I figured he met up with some sugar-daddy (or sponsor, as it's called today by some muscle-boys) who had more to offer (you know . . . a bigger house, car, wallet) and packed up.

Almost right. After the gym he filled me in.

He was banging another guy on the side of me. *Says* he was whoring for bullshit cash. Now, that wouldn't have bothered me and he knew that. But they were partying big time and he knew THAT would've bothered me. Says that it was getting hard for him to keep that info from me. I reminded him that I remember asking him about crystal (which he denied doing). Anyway, the crystal became more important than anything (ain't that a sad truth) and this "other" guy was the supply. So he bailed . . . with the other guy.

I interrupted, "So you were doing him for more than dollars?"

He smiles and nods. "Yeah, man." (Damn, he's grown into such a hot fucking man. For an instant I wonder how he'd feel wrapped inside my arms again. Safe.)

Anyway, to make a long story short (yeah I know – too late), after a while they had to start dealing to support their habits. Crystal led to coke; coke led to crack; crack lead to jail and the rest is history.

Somewhere in this tale I asked, "You didn't come back to me?"

"Would you have taken me?"

I didn't answer. I don't know if I would've. Anyway, it was too late by the time the shit came down on him. I was already heavily involved with Greg (one of my life-partners).

So he got busted and ended up in jail for several years.

Now he's bigger, meaner, covered with tattoos and selling his dick in the back of HotSpots (a local gay bar rag).

On the way to my car, "So how'd you pick my gym?" I asked. "All the hot men go here, man."

Figures.

That horny nineteen-year-old I blogged about is still sending me pics of his butt. Man, I must be good, cause he's begging to pop on over and "bust some nuts". Ah the taste of sweet young come and butt.

Monday 29 September 2003

So, after weeks of being this huge bottom, I FINALLY get back to my usual Friday night of "finding me some boy butt".

Wearing tight 501 jeans, black suspenders, fifteen- year-old jump boots, no shirt; I steal a cigar and hit the Ramrod (a local "leather" bar). I'm in a serious mood. I know exactly what I'm looking for: a bucktooth, skinny (compared to me) white boy who wants a hairy muscle daddy tearing apart his butt. Plenty of them jumping around, especially in Florida. But, not tonight. The Ramrod's dead. I spot my usual bartender; he's a fighting buddy from way back.

"You Dogboy, sup?"

He tosses me a beer. "You're in *that* mood." He laughs.

The fucker can tell, too. The jump boots give it away. I ONLY bring these bitches out when there's serious business on the horizon.

I feel like chewing the bottle. I'm that worked up. "Yeah, I need it bad."

"And that's new?" the fucker asked.

We chat some more, throw a few punches, and speak the usual game. It really is dead. He *rarely* has time to shoot the shit on a Friday night. I ask,

"Eagle got a big dick contest going on or something?" I ain't heard of it and I don't miss something like that.

"Nahh, everyone's dead."

Another bartender jumps in, "It's Folsom and the Jewish New Year."

"Oh, shit, I forgot," I say. It's Folsom. Everybody figures nobody's out so everyone stays in.

I say my goodbyes and head for home. I hit the Net.

12.30 a.m., Manhunt

Usually the bottom-to-top ratio is like 500-to-1 but Friday night the site is loaded with tops. Shocking. It's a crying goddamn shame when Manhunt has more tops online than bottoms. I mean, "God, throw me a fucking bone here!"

Anyway, I'm about to pack-it when BAMM, I get a message from this cute boy whose profile has a picture of him riding a skateboard. PERFECT! I reply, he replies and we both pass our private pictures (the ones that show face, dick and ass). He's 22, 6 foot 1, 165 pounds, strawberry blond and his butt pictures are just mouth watering. More messages, back and forth and FINALLY I message my number.

He calls. We do the HIV thang, the top/bottom thang, blah, blah and before I know it I'm standing at his door (got a tank top on now).

I knock. He opens the door. He's naked and looks strung out but man his pictures were right on. He smiles. I walk in and close the door.

"Steve," I bark while holding my hand out. He shakes it and looks down.

"Can I unlace your boots?"

"Sure, get to it."

He practically falls to the floor and starts with the laces and I notice the shape of his apartment. Boxes and dirt and stale old food and just shit everywhere.

I slip my boots off. He's looking up at me. His eyes, they're a beautiful blue.

I pick him up and kiss him hard. He's surprised but we get into a serious flow of swapping spit back and forth. He's holding onto my whole body while my eyes are closed, tasting him. God. He rubs my nipples. I start to get hard.

"Show me the bedroom." He turns, walks and like a good dog I follow (with an eye on his butt) him in and out and around all the crap that's laid out on the floor. It's like treading though a fucking maze.

He says, "I just moved in."

I go, "Yeah, right."

Find his notebook (computer) and his cell phone, both are sitting on a small desk. His bed's a cheap thin mattress lying in the middle of the room. I throw him down hard and slide my jeans off. I'm standing there, half-hard dick in hand, about to pounce when he slowly gets up on all fours and *presents* his perfect white butt to me. I take what I want. I lose myself. Finally we got into a sort-of 69; him on top pressing his butt on my face while bent sucking my dick. We do this for a while.

I push him off and announce, "It's hammering time."

I lift his legs on to my shoulders, he grabs onto my arms and I slam home. Not a peep out of him, just a lazy smile on his face and some soft moans. I'm hammering away when I notice his arm is floppily slapping the bed at an odd angle to his body. Damn, he's joansing.

I pull out, put him down and sit cross-legged in front of him. "You high?" I ask.

"Huh?"

I quickly look for track marks. His arm is still slapping the bed, softly this time. I'm kicking myself cause I can't believe I missed this.

"What are you on?" I ask.

He suddenly lights up. "What happened?"

"What are you on?" I ask again.

He lists various chemicals he's taken into his body. Jesus, what the fuck is a matter with these boys? Then he blurts out how hungry he is.

"When was the last time you ate?"

"I don't have any money," he says.

I roll my eyes. Part of me just wants to leave. But I see his eyes, again.

"My treat." I wipe my dick off and get dressed. He just flops there, on the bed.

"Cm'on, LET'S GO, NOW!" I yell.

We hit the Floridian, a decent 24-hour diner.

We sit. He just stares. The waitress comes over.

"Drink?" she asks.

I order a Diet Coke; he just looks at the table.

"He'll have the same. Oh, I'll order for both of us. OK?" I said.

"Sure, be right back." She dances off to fetch the drinks.

"Oh, shit" the boy blurts out. A line of clear liquid snot flows/ slides out of his nose. Shit.

"Here." I hand him my napkin while signaling the waitress for more. She sees and has it covered.

I order. We eat. We don't speak much.

After, "So how do you pay the fucking rent?" I ask.

"It's not mine."

Oh, that figures. He's using his friend's place to trick and crash. We talk a little more. The usual shit. I mean what the fuck can he say? And me? What the fuck am I supposed to say? I could lecture him but he's 22, he won't hear me. Anyway, he's just another kid who cruises a main strip (US1 – off Sunrise Blvd) for old men to suck off and roll. And sometimes he works it online (I doubt that's his notebook) to find something he actually likes (me).

So he's getting high like all the time to escape a reality that he's created and continues to recreate every night. What a hole, and South Florida is filled with them. They have no address, no credit, nothing that our society considers to be important except ass and cock. Shit, man, his fucking pre-paid cell phone is more important to him than food, cause he makes sure that is paid up.

But man, what the fuck am I supposed to do?

I take him back to the apartment. He offers to get me off, offers more of his butt.

"That's allright man." I actually came close to taking him up. I had the upper hand now. He owed me. I didn't play that card, though. I didn't want to. So I gave him money.

"Here, buy some food."

He thanks me and gets out. I watch him go inside and then drive off. I doubt he'll use the cash for food. I felt like running after him. Taking him home. But that would expose *me*. But I'm thinking about him, a lot.

Wednesday 22 October 2003

So last night I had a wet dream. Woke up at four in the morning with a raging hard-on, dripping pre-come and piss. Man. I remember flashes, sort of. There was a girl sitting in my lap, her legs wrapped locked around me and she was sucking on my neck while rubbing her whole crotch against my dick and then BAMM. I woke up. DAMN.

I don't need a house to fall on me. I need some girl on guy action. Mindy comes to mind. She's a hot fine-ass Latina slut I fuck with now and then, who enjoys getting it as much as I dig giving it. She tastes good, she's always soaked and she's loud. I love loud chicks. God, does she moan. Anyway, last time I saw her she was telling me about her husband who's been serving time for robbery.

I ask, "You gonna tell him about us?" I step out of the shower and she hands me a towel.

"He loves hearing all my dirt."

"Shit. He's gonna gun for me when he gets out?" I ask. I'd like to know now.

She reassures me he's cool with it all. I believe her too. Plus her man is FUCKING HOT. I'd love to do a three-way with them. I don't know if he's straight, bi or what. I don't ask. I'll find out soon enough. I mean, I know he's getting out on parole at some point in the near future, cause Mindy is still hanging around. I mean, sure she's rolling her oats now, but I could tell she loves him. She's a nympho (and so am I) and I doubt her man doesn't know that. So he can't be holding any stupid jealousy inside. Mindy's a chick who needs to get nailed every day, at least. Judging from what she says, her man knows that and took care of *business* when he was free. DAMN, I can't wait to meet the man who was able to keep up with this chick. [BIG SMILE]

Back to men.

Since I've been lying low, not much happened save for the usual beating off (so much my dick is sore) and rescheduling of my usual crew. I'm, like, now all booked up. My whole weekend is jammed with men/boys and I still gotta give some up to Da Piece and crew. Ah, life is so hard.

Earlier, something fun happened. I was beating off, in my favorite chair, left leg thrown over its left arm to some decent bi porn when the phone rings.

"Yeah?" I ask.

"Yo Steve, Redge."

"Yo, man, I'm kind of *busy*."

"Yeah, doing what?" he fucking asks. Just like him.

"Beating off, man," I yell.

"You thinking of me?"

I wasn't. But I couldn't let him down, plus NOW I was. "Yeah, man. Your fat cock dripping juice down my throat."

From there we had some of the hottest phone sex I ever had. I shot a HUGE load way in the air, landed on my stomach, chest and face. Damn.

"Save some for me."

"Save what? My come?" I ask, panting.

"Yeah, freeze it."

I've played this game before, so I have no problems freezing my come. Used to keep a decent amount stored in a "special" freezer tray. When I had someone special over, I wedge some out, slam it up his butt or mine, let it melt and go to fucking town. Makes EXCELLENT lube. And *trust*, any bottom come pig will go nuts if you use come as lube. This reminds me about Larry, a Staff Sergeant I knew in the Army.

This fucker wasn't pretty but, man, could he come. I'm not kidding; he'd fill up a shot glass every fucking time. And he could do it like two-three times a day. Amazing. We used to work out together and then go to his place, watch porn and just jack off. We'd usually stand up and see who shot the most and how far. I'd ALWAYS shoot further (I had great ballistics) but he'd shoot so much fucking come it'd just river out of his dick, forming a pool on the floor. I used to draw faces in it. I always wanted him to fuck me and come up my ass. Never did, though.

Last I heard, he was doing some amateur porn shit. You know, the "Still in the Army and I'm straight" bullshit. Hate to burst your bubble, but these guys are not active duty. Not that it matters, cause most are hot as shit and I'd do 'em (and have) in a heartbeat. Larry, though, man, if I ever meet up with him again, he's fucking me till he comes BIG TIME. Period.

Monday 17 November 2003

I was gonna blog about this chick I scored the other day. Nothing unusual. Just some slut Mindy turned me on to. I whaled out on her for an hour or so. Then I paid her and watched her bounce out the door. I was happy, she was happy and I'll probably call her again in a few weeks or so.

Instead . . .

Man, SO many New Yorkers are relocating here [Ft. Lauderdale]. It's beginning to look like fucking Brooklyn outside. People I haven't seen in years are contacting me out of the blue. Opening up memories in my head.

Max (52, 6'3", about 210 lbs and a dick of death that he's been threatening to fuck me with for years). He calls me up out of the blue. Haven't heard from him in months. And last time I saw him was 1997 New Year's day. He scoped me out, lying on the beach with some of my old Fire Island housemates. It was our last blast as a gang together so everyone who could . . . made the trip. I was still sick but the chemotherapy and radiation that the VA was blasting me with had destroyed most of the KS in/on my body. And, save for a port sticking out of my upper chest, I looked fine. Thin, but fine. He was surprised to see me. For some odd reason we kept in loose contact over the years. And he reads this blog (I now know).

"Hey, I'm here," he proclaims.

"Here?" I ask.

"Didn't I tell you?"

"Tell me what?" I ask.

"I'm in WPB now." [WPB = West Palm Beach].

"Wait . . . you moved down?" I ask and add. "Shit, you dog."

We work out the details for a meet the next day.

I met Max through his boy, Louie. Louie was a beautiful little redheaded punk boy I met at the 23rd Street YMCA gym. I have a MAJOR thing for redheads so of course we started fucking around. Usually at his place, cause he and Max were very open about fucking around. I was not so open with Tom, my BF (more on him later) at the time.

The sex was hot and with the added attraction of Max catching us in the "act" now and then (he'd sit and watch – the pig) made it even hotter. I used to beg Louie to get Max to join in (I wanted his dick up my ass) but he never touched me. He'd just sit, jerk his big fat dick and watch us piss, fuck and suck our brains out. Sometimes he'd direct the action (which was HOT). You know, tell Louie to fuck me hard or throw a dildo into the mix (I'd usually push it up Louie's butt while he was fucking me). Shit like that, but that was rare. (If this type of action was going down today I'd look for a webcam.)

Anyway Louie and I fucked like bunnies till he got really sick. Then we did [an AIDS] support group together. I wasn't as sick as he was. I mean, when Louie was getting very sick I was just starting my trip down that road.

The last time I saw Louie alive was when our support group held its weekly meeting in his apartment. The group did this sometimes when a brother-in-arms was too sick to travel (they did it for me too). Louie was thin, yellow, weak and on TPN (feeding tube). But he could smile and talk slowly. He was also blind. CMV had destroyed his eyes. Blindness. You know, that's what scared me the most. I came VERY close to blindness. I was lucky, though.

The last I saw Louie *period* was at his funeral. Not his body, but his picture. It was March 1995. I was well on my way to being sick. But not close enough to quit crystal or the circuit (I collapsed in June of 95). I had KS lesions on my legs, chest, and face. I covered the lesions on my face with make-up (didn't work too well). I was still holding down a job. But life was getting harder and harder.

The funeral was at 6 p.m. I arrived 30 minutes late (on purpose) and slipped into the back row unnoticed. I didn't want to be *seen*. I was embarrassed by the lesions and swelling they caused. You know, illness has a way of kicking you right where it hurts the most. My vanity was the first thing AIDS hit.

Soon that part of the funeral when friends and family of the dead wander up to the podium and say their piece came. While I watched Louie's family, Max, and a couple of others testify, I stay glued to my seat.

When the service was over, I tried to slip out unnoticed. But I caught Max watching me out of the corner of my eye. He waved; I nodded, grabbed a cab and fought back tears all the way home.

Louie was 26.

Back to the current . . .

Drove up to WPB to meet Max. He lives in one of those housing developments built around a golf course (a big change after living on the Upper West Side). After the greet-n-meet he shows me around his place. Being the horn-dog that I am I'm thinking of finding the bedroom and sitting on his cock. We pass by the bedroom and head out back.

"You wanna jump in the tub?"

You kidding? I play it cool, though. "Yeah, sure."

I strip, he strips and I watch his dick swing as he climbs in. The water is already hot. I go, "You had something planned?"

"Figured YOU'D want to check out the hot tub," he jokes. He was right.

We talk about shit. How NYC has changed, politics, this blog, boys – you know, just shit that fags chitchat about. Then he goes, "You're going grey."

I go, "Yeah . . . thanks for pointing that out."

He goes, "Your body is incredible. What are you doing?"

We get into a conversation about the gym, yoga and his running. Then the big game starts . . . the game I hosed out my butt for.

"So, horny?" I ask.

He laughs. "Direct approach, hey?"

"I'm not getting any younger, man," I joke.

He floats his body up on top of the running water and flops his dick around, splashing my face with water. I'm like, "Show off."

Then he sinks back down and just looks at me for a long moment. His eyes swell up, "When I look at you I see Louie."

Now my eyes swell up. I slide across the tub next to him, find his hand and hold it. We just sit, looking at the puffy clouds for a while.

Wednesday 25 February 2004

First the sex party.

BORING. Are all twinks in Ft Lauderdale cracked out? Me and this tall, good-looking (smooth tight swimmer's body) 36-year-old had the only hard cocks in the joint. So we, of course, fucked around with each other for while.

In the middle of this, this 24-year-old "porn star" (the usual body, nice big dick, sweet juicy butt) I know comes over and drops to his knees. He goes at me and this other guy for a bit. He's OK, not good, just OK. I pull him up and drop to my knees and swallow his cock and stick three fingers up his ass. He's like, "I hardly get fucked." Sure. Whatever.

A few minutes later Porn Star is in the sling, legs strapped in the air and the 36-year-old is opening up his hole with fingers and a large black butt plug. Porn Star is twisting and pulling on his dick really hard, trying to get it hard. He can't. He's tweaked.

Even though I was told this party was bareback, I ask, "You poz?"

Porn Star goes, "No, but I fuck raw. Just no come up my ass." I *almost* laugh.

Soon most of the boys are wrapped around us three, glazing, threshing their cocks about, trying to get excited. They're bored. Sex, feeling – it's all meaningless to them. It's easy to get and crystal removes the connections . . . the strings that help us merge. Anonymous sex *has* feeling and passion. It's fun and healthy for most queer men. But crystal has made it a trashing trance of cock and butt . . . All looking for love, seeking to blow that big orgasm that will satisfy their bleakness.

Sober, you'd stand a better chance of filling THAT void. But how do I tell these boys this? They don't hear me.

One thing though, NO MORE cracked out crystal bottoms for me. From now on, I'm passing on that sadness.

Now the chick.

Mindy turns me on to some poz broad. She wasn't a 300-pound broad . . . just a big hipped girl with ass for days and tits to match. My favorite type.

So we're rocking, my face is buried in her cleavage and I'm kissing her everywhere. And she's squirming up a storm, loving all the attention. I had already juiced her up by chewing on her clit and smacking her butt till it glowed pink. So, man, we were ready to roll when I pushed her down and lifted her legs up. I was about to pounce when she stops me flat.

"My *behind* is off limits."

"OK." I really don't mind. I'm not one of those guys who feels the need to fuck *every* girl in the ass.

Fast forward a few, I'm on top humping away. She's squeaking. (Yeah, she's a squeaker.) Over and over and over – TRUST me it's funny and it's all I can do to keep from giggling. So in between squeaks I ask her to rub my nipples [it makes me come faster].

Nothing. I stop humping, inside her, and go, "You OK?"

She says nothing, just looks at me, breathing hard. She wiggles, pushes out from under me and starts to roll over. (**Roll** being the word of the hour.) I'm thinking, "OK, what the fuck does this chick have in mind?"

She stands up and bends over the edge of the bed, ass jammed up in the air. And when I say ass . . . I mean *ass*. This chick has a fucking booty, the type that starts *way* up on the shoulders.

Anyway I angle myself behind her and get back to business. After a few, I forget about her and rub my own nipples. Sure enough, minutes later I pull out and unload all over the carpet.

I lean back to rest and she hits the shower. After, she gets dressed; I pay her (a nice tip too), and walk her to the door. And I kiss her goodbye.

Fisting

Me and this HOT muscle-boy have been circling each other for MONTHS. At the gym, online, clubs. Finally we hook up and in a span of 30 minutes I got half my arm up his butt, slamming him so hard he just moans and comes. After, we both lean back, he goes . . . "Whoa. I gotta come down. Got work."

He wasn't tweaking, just high on poppers, pot and the sexual boom you get when you've been going at it hard.

I go, "We got time to go at it again."

He goes, "I don't know . . ."

Pauses a few minutes. He's thinking about it and I'm egging him on. He smokes another bowl and 15 minutes later I got more of my arm up his ass, plowing him hard. Long strokes, pulling most of me arm out and slamming it all the way back in. He's shaking and rock hard. So am I.

He comes. I come. We shower and bail for a late lunch. Talk, circle each other more and both decide we want more of each other. He's got a hot BF too who wants to jump in. Fine by me.

YOU SILLY GIRL:
LITTLE EXORCISMS

Katie

http://yousillygirl.blogspot.com

17 April 2003

The Resurrection

Jesus appeared on my doorstep a few days ago. Elvis sent him.
Actually, it was Elvis Furniture; a major appliance store in the
notoriously tacky east end of the city. When my dryer stopped
effectively drying my clothes, I called the store to send a repairman.
The man who answered the phone cautioned me that the chosen
man would be a "*petit immigré qui s'appelle Jesus.*" Loose translation: a little immigrant named Jesus. The way he said it, I could
only assume that he intended to stay true to the themes of discrimination and persecution historically associated with the name.

In any case, Jesus rang my doorbell and if he hadn't been
carrying a paper with the word "Elvis" on it, I wouldn't have
let him in. He looked like he'd been brought back from the dead.
His hair was matted in four enormous, unintentional dreadlocks
which stood atop his massive skull. Jesus's face was smudged with
grease and he was coated head-to-toe in a brown, powdery substance. Had he just emerged from the fabled cave?

In any case, I greeted him as I would anyone who had come to
help me out of a soggy situation. He approached my ailing appliance with familiarity and said, "There is nothing wrong with this
dryer."

"What do you mean? It doesn't work!" I insisted, certain it was an evil plot from Elvis headquarters to avoid honouring the King's guarantee. But, he simply laid his hands on the machine, turned the dial and pressed the start button. Behold! I heard a great rumble of another dry cycle beginning. In days like these, perhaps God has to get a word in when he can. Those of us who aren't especially "religious" can benefit from little miracles should we choose to believe in them.

21 May 2003

Educational Gaming

I love playing games. I learned most of my math skills as a little girl while sitting on my Dad's lap during cribbage games. When I was old enough to remember the rules, I got to play against him. It was my chance to prove myself to him, I had to be able to not only count my own points, but to double-check his – just in case he tested me to see if I was playing *seriously*. I am 25 now, and just last year he finally did it. I had been nervously, obsessively checking his points for 15 years before the time had come. He takes his time.

Games are naturally associated with good times, and I have some very special memories. I played a variety of games with an assortment of people. My grandmother taught me to play Rummy. This always seemed a little out of character for her as the pacifist, naturalist sage she was, but then again, over the years a lot about my grandmother surprised me. I enjoyed every tidbit. Scrabble © was always a big event at her house. My grandmother, as the most highly educated person in our family (both formally and informally), it was just understood that no one would *ever* outscore her.

When I did start winning rounds of Scrabble ©, it was very distressing.

My mother's side of the family is Polish and proud of it in a very self-deprecating manner. It's hard for me to understand their penchant for Polish jokes, but I suppose the older generation actually endured discrimination, and they're just trying to make light of it. As a third-generation Canadian, I'm removed from all that – except for what my family subjects me to. Most of my extended family lives a 25-hour drive from where I grew up, so when we all get together, it's a special event. They're all very witty and cheerful, and all-in-all the gatherings are refreshing reunions where alcoholism is thinly veiled under the guise of "Polish tradition". We're talking about people who'll drink Caesars for breakfast because they're healthy. *Nazdrowie!*

This ubiquitous alcoholism makes for entertaining game-playing. Usually we play cards for money. Any game will do really, as long as it's for money. I have fond memories of being very young and winning my first bowl full of dimes. I flaunted my loot for a day or two and then lost it all playing Thirty-one. One rule that applies to all family games is: no mercy for anyone over the age of five. I think this provided me with some valuable life experience.

I hear that in Poland, when a guest arrives the house bottle of vodka is brought out and consecutive shots are poured for everyone present until the bottle is emptied. And *then* the drinking begins. That's just the toast. Again, *nazdrowie!*

Now that I am grown and living in a province sandwiched between my immediate and extended family, there is a shortage of people willing to play cards with me. No one wants to lose their money, and no one wants to put up with the heckling involved in a rowdy game. Every so often I can convince my boyfriend to play Shithead with me. While there is no betting, the level of permissible heckling makes up for it. More often than not, I am left to play my own games. Today I developed a new one.

My home is positioned in one of those city areas where men can sense a quiet corner and immediately develop an urge to mark their territory. This drives my neighbor crazy and several times she's called the police to ward off the extremely common species we've come to call: The Urinators. There are variations: a) the high rollers who will whip down their drawers in the middle of the park because they just don't give a damn; b) the elderly; c) raving drunkards who've already been warned.

Today, I witnessed a Type "C" approaching the corner. He looked over his shoulder to see if anyone was behind him. He looked toward my neighbor's house to see if she was watching. He took the pre-pee stance (legs apart and ready to unzip), and at precisely that moment I banged loudly on my window. I watched him panic and try to determine where the noise came from. Then he ran. He was gone for a full hour before he came back to the park to sleep off the Aqua Velva.

One point for me, zero for The Urinators.
I'm in the lead.

16 May 2003

Let's get physical, physical!

I've recently learned how to go to the gym. All my life I have avoided physical activity; going so far as to be a real pain in the ass about it in elementary school. My poor teachers must've cursed my parents for telling me not to let adults make me do *anything* I didn't want to do. I reinterpreted that safety lesson to work in my favour during Phys. Ed. When forced to play soccer at the tender age of nine, I protested by running *away* from the ball. I am not sure if I was upset because I was picked last for the team, or if the team picked me last because of that. In any case, I found the whole matter to be entirely unfair. Again, I pity the underpaid teaching staff.

I did try intramural soccer once more in high school, but I snapped my wrist during the first game and ended up in a cast; forbidden by my doctor to play again that year. I would have the cast for eight weeks, and it was exactly eight weeks until the prom. I took that as a sign from the PE powers that be. I wouldn't tempt the heathen gods again.

While growing up, I was told over and over (by chubby people and chubby people's mothers) that I was "too skinny". By the time I reached junior high, I had developed a complex. I started eating twice as much, and most of that would be just before bedtime, partly in fear that I'd accidentally burn some calories if I stayed awake and partly to taunt my metabolically challenged friends. I was convinced that if I could just again a little weight, my breasts would grow. I was wrong. I'm still playing for the A-Team.

I did reach a whopping 125 lbs. When I got there, I realized I didn't want to be there at all. Now it's not that I think 125 lbs is a lot, but it looks weird when it is only on your belly and you still have skinny arms and legs. I didn't want to be a chicken lady. I just wanted boobs.

At some point during university, I decided that – since boobs aren't in the stars for me – I might as well get other cooler body stuff, like muscles! Then, I realized that would involve physical activity. I thought maybe I could start slow. Maybe I would join a contemporary dance class. I thought that was a great idea! It wasn't.

After the first class of "freeing my body" and "letting it speak" and "being a tree" and "walking without bones" I was too degraded to go on. If that was what physical activity was all about, I wanted none of it! I decided the muscle idea could get nice and comfy on the back burner.

A few years later, a combination of things motivated me to actually commit to training. Mostly it was instinctive competition; survival of the fittest. Buying the $600 membership was the clamp on the dumbbell. After weeks of doing 50 minutes of cardio and an hour of weights, I still find that my self-perception is totally screwy. I have no idea what I really look like. I don't own a scale and, after visiting someone who does, I'm happy not to. I learned something about myself by stepping on it several times in a 24 hour period: I weigh 115 lbs pre-buffet and 120 lbs post-buffet. I am not joking.

11 May 2003

Rockin' Out (of character)

To say it in my native Canadian Maritimes dialect, last night I "got raight out uff 'er". This translates into: ripped, wasted or trashed. Not just one of those words, I mean all of them together. So, it is something like being inebriated to the power of three. It's been a long time since I've allowed this to happen. Since Halloween to be specific, when I met a fellow Maritimer at a house party in Vancouver and together we practiced this self-defeating ritual. While I am certain it poisons my body, it has a way of clearing my mind. It's as though stress is expelled in one enormous obnoxious outburst. Be warned my friends, such an exorcism can last for hours and it's not "perty".

I bought two tickets to a rock show and I was really looking forward to going. I hadn't been spending any quality time with my live-in buddy, so I thought a Saturday night on the town together might do the trick to get us back in the groove. As the sun started to set, we wandered to a restaurant with a sidewalk terrace, so we could enjoy the last bit of the almost-as-nice-as-summer day. We opted for the "moules et frites" (a popular mussels and chips combo) and an ostrich burger with jalapeno sauce. It was delicious, but sitting in the hot sun, the beer was better. We started out with imported beer but soon moved on to a local beer which really can hold its own anyway. The salty, spicy and exotic food made us thirsty; we needed to be refreshed. You see then, how innocently it all started.

We realized the venue's doors were opening for the show and we still had a fifteen-minute walk ahead of us. We paid our bill and giddily headed out in pursuit of entertainment. Upon arriving, however, I realized I had grossly overestimated the popularity of the bands. There wouldn't be a line-up. The door man joked with us that people usually prefer to be fashionably late. There we were, unfashionably eager. We decided maybe instead of waiting inside the venue with the estimated ten other Unfashionables, that we'd grab a drink at a local watering hole.

It just so happens that it was Happy Hour, or as we say in Quebec "le 5 à 7." It wasn't *my* fault bottles were only $2. We felt it was our duty to stock up before we reached the concert venue where the drinks would surely cost at least twice that! We thought this was being responsible. An hour passed and the show was supposedly starting, so we giggled our way back to the club. I had forgotten it was an all-ages show and soon became nostalgic about gigs I attended while in high school. We'd sit on the floor in front of the stage and wait for the no-talent bands to emerge, scream into the microphones and eventually spit on the crowd.

We casually sipped another drink while we waited for the bands to appear. When they finally did, I began wishing they'd go away and practice more. By the time the third group took to the stage, the crowd was desperate to party. People were dancing, screaming, pushing each other and taking off their clothes – like a concert should be. Then the headliners came.

Now you see how I totally forgot about the drinking? And how I got all excited about the music? Well, that is what happened there, too, except I was still drinking because I was thirsty. I just wasn't noticing that I was. My date, who can't handle his liquor at the best of times, was buying me beer. He bought so much that I often had two bottles in my hand, eager to give them away to any taker. As it turns out, he was pacing his intake according to the amount I could consume. Since I seemed to be drinking it all, he figured he must be in the clear. It became apparent that I would have to chaperone him when he started buying drinks for his sworn enemy. The night rocked on.

After the concert, as I was saying good-bye to a friend, she suggested I take my date straight home. "Why?" I asked, thinking the answer would be: "Because he is wasted." Instead she said: "Because he just did a cartwheel and now he's on the floor."

"Oh . . ."

At some point, walking back to our neighborhood, I started talking about how I would like to take self defense lessons. Somehow this led to my date saying: "Punch me." Lacking rational thought, forethought specifically, I punched my date in the arm. It reminded me of living with my sisters, just a cheap jab, to hear the other person say, "Ow!" But, I don't think he expected me to hit him that hard, or maybe I didn't know how hard I was jabbing. He retaliated with a jab to mine. So I retaliated. So he retaliated again. And so on. Somewhere among the laughter and cheap shots I opted for a sideways elbow jab. I didn't direct it. I didn't plan it. I didn't think about it. But, it was at that point my date vomited.

I would have apologized, but I was pretty sure he would have vomited anyway – and I told him that. In its truest sense, *THIS* is what "raight out uff 'er" means.

The beauty of the occasional "raight out uff 'er" night in traditional Maritime style is that you can still be friends in the morning.

4 May 2003

Trust me

My parents always told me I shouldn't trust people who can't look me in the eye. This came along with other useful tips like: "Never trust someone with a weak/cold/clammy or complicated handshake" and "Never trust someone who has to tell you, you can trust them." You'd think there were trust issues when I was growing up, but we all trusted each other so much in my house, that even as a teenager I didn't bother to hide my diary. I didn't even question how my sister might know about the secret-sinful things I'd done. I thought maybe we were just really close and had developed some sort of sibling ESP.

I've kept diaries ever since I ran out of metaphors for teen-angst poetry, so I have excellent documentation of the most embarrassing period of my life. I love rereading entries describing break-ups, make-outs and substance abuse. I am appalled by my terrible handwriting. I am fascinated I survived those years, and amused by every painful second of them. I made the mistake of thinking it would amuse my friends, too.

I decided to make my diary (a gift from my older, drug-using, fast driving, cigarette smoking, son-of-a-lawyer boyfriend) recounting my sweet sixteenth year, public. I placed it on the coffee table and announced that everyone was welcome to read it. I had even returned torn out "pages-of-shame" to their rightful place inside the book. I couldn't wait to sit around and joke about the person I was. I thought it would be hilarious for my ex-boyfriend to read about how madly in love I claimed to be. I thought my best friend would laugh when she read how I *really* felt when she kissed my boyfriend during a mononucleosis outbreak in our high school. Not so.

The book was left untouched and they eventually asked me to put it away because it made them uncomfortable. I suppose we are tied so intimately to our past that, in other people's eyes, it's hard for them to recognize that we've undergone complete cerebral overhauls. I simply am not capable of doing, saying or thinking most of the things I'd written about almost a decade earlier. It then occurred to me that maybe when people can't look you straight in the eye, it's because they don't trust you.

This all came to mind when my ex-boyfriend, the one who provided much of the drama in the diary in question, emailed to ask if he could spend the night at my house on his way through the city. I mentioned it to my current live-in love and we supposed we wouldn't mind. I said, "Well it won't be that bad . . . it's not like he'd steal from us or anything." As the words left my mouth, I remembered who he was and began questioning whether he really might.

We'll see if I'll be able to look him in the eye when he gets here. I might have to keep my eyes on my stuff instead.

12 June 2003

Spreading bad vibes, one inconsiderate act at a time

I am drying my hair in my "*salle de bain*," and I look out my window to see a stylishly dressed 25-year-old pissing outside. Recently, the technique of suggesting an alternative location to piss has been quite effective in getting them to go elsewhere. The drunks, surprisingly, are polite and apologetic for the most part. Dealing with stylishly dressed 25-year-olds is an entirely different matter. I called out of my little window: "There is a washroom at the cafe around the corner!" He looked around and located me, zipped and approached my window asking, "What?!" I repeated myself and he responded in the way only someone who recently emerged from adolescence could, "Well, I wasn't AT the cafe . . . WAS I!?"

Well, he had me there. He certainly wasn't. He no longer had to pee either, so I acknowledged that there isn't much else I could do. He kept standing there, though . . . so I felt inclined to say *something*.

"It's illegal," I said.

"So call the police," he answered. Then he hurried from the park.

The problem with reporting public pissers is that they leave when they get the job done. Well, except for the drunks. But, they are already "gone".

After this little interaction, I started brainstorming again. I reminded myself of my plan to take photos of these pissers. I reminded myself of my plan to arm myself with a "super soaker" filled with vinegar. I reminded myself of a poster campaign that could plant a seed of paranoia in the minds of The Urinators. It would suggest that a violent man often hides in those same bushes and had been known to attack unsuspecting Urinators when the have their pants down. Or perhaps I could just spread some disgusting concoction all over the grass, something not even Urinators would walk on. Then I reminded myself that this is a losing battle. No matter how hard I try to dissuade these men, they'll always be full of piss.

The feeling that was left with me was absolute frustration. I was actually shaking. I wanted to follow him and take his picture and find out where he lives, and piss on his doorstep. I *did* make a mental note of his face. I like to think we'll cross paths again. When we do, I am hoping he'll make a pass at me – at which point I will mention that I have already seen him with his pants down, and wasn't very impressed.

26 July 2003

Patron Saints of Carnal Desire

There are several authors' works by which I live. None of them include any critically acclaimed holy books. I applaud you if you have found a way to interpret them that satisfies your intellectual and spiritual needs, but I simply haven't the patience.

When I was a young girl, my mother regularly sent me to Sunday school in my little, black patent leather shoes. They clicked all the way down the street to the Baptist church where I would spend the following hour colouring pictures of Jesus. I don't remember actually attending any actual church services, but I do remember when I reached a reasonable age to serve at church luncheons – all of a sudden I was in high demand.

I learned from these luncheons that Nova Scotian Baptists like to eat cream cheese and maraschino cherry sandwiches. Baptists, I concluded after serving a second round, do *not* believe in crusts. Coming from a household that offered only homemade 100 percent whole grain bread, this was heresy!

Actually, I was baptized Anglican. I still haven't a clue how that distinguishes me from Baptists. The church ladies were never very particular when they called on youth for finger food servitude.

By the time I reached Junior High School, I realized it wasn't cool to serve at luncheons. The church ladies gave up on me after a year of phone calls and ultimately mentioned my excommunication to my mother. My mother was unable to pressure me into volunteering. Not even she wanted to attend these socials.

While in Junior High, my best friend joined a Christian youth group at the prompting of her otherwise emotionally absent father. They would help keep her on the right track, he thought. How could she refuse an opportunity like that? She begged me to attend. I avoided the youth group like the plague for several weeks.

Another friend, born Jewish – and otherwise atheist – and I had spent the entire summer trying to make her question her faith. How could I shame myself by hanging out with God's groupies?

Well, I did. I realized quickly it was an untapped social resource. It was fantastic! Here I was, meeting ten other kids – all my senior – willing to take me under their wing. I was positive we could get one of them to buy us beer. Well, as it turns out, we couldn't. They really honestly believed, and I found that fascinating. They were just like other kids, but looked a little glazed over.

It took a while for me to realize they were stoners. Pot was not something I'd considered doing, but at the tender age of fourteen, it was certainly something I wanted to know about. The minister's son seemed to be the baddest apple, so I naturally set my sights on him. I thirsted for knowledge of the seedy underbelly of Christian youth groups. I sat next to him at every opportunity, my stream of daydreaming broken only by the nightly question: "Are you ready to accept Jesus into your heart?"

There I sat – having lustful thoughts of the minister's son, yearning to hear tales of the illegal acts he'd surely committed. The minister often alluded to such sins, and thanked the Lord he was able to save his son from such vices. Thank the Lord he has a hot son, I thought.

That is why, when they'd asked me to accept Jesus into my heart, I was pretty sure I wasn't ready. As a teen, I was aware of my wild oats and fully intended to sow them. "Not yet," I'd say. There was always a group frown before they moved along to someone more pure of heart. One by one they were all "saved". Soon, I was the only bad seed after the minister's deliciously rotten eighteen-year-old apple.

Eventually, I took a nibble and was expelled from the Garden of Eden that was the youth group. It was my first kiss; a long, passionate, sloppy, gag-me-with-your-tongue kiss. The unfortunate detail is that it occurred at 4 a.m. after my parents had already notified the police that I was missing, searched the highways and prepared to be devastated. They found me, immediately post-kiss, sitting in the rotten apple's car on the pier. It was all very romantic, but persecution followed.

Soon after the incident, I was taken aside at the weekly youth group gathering. The leader had prepared a large piece of Bristol board on an easel. While he drew a cluster of Xs he said, "THIS is the youth group." Then he drew a lone X on the opposite edge of the paper and said, "THIS is you. We don't want THIS to happen." He circled the cluster of Xs and drew an arrow toward the one that represented me. "So, we're going to have to ask you to leave."

That was it. They were scared I was leading people away from Jesus. I was the Anti-Christ.

Friends stick together, though, so my two closest girlfriends left the group with me. We were just going to have to develop a new plan for meeting older guys.

That summer, it just so happened there was a new candidate in town. I spotted him immediately. He was driving with the minister's son and I thought that made him seem all the more tasty. The rotten apple stopped his car and started to chat, and introduced his friend.

This boy was a Francophone angel sent from Quebec; boarding at the minister's house to practice his English skills. His accent made me weak. Over the course of the summer, he became my first love. Each day was spent together at the beach, often in silence. We would hold hands and gaze into each other's eyes and share little dreams and compliments. We kissed, but never more. It was so fulfilling, so perfect and pure, that nothing more was necessary. His name was Emmanuel.

If I had known him just months earlier, I would have been able to tell the leaders of the youth group that I would accept him into my heart readily. In fact, I would lay it on the table. I would be willing to crumble it into bits in his honour.

As the end of August approached, this young Adonis prepared to return to his homeland, thousands of kilometers from my Anglophone oasis. The day he parted in his K-car, I was crushed. CRUSHED; how only a first love can do. It ended sweetly, though, because he left while I still worshipped him like a god. We wrote love letters for a full year, and when he started dating someone else, he broke the news to me so gently I could only be happy for him. He assured me I had a special and permanent place in his heart. He set a precedent. Each and every potential boyfriend would later be compared to this hot, young man chiseled in the image of God. I knew how I wanted to be treated. I wanted to be a goddess. I lived by this model as best I could. Jesus, Emmanuel saved me from my adolescent soul.

When I moved to Quebec for university studies nearly four years later, he called and left a message on my answering machine. We were finally living in the same city, but a lot changes in four years, and I didn't want to risk devaluing my memories. I never returned his call. I wanted to keep my faith just as it was.

Everyone wants a little redemption

When I was about four years old, I had not a single friend. We'd just moved to Nova Scotia and my sixteen-year-old sisters seemed to have a ton of them. Sure they were all guys, and according to my parents, were more like loiterers and sexual opportunists, but still my sisters were sought after.

I, on the other hand, had periodic playmates when my mother distributed popsicles. It was revealed to me, twenty years after the fact, that she had lured children into our yard to play with me by bribing them with treats. My sisters ensured me that the tactic was effective, until the popsicles were gone. Perhaps, if I'd grown to be a socially inept adult, they wouldn't find this as funny as they do. As it stands, I'm only partially inept and they think it's hilarious.

To be fair, I was the only child my age within walking distance. The boy closest to my age was an adorable olive-skinned latch-key child with snot in his nose and scabs on his knees. He had little interest in paper dolls and Cabbage Patch Kids ©. His hobbies involved collecting choke cherries, bottling swamp water and breaking erasers into bits – all of which were to be thrown at me at a later date. This wouldn't have been quite as annoying if he didn't have a little brother and emotionally unstable neighbor to rally against me as well.

You can imagine my dismay when, returning from school one afternoon, my mother informed me she'd agreed to care for them until 5 o'clock every day when their parents arrived home from work. It's not as if she didn't know how they treated me. I think this was a psychological experiment. I think she actually believed that with the guidance she could offer during those two hours/day, these boys might stop acting out, and therefore leave ME the hell alone. Perhaps she thought we'd actually play together.

Things went smoothly for a while. I tiptoed around my house, stopped speaking and made sure never to blink both eyes at the same time. When I watched after school TV programs, my peripheral vision was always tuned in. I was afraid they'd imported choke cherries. What really frustrated me was that they were always so careful to never get *caught* harassing me. Someday, someday they'd get their just desserts – and it wouldn't be a Popsicle ©, damn it.

One sunny day in my living room, I walked in on these two boys dissecting my fuzzy, stuffed frog toy. Perhaps they were biology prodigies. Perhaps they were assholes. This, I thought, is exactly the evidence I'd need to get them kicked out of my house forever!! The TV would be mine, and only mine, between 3 p.m. and 5 p.m.!

Again, you can imagine my frustration when my mother gave them a second chance. She thought it would be effective to leave the toy on the table the next time they came over, so they could remember the bad thing they'd done and repent. She forgot she was dealing with the spawn of the devil.

I realized I was going to have to play as dirty as they did. I falsified evidence to have them expelled from my house. If I remember clearly, it involved spreading talcum powder all over the playroom. Sure they were telling the truth when they said, "I didn't do it," but no one was going to believe them. I was a child genius!

This untruth, however, was repaid with an ambush. I was pushed off my bicycle on the way to the place where all the stray cats lived. I bagged my leftover dinner nightly and carried it there to feed them, thinking I was helping, as opposed to perpetuating the stray cat epidemic. All that swamp water they'd saved up was poured over me and my bike; the cat food strewn all over the pavement. I ran home, hyperventilating. When I walked into my house, my mother rushed out of it. She was gone for about ten minutes. I was feeling sorry for myself in the bathroom when my mother returned to comfort me. I haven't a clue what she said to the boys or their parents, but no one bothered me again. Mother's instinct for protection can be very powerful. It can conquer the devil.

Years passed and friends came and went. They were angels in my life who moved to heavenly places like Bolivia, Mexico, British

Columbia and Holland while I wasted away in rural Nova Scotia. Eventually I turned seventeen, and was confident enough to go to parties attended by people who tormented me when I was small. We politely ignored each other and went on with our good times.

One night, the boy who tormented me most, approached. Even after a beer or two, my knees tingled and I considered running. We were neighbors, but not a peaceful word had ever been shared between us without an adult offering an ultimatum: "Say you're sorry or you'll get a detention."

This particular night, however, he told me I was beautiful. He flexed for me and cried. He said he'd been trying to get me to notice him for years. I felt like saying: "I was just trying to avoid an ambush." He *did* clarify that I wasn't as beautiful as my sister, but I was close. I was speechless.

A few years later, he tried to burn his parent's house down. He's since been institutionalized.

Compliments can come from some of the most unexpected places. I try not to judge mean people too harshly, because meanness is almost always misdirected self-hatred.

Thank you goes out to the dry cleaning technician, to the elderly Polish man who invited me out for borscht, to the bank manager who never makes me stand in line, to the girl in my class who said I have nice eyes, to the women who took a picture of me on campus, to the flight attendant who said my smile was contagious, to my beloved who never fails to love me, and say it, even when I am feeling conflicted. And, thank you to the poor tormented boy from my childhood for trying, even if it was a little too late.

18 February 2004

A tale of bruised hearts, puppetry and wrestling

On Valentine's Day, one of my closest single friends came to my house to indulge. We claimed the day as our own and gave ourselves permission to drink red wine and gorge ourselves on freshly made brownies laden with Hershey Kisses ©. The "pity party" became a "piggy party". What could be more appropriate?

All around university campuses there have been posters advertising V-Days. Should you notice one of these and read the not-so-fine print, you'll realize this is a reappropriation celebration of the day that makes so many lovers-scorned mournful.

V-Day, as opposed to Valentine's Day, doesn't take Cupid's shot lying down. Activities planned included renditions of the Vagina Monologues and puppet-making workshops. Such workshops advertised the opportunity to show your vagina's true personality, but alas, I already had plans.

Arriving at my house with craft supplies, my friend suggested we have a do-it-yourself puppet conception session. And so it was.

After consuming a pan of brownies and polishing off a nice bottle of one of my favourite economy-reds, we created said puppets. Giggling and certain the night could not possibly be dull, we donned our winter gear, puppets on hand, and set out for a Rockabilly show.

First, we stopped at a store near the bus stop to use the ATM. While there, a nice-looking, preppy, clean-cut guy in a shiny black leather jacket and manicured everything dropped a coin.

We heard the clink. We all watched it roll and ultimately find a new home for itself under the ice cream freezer. The man, obviously concerned about his image, looked up at my friend and me. We could see the desire in his eyes; the desire for that damn dollar he dropped. There he stood with a decision to be made. He shifted his weight, and leaned in the direction of the freezer. Finally, he left with his pride intact and the dollar coin lodged under the unit.

Without hesitation, as the door swung shut behind the preppy man, a truck driver who had been perusing the map section of the convenience store was heard to mumble, "I'll get the damn thing." With relative ease this man lifted the freezer, exposed the soiled coin and told my friend to fetch it. She did. When she straightened herself out she motioned to hand it to him. He told her, with a smile and a wink, "Keep it."

I was tempted to thank him with my vagina.

Cheerful and feeling like this was the kind of night strange men would lift large appliances for us, we caught the bus. The thirty-minute ride passed quickly as we giggled, for only we knew what we had up our sleeves.

The bar scene was perfect. There was a mix of young and old. Each table wore a faux lace tablecloth, the wallpaper was flowery and wilted roses adorned all flat surfaces. The bartender, aged 80, called everyone "*dear*" and poured pitchers of flat draft like a true pro. It was delightfully ridiculous and I didn't know anyone there.

My friend introduced me to her boss and some acquaintances. There were several girls who personified "indifference", even when they danced and some guys who entertained me just enough. I was having a good time. My vagina was getting a lot of attention and, to my surprise, other women borrowed it to make it talk and growl. My friend's vagina was eventually clamped to the Rockabilly singer's face. He wore it well.

There were lots of laughs and I was having a good time when I was smacked in the head with a thorny rose. Even in my warm and fuzzy brain I knew it left a mark.

Now, I know a lot of people have issues with Valentine's Day and I know some people have issues with the opposite sex in general, but c'mon. I'm not exactly sure what events led to this, or whether it was before or after the same guy sprayed beer from his mouth onto me, but I do remember acknowledging that enough was enough. I had been sitting behind him and after I wiped my shirt dry on his, I stood. And then he stood.

A small part of my brain recognized him as the same guy at the last Rockabilly show who was being an ass to a different cute girl. Almost at that same instant, he pushed me. Later I realized he poked me with his thumb hard enough to leave a small bruise on my left breast, just over my heart.

True, I only did it because my brain was warm and fuzzy enough to allow for my body to react instinctively, but the singular most empowering move my self-defence instructor taught me nearly ten years ago, resurfaced. With relative ease, I swung him to the floor. Then, I literally (and just once) kicked his ass. Not to hurt him of course, just to humiliate.

I was surprised, when my brain finally caught up with me, that he was lying on his back on the floor beneath me. His eyes were glassy and he looked mad – like a dog. I realized this might be the first Valentine's Day I'd be receiving a black eye. Instead of waiting for this to happen, I grabbed a chair and used it to pin him to the floor.

With my vagina somewhere else in the bar, I had the balls to say, "Do you wanna go at it like THIS? Or you wanna call a truce?"

He called a truce, and I took a cab back to town with his

girlfriend, who said he probably deserved it, and some guy who had a penchant for female wrestling.

You see, Valentine's Day is one thing when you wear your heart on your sleeve, and something completely outrageous when you wear your vagina in its place.

What is Valentine's Day if not for the hottest guy in the bar to be falling at your feet?

10 May 2004

The San(ct)ity of Marriage

They popped the question again.

We were in Ottawa, celebrating my boyfriend's mother's birthday. His family would have preferred that we were there to celebrate my mother-IN-LAW's birthday, though, and they made that clear.

After a nice lunch hosted by the "Uncles" (two men who've been living, traveling and presumably sleeping together for more than thirty years now), we bought some shitty gelato and went for a stroll along the Ottawa canal. The city is currently hosting the tulip festival – a colourful, yet painfully dull annual event.

The city itself breeds mediocrity.

Sure it's multicultural and has lots of government funding. Sure everyone there has a job and a multi-level brick house with stone pathways leading to frosted glass and brass front doors and loon-print welcome mats, but I'm not ready for my 2.5 kids. I'm just not interested.

My boyfriend and I walked hand-in-hand and his brother walked alone. My Un-in-laws also walked together. Surely they'd have held hands if my boyfriend's dad had been able to stop taking pictures. The Uncles never walk too close to each other, and never hold hands in public.

It was later that night, following another meal of so-so Vietnamese food, that the Unfather-in-law cornered me.

"Soooooooooooooooooooo . . ."

The way he drew the word out was meant to prepare me, I think. "Have you two made any DECISIONS about your relationship yet?" he asked.

I was relieved that my boyfriend was there to share the pressure with me. Last time they tried to get me to confess that I craved stability and the only way to really get it would be to convince my boyfriend to marry me. Until then, I don't think it had occurred to them that I didn't *want* to have a wedding either.

That first conversation was almost as uncomfortable as when the aunts referred to their non-Catholic nephew as an "idiot" and then remembered I was there. This time, I shared the stage. My boyfriend's mother laughed nervously and his brother cackled with amusement.

I considered sharing my reasons for not wanting to get married. I thought of pointing out that the fact that two men who've loved each other for more than three decades aren't legally able to marry, and that if marriage isn't about *love* it must be about economics.

Considering my priorities – the things I believe will make me happy – if I spend a few thousand dollars a wedding, that would make me a moron.

To those of you who *are* married, I respect that. It was a priority for you. But, this is more in line with how *I* feel:

Traveling somewhere tropical, enduring 19-hour flight delays; helping each other through long nights of the shits because we ate the "special" meat on some remote island; almost being arrested while driving through the mountains in BC because of mistaken identity; being sponge-bathed to bring down a three-day fever of 104° F-and-rising in NYC during 9–11; having the air let out of someone's bike tires because they disrespected me; having my '67 Schwinn fitted with the original grips of my dreams; having the house filled with ginger flowers when I return from a trip; choosing the perfect tiki lanterns together on Ebay . . . those things hold more weight for me as a symbol of everlasting love and affection than trying not to get too drunk on bubbly before the white-dress ceremony.

It's just hard to tell *that* to the Filipino-Catholic not-yet-relatives. They are so big on symbols of commitment – on official contracts.

And, that's exactly why we settled for life insurance policies instead.

5 May 2004

Special treatment: more than just your average transaction

Starting this May, I'm going to have to stand in line at the bank just like the rest of you. I don't expect sympathy, but it's going to take some getting used to. I'm really not sure how it began, but for several years I've been getting secret, special treatment thanks to a flirtatious young employee.

Starting out as a simple, chubby teller, he had a bright smile and plenty of enthusiasm, when I'd arrive to cash my weekly paycheques. At first I noticed that he'd put up a "Next Teller Please" sign when he'd spot me in line. When I'd near the front of the line, he'd lift the sign and motion me to his booth. This went on for months. I was polite enough not to mention how painfully obvious he was. Besides, talking about his possible attraction to me was right at the top of my "things to avoid" list.

The first real favour involved making a note in my account that there should be no holds placed on my foreign currency cheques. I thanked him sincerely. Other people have to wait 40 days to get their cash.

Then it started to happen. He began losing weight, tanning, and wearing tighter shirts. He unbuttoned those silky atrocities just enough to allow for an occasional glimpse of a two-inch gold cross, nestled awkwardly among his chest hairs. I knew what was coming. It was inevitable.

The managers were pleased with his *way* with the customers and soon promoted this aspiring Greek God of Finance. With his very own office, his confidence skyrocketed. From that point on, when I'd stand in line with the good citizens of Montreal, he'd emerge from his office, adjust his suit jacket and ask me in a very professional tone, "Are you here to seek advice about a Retirement Savings Fund, Miss?" Just so I wouldn't miss the cue, he'd wink – every time.

From this point on, I would be escorted to his private office immediately upon arrival and, in exchange for a little small talk, I could avoid standing in line.

This interaction wasn't without weirdness, though. I soon learned that this fine young Momma's boy was looking for a spicy-yet-innocent, young wife to appease his traditional Greek family. Pictures of his siblings' 15 children decorated his office and his dark eyelashes waved at me for the duration of the transaction. You see, he wanted a "nice" girl who could still be "naughty".

He was nice enough, but gee, his "professionalism" was astounding.

I started weighing the pros and cons of this "special treatment". Sometimes "special" isn't so great. Sometimes it just means "weird".

Each visit to the bank became more and more awkward. I began timing my visits with his lunch hour – hoping to avoid the inevitable. I had also developed a minor guilt complex. I mean, what makes me *so* special? Why shouldn't I have to wait in line like everyone else? I mean, he'd pull me out of line when there were frail old ladies wavering on their canes ahead of me. Ultimately, I decided to smother my internal Socialist . . . after all, a bank is no place for Socialism.

Then, one night, I bumped into the banker downtown. He was in one of his silky suits and I was riding my old beater bike with sneakers and a messy ponytail. I had to break the news to him, "I have a boyfriend."

(What I really wanted to say was: "How can you possibly think I am your type????")

I really thought that might scare him away – and I wasn't sure I'd mind. I shouldn't have been so naive. For the following three years, he continued asking me if I was there "seeking advice about a Retirement Savings Fund" and winking so I'd know to follow him to his office, but there was this addendum: "You still got a boyfriend?" I still always blush when I say, "Yes." After several years of this, with only nine days until his departure for the greener pastures of the downtown financial district, I don't think my answer is going to change.

9 June 2004

Your very, very friendly neighborhood policemen

My interactions with police are unconventional.

Growing up, police were for "other" people, and television, only. In a town as small as the one where I was raised, men of law only appeared on Halloween to catch vandals – and they never succeeded.

As a teen – drunk and disorderly – police were the guys you avoided. They were the only people in town you couldn't ask to go to the Liquor Store for you.

In the city, I realized that interactions with the police simply can't be avoided. I'm just happy none have been scary. In fact, my personal experience has been that the police are far more pleasant with me than I am interested in being with them.

In 2001, when two friends and I were mugged at three o'clock in the morning – on a quiet street in front of the wimpiest hotel security guard ever – I called the police for the first time. Actually, I just yelled at the dumbfounded security guard until he called the police for me.

Actually, he ran away from me and locked himself in his car and rolled up the window. It was while he was in the car that I convinced him to call the police.

We waited for nearly 45 minutes before the policemen showed up. By that time, we were starting to sober up, and boredom filled the gaps where adrenaline waned. Then, with renewed fervor, we all yelled our story to the two, young officers, simultaneously. They did the usual run-through. They asked for a description of the muggers (all three of them) and then we signed our statements.

The night could have ended there, but there was a twist! They offered to drive us around while they looked for those nasty criminals. As drunk as we were, even WE knew the muggers were long gone. But still, who can say no to a ride in the back of a cop car?

So we piled in – three drunken girls on a Friday night in the back of a cop car. The seats were surprisingly comfortable – well broken in. We really wanted to drive by people we knew, and there was a good chance of that, seeing as we were essentially taking a tour of the party district. We weren't subtle; the lights were flashing. I had always suspected police to be a little trigger happy with the light switch.

Then the car sped through the middle of a busy park, past kids rolling joints, past people drinking in public and making out, and screeched to halt in front of the only black man in the park. The officers lowered their window to question him.

You see, the description we gave the police included: Three

fairly good-looking teenaged guys in sweatshirts, big jeans and nice sneakers . . . oh . . . and they were Anglophone . . . and black.

Yeah, I know it's vague. And I am sure you are thinking, "Well, that could be anybody."

And you're right. It *could* be anybody. That is, anybody other than a 60-year-old homeless guy – they were harassing him for our benefit.

But, what were we supposed to do? There we were, drunk and disorderly ourselves, in the back of a cop car, witnessing racial profiling and injustice. Well, I'm not sure what the exact right thing to do would be, but we were too inebriated to care. So we just started screaming. And then they screamed at us to shut up. And, we did.

The bum was left to pass out on the bench in peace, and all was quiet in the back of the car for a minute. A little later, the police asked us where we lived, so they could drop us off at home. What a nice offer! Except we didn't want to go home – we had been heading to an after-hours party when we were mugged – and we thought we might as well go out and use our adrenaline. By this time, the officers were more than happy to drop us off.

They parked the car and got out to give us all a proper good-bye. We "kiss-kiss" our friends here in Montreal . . . and since I'd never kissed a cop before . . . I . . . well . . . anyway . . . ethics, principles and morals be damned!

We got into the party for free. There are perks to having police escort. Policemen really are our friends – if you're a damsel in distress, that is.

And it just so happens that I am, on occasion, a damsel in distress.

TWIDDLY BITS

http://twiddlybits.net

25 July 2003

Introduction
(Posted by **TwiddlyBits**)

I've decided to start a sex blog. Why? Aren't there enough sex blogs out there already? There certainly are a lot of them out there, it's true, but none of them are about *me*!:-)

Anyway, a little about me: I'm your host, Twiddly Bits. I'm female, in my mid-30s, married to a wonderful man, and voracious about sex. (My husband often says that he's living a Penthouse Letter.)

Hold the 'phone! Did you say 'married'?

Yes, I did, but that doesn't necessarily mean "monogamous", does it?;-)

My husband & I have a very committed and intimate relationship, but neither of us sees anything wrong with fun sex with other people, *provided* that we both know about it. We prefer to participate together (and always have, so far), but as long as neither of us keeps any secrets from the other or lies about anything, it's all good.

In the interest of privacy, no real names or identifying details will be used in this blog, ever.

So, that's about it for now. I hope to keep this blog regularly updated with all kinds of adventures and sexy things. We had quite an adventure last week and I plan to write about it very soon. Meanwhile, be sexy, sane and safe!

30 July 2003

A Visit from Friends
(Posted by **TwiddlyBits**)

Back in the Introduction post, I promised I'd tell y'all about a recent adventure my husband & I had.

We were paid a 9-day visit from 2 friends who we used to live near. The male half of the couple (male & female, newly-engaged) & I used to work together for about 5 years, so we were pretty good friends. He & I had been IM'ing fairly regularly since we moved away and all 4 of us were looking forward to their visit. During our IM sessions, the subject of sex came up (doesn't it always? *grin*) and H & I decided that, if "something" were to happen, that'd be just fine by us, and if not, that's cool, too. Fortunately, we both have very open-minded and easy-going partners who didn't mind if "something" were to happen between H & me – or even between the 2 of them. H confided in me that nothing makes him more aroused than knowing that W is enjoying herself. So, H and W came to visit. We planned to do a bunch of touristy stuff – there's plenty to do in this area – and hang out & catch up on old times. H turned out to be even more shy than he had warned me of via IM! After 4 days & nights, the only "something" that had happened was shower-swapping (i.e. I showered with H, my husband showered with W, we fondled each other & kissed, W sucked my husband's cock a little, nothing more). *hmph*

That changed on the 5th day. Exhausted and badly sunburned, H, W, & I decided to stay home for the day and rest (my husband had to go to work). While lounging nude about the living room, I was lying on the couch while H & W were lounging on the floor (H leaning up against the couch). W starts to lightly stroke H's cock, which appreciates the attention.;-) H leans back to kiss me while W snuggles under his arm. Eventually I say, "If y'all scoot over just a little bit, there'll be room for me down there, too." They scooted over, so I joined them on the floor. I spoon behind H, kissing his ears, neck, shoulders, etc. I sidle my way down his arm and onto his belly and end up with his lovely cock in my mouth. Such soft and tender skin! He keeps the whole area shaved, too. *chuckle* In all the years I've known him, I've never heard him whimper like that.;-)

He seemed to appreciate my ministrations and I know that W was kissing him quite passionately, too, which just fueled his fire. It must have been very intense for him because he cried out, "Oh, God, please let me come!" which, unfortunately, had the effect of making W & I break out in giggles, so the end result was that we slowly stopped what we were doing.

We had to leave in a few minutes anyway to keep an appointment we'd made.

That night, W wasn't feeling well – probably something she ate at dinner – so we all ended up just going to sleep.

The *next* night, however, after we'd had this *ahem* taste, we went to dinner at a local British pub & got pretty drunk. On the way home, I distracted H from the scenery by kissing him and fondling his cock through his pants. Once we were at home, we put in a porn flick (*Edge Play* with Marilyn Chambers) and the 4 of us got distracted some more.

The 4 of us sat on the couch with glasses of wine. My husband (hereinafter labelled "P") started caressing W's magnificent breasts and while she moaned, H & I started kissing and caressing each other. Soon, P was on the floor in front of W eating her tight pussy while I encouraged H to watch her writhe and listen to her moan while I gently nibbled on him. Eventually H tickled my clit with his tongue before I pushed him backwards onto the floor and climbed on, sliding his dick into me. After several orgasms on my part, he came and we snuggled a little bit. By this time, W was on the floor in front of P giving him what sounded like a very pleasing blow-job. I excused myself to go to the bathroom & when I returned, H followed suit. While he was gone, I curled up on the couch next to P and started teasing his nipples while W continued to suck his cock most enthusiastically. I kissed him & whispered in his ear things like "Oh, isn't she beautiful sucking your cock like that? Don't you just love the feel of it?" etc., to which he moaned and groaned his agreement. H came back in while the 3 of us were so engaged and ended up on the floor behind W and slid his cock into her. Boy, *her* moaning sure kicked up a notch! :-)

We carried on like this for a little while, then H stopped fucking W and turned to me. I kissed P one more time and joined H on the floor, where he entered me again and made me squiggle in delight before coming again. Meanwhile, W climbed up onto P's cock and rode him until he came.

Afterwards, we all got cleaned up, snuggled and drank some more wine. We commented that we'd missed most of the porn movie! LOL

Eventually, we retired for the night.

P took the next day off of work and we planned to do more tourist things together, but afterwards . . ., well, I'll save that for another post. Maybe tomorrow . . .

12 August 2003

TwiddlyBits gets interviewed
(Posted by **TwiddlyBits**)

Married But Lonely posted a response to 5 interview questions that **Sophia** asked him. As part of the agreement, he asked if others wanted to be interviewed by him. I replied & here are the questions that he asked me and my answers:

1. Due to the anonymous nature of our blogs, we tend to let it all hang out. So I'll ask you the same question I asked Sophia. Describe how your "everyday" persona varies from the one who writes in your blog.

As far as my "voice" and style goes, my IRL persona is pretty close to my on-line one. I've always managed to project the "real me" on-line, but it's only been since my marriage to Dangly that my IRL persona has started to be the "real me", too. My first marriage was characterized by the squashing of my personality. I became mousy and "librarianesque" and emotionally restricted. Dangly lets me be *me*, so I am free to express myself & my personality has opened up as a result. Now, because of the nature of my job, I can't talk about my sexual adventures in public – that's why my blog is anonymous. I do have to hide some aspects of my personality in my everyday life. But, my close friends know me for who and what I am and love me. So, I am able to tolerate that small amount of "hiding" myself because I know that with the people who I care for, I can truly be myself.

2. Describe the circumstances under which you first discovered that DanglyBits was a cross-dresser. What was your reaction?

Good question! Dangly & I met at a business conference in a state far from both of our homes. After returning home, we continued our developing relationship via email. Very early it was apparent that we were falling in love and Dangly decided that he needed to tell me about his TV-ism right away rather than either hiding it from me (which too many TVs do) or wait to tell me until it was "too late". It was at a point that, if I had been unable to take the news, we could have broken off our relationship without having invested too much emotional energy into it. In his email he asked if I had noticed that both of his ears were pierced (I had) and that when people asked him about it, his standard response was, "I got tired of wearing clip-ons." (This is usually said with an edge of sarcasm, so people take it as a joke, but it's the truth.) He then told me that he is a transvestite. At first, I was a bit confused. I was unsure whether my new friend was genetically a man who wears women's clothing, or vice versa! So, after getting that straightened out, I thought about it for a little bit (just a few hours) and reflected that, in the course of our conversations, I had discovered a man who understood my soul and who connected with me in ways that I had never dreamt possible. Then he tells me that he likes to wear women's clothing. He had been a TV all along, I was just unaware of it. So, what did this revelation really change? I realized that it changed nothing. I told him that I wanted to continue our relationship, but that I had questions. He told me he'd answer any questions I had, and he did. Over the course of time, I've come to cherish his feminine side. **As he wrote in the blog**, it's like having a girlfriend, husband and lover all in one package. He understands the way I think, the way I feel, the way I *am*. I can ask him about clothing, hair & make-up and know that he is knowledgeable and interested in it, yet he is still a "car guy" who likes hotrods. We can giggle together like girls, yet he can sweep me in his arms and carry me off to the bedroom and be "the man" in bed when that's what I need.

This is not to say that I "tolerate" his cross-dressing simply so I can have a sensitive & understanding husband. Quite the contrary!

I simply adore my husband. I've discovered that marriage is about giving the other person as many opportunities as possible to be able to express his full personality however he wants to. Unfortunately, our society looks askance at people who don't follow the rigid gender roles. It seems to me that the transgendered community is one of the last groups that it's still socially acceptable to openly mock and ridicule. *sad sigh* Still, I want our home to be a safe haven for Dangly so that he's comfortable being himself, even when he's being "herself".

And what was the first outfit he wore for you?

About 2 months after we met, Dangly came to visit me and brought some of his femme attire. He is actually quite good at picking out clothing that suits his figure (he is tall and thin), rather than dressing like a prostitute, which is what a lot of TVs end up doing. (Mostly because they aren't given an outlet for their TVism and so never learn how to dress like a "real" woman.)

He wore big, dangly earrings, a nice white shirt with a light flower print, and a long denim strapped dress with some low heels. Under that, he had pantyhose, panties, and bra (with the tits he was fixing the other day), as well as padding for his hips and a waist cincher. I spent the day totally nude and we ended up in bed, him eating me out, his earrings brushing my thighs. It was the first time he'd ever made love with a woman while "dressed" – and it was the first time I'd ever been with a cross-dressed man, too.

I'll also answer an unasked question and say that nowadays, a few years into our relationship, Dangly sleeps in a silky nightgown every night. He wears panties every day and most of his everyday clothes is "women's clothing", even though most people don't realize it. He likes to wear bras when he can (mostly at home &/or on the weekends) and has women's slippers that he wears around the house. He does have some lingerie – some of which I have bought for him – and I enjoy it when he wears it. I think it's important to make the distinction that this is *not* a fetish in the sense that he needs women's clothing to function in a sexual manner; it really has nothing (or very little) to do with sexuality. It is just simply an aspect of his personality.

3. Would you describe yourself as the dominant or submissive in your relationship, or is it not that simple? How do those sex roles figure into your everyday marriage as a whole, or do they?

That's a tough one. I'm not sure we have such clearly defined roles. I've already mentioned that I appreciate Dangly's feminine side. I've always been an aggressive lover, in that I'm not afraid to make the first move or flat out ask for what I want. Dangly has no problem letting me be the "dominant" one in that case (and that has no bearing on sexual positions – I can be "dominant" and still be on the bottom). He likes to feel cherished and protected sometimes, too. OTOH, sometimes *I* am the one who is feeling all feminine and shy and want to be wooed and romanced, and I think *because* I allow him to be fully himself, he has no problem stepping into the dominant role himself from time to time. If I had to chart it, I'd say that as far as sex goes, I'm probably the agressor 75–80 per cent of the time, which suits us both fine. For other things, I think we're pretty evenly matched. We are each capable of making everyday decisions on our own, yet consult with each other for all major decisions. Neither of us has "the final say-so". Of course, it helps that we think so much alike, too.

DanglyBits once said to me, "I think we have the same mix of yin and yang as other couples do, it's just distributed a little differently."

4. You get to plan the perfect sex related experience. Describe it.

chuckle I think I live that experience every day!:-) Seriously, I am so happy with my relationship with Dangly that I really can't imagine anything more perfect than our life together. He goes out of his way to help me realize my fantasies and desires. I still have a couple of fantasies that haven't been fulfilled yet, but he's willing to help me do so when the opportunity arises. I know this sounds like a cop-out, but it really isn't . . .

5. Do you and DanglyBits plan on having kids one day? If so, do you think that you'll be able to keep up your "alternative lifestyles" while parenting?

This is actually an easy question to answer. Dangly & I do not plan to have children. I have had a Tubal Ligation. Some people think that's selfish of me/us, but we don't think so. Here's why: I have very specific opinions about how children should be raised and I am simply not willing to make the sacrifices that I think are necessary to do so. If I'm not willing to make those sacrifices, why bring a child into the world? I'd only end up resenting the child and that's not fair to either of us. So, we intend to remain blessedly child-free.

14 August 2003

My recent business trip
(Posted by **TwiddlyBits**)

I've been **promising** to tell all of you about the happenings on my recent business trip. I haven't forgotten, I've just been formulating my thoughts & have been wondering where to start. So, last night while Dangly was **shaving me**, I decided that you need the back-story, so here it is:

The Back Story

2 summers ago, about a month after Dangly & I were married, I went on a business trip for a week. I was going to be rooming with M, a woman that I'd only met via email. We got along great and had a wonderful time hanging out during the conference and socializing. We went out with one of her male friends who was also attending the conference, had some wine and teased him unmercifully over dinner, poor guy. She was also the first person I told about my **piercing**.

I thought I sensed some sexual tension between us, but being the highly-sexed individual I am, I thought I might have been imagining it. More on that later . . .

Anyway, when I got home, the very first thing Dangly did was pick me up & carry me into the bedroom where he proceeded to undress me and bury his face in my pussy. What a homecoming! *grin* After I came all over his face, we cuddled and he asked me how my trip had been. I told him all about M and how much I liked her.

He asked, "Did you *play*?"

I stopped dead in my tracks, speechless. Dangly & I hadn't discussed any sort of "open" arrangement in our marriage or anything, so he caught me completely by surprise.

I answered, hesitantly, "Um, no. Why do you ask?" and we proceeded to have a discussion, the end result of which was a set of "rules" by which we'd agreed to conduct ourselves in our possible future sexual relations with people outside of our marriage. We had no firm plans, but we were opening ourselves up to the possibility – the results of which you see in this blog.

Of course, these "rules" have since evolved, but that's OK – relationships evolve & grow & that's A Good Thing.

Flash Forward to the Present

M was at this conference, too, although we didn't room together this time. One night, she & I went out to dinner with one of her female companions (who ended up being the Designated Driver for the evening). I had a couple of beers & so did she (plus a couple of margaritas). After dinner, her friend had to run an errand, so she & I went to a bar & each had another beer & talked about things. I ended up telling her about this blog & some of the things it contains. She said that she could see herself being with someone like me, but wasn't so sure about being with another man (she is also married).

After her friend got back from the errand, the 3 of us plus another female friend went to another bar. Man, the bouncers were HOT! I found out their names from another bar employee while waiting in line for the bathroom. Teddy & Roger. Teddy, especially, had SUCH a nice ass! I wanted to just squeeze it over and over again. Of course, I took every opportunity to go outside and talk to them and compliment them on their physiques and tell them about all the naughty things I wanted to do to them. They didn't get off work until 3.00 a.m., though, which was too late for me since I had to be up at 7.00 a.m., but I told them that if I hadn't been rooming with 3 other ladies, they'd *BOTH* have been coming home with me – and think of the **Penthouse Letters** they could have written! LOL!

But I digress . . .

At one point, our 2 party companions had to run another errand, leaving M & me alone together. Now, we were not in a booth or hidden in any way. We had the front table, by the door (hence my easy access to Teddy & Roger!), in front of the big front windows, practically rubbing elbows with the tables around us.

The music was loud, so we had to lean in close to each other to carry on a conversation. M pressed her forehead to mine & nuzzled me, then kissed me. (*So, I guess I wasn't imagining the sexual tension last time, huh?*) I returned the kiss and she asked, "Why didn't we do this a long time ago?" I chuckled and kissed her again, placing my hand on her thigh. She took my hand and put it up her skirt, between her legs, on her pussy – she wasn't wearing any panties. I fingered her a little and stroked the insides of her thighs and up under her shirt to her breasts, tweaking her nipple before letting my hand fall back to her pussy and fingering her some more.

She asked me what it was like to be with a woman. I told her that women are snuggly, soft and warm, and wonderful to be with.

Whenever the door would open, we'd turn our heads to look out and grin at Teddy & Roger – I'm sure they were getting *quite* a show! We carried on this way for a good while, then broke apart when our friends returned. A few more beers later and we decided to all call it a night. I said my good-byes to Teddy & Roger and we left.

They drove me back to my room – sort of a 4 bedroom 2-story townhouse on the campus where the conference was held (M was staying with friends off-campus) – and M came inside "just to see the place". After greeting my roommates downstairs, M & I headed up to my bedroom where she quickly closed the door & threw herself down on my bed, holding me to her and kissing me. I caressed her breasts and touched her thighs and had my fingers in her dripping wet pussy and was about to head south when one of my roommates (who is an acquaintance of M) called up to her to ask her a question.

So, we decided to break it up – besides our other 2 friends were still waiting for her in the car! – but I made sure to look her straight in the eyes while licking her sweet juices off of my fingers. She looked like she was going to melt when I did that!

We went downstairs, I showed her to the door, then chatted a bit with my roommates before having a shower (to wash off the smell of smoke from the bar) and heading off to bed to masturbate. I had to relieve the tension somehow! We'd been *so close*!! I just know she'd have creamed all over my face if I'd gone down on her – I really think she would have enjoyed that.

Unfortunately, we had no other opportunities to finish our "business" for the rest of the conference. I can only hope that we see each other again soon at another event and don't have to wait another 2 years for the next conference.

13 August 2003

Tired and cranky . . .
(Posted by **DanglyBits**)

. . . is what I am. Work was a trial today – no real reason why, it was just a trial to get through it. The people I dealt with were no stupider than on any other day, and the technology I deal with wasn't any more truculent than on any other day. Just one of those days, I guess.

Coming home was definitely the best pat of the day. Traffic was good and line at the grocery store was short and moved quickly. The best part of coming home, though, was being met at the door by a naked Twiddlybits. She is soooo sexy – and she doesn't even know it. I put my stuff down, kissed Twiddlybits, then went out to check the mail. When I got back, I snuggled with Twiddlybits at the door – she snuggles delightfully. Mmmmmmmm I caressed her from top to bottom (well, I didn't reach down and do her feet and calves, but I think you know what I mean) and nibbled on her neck a bit. She purred and squiggled charmingly and then started to undress me. Right at the door. I barely had time to kick my shoes off. Not that I'm complaining, tho. She stopped after undoing my shirt, tho, and snuggled her bare skin against my bare skin. Lovely. It was a good start along the way to forgetting about the day.

We went into the bedroom and I finished what Twiddlybits started. I noticed three vibrators on the bed. (Twiddlybits has written about what she did with them in **a separate entry**) I commented that she had played and that she had been quite a busy girl. She cheerfully admitted it and put the vibes away from where she had left them "to dry". Uh-huh. I think she left them out just to tantalize me. And it worked. I started getting hard just seeing them there and imaging how she used them all on herself. I could just imagine her sliding the thick pink one in and out of her beautiful ass while she held the other two on her wet, throbbing pussy.

I cleaned up, got the residue of the day off me and decided to let my feminine half out for a while. I got out a midi-length pink skirt, a light shirt with bright splashes of colour on a white background, and then got out my tits. I am happy to say that the surgery I performed on them was completely successful. They are once again fully functional and proudly in their rightful place – in a bra that's wrapped around my silky smooth body. When I got out my tits, Twiddlybits said, "Oh, good, you're going to dress!" and then proceeded to tell me which bra and panty set she wanted to see me in. Not so amazingly, given how much alike we think, it was the same set I was thinking of wearing. I kissed her naked ass a few times, then got dressed, ever so carefully placing my tits into my bra and then pulling up what little chest I have to try to form something resembling cleavage. I completed the ensemble with a set of dangly earrings, something I don't get to wear regularly.

It's amazing the transformation that comes over me when I'm "dressed". I become calmer, softer spoken, less hurried – more feminine, really. But then, that's the reality of being a TV. I'm very fortunate (as was commented privately by another TV) to have a life partner that understands and appreciates that my feminine side is just that – another side of who "I" am. Putting on a skirt doesn't turn me into someone else. I'm still fundamentally me.

Well, we've had dinner, I'm still sipping on my beer, and I'm doing some evening work while Twiddlybits peruses blogs by the dozen. Ah, the curse of technology that lets us work from home . . . Hopefully I'll be done with my work soon enough that Twiddlybits and I can go and explore each other's bodies in some intimate detail with lips, finger, and other appendages natural and otherwise. I'll leave the details for the reader to put in place.

Good night, all.

15 August 2003

Sucking cock . . .
(Posted by **DanglyBits**)

. . . has got to be one of the simple pleasures in life. Twiddlybits certainly enjoys it. It's something I've never done – at least, not for any length of time. I've often lusted for the feeling of that silky skin sliding along my tongue and past my lips, feeling the softhard head gently nudging the back of my throat as I try to take the full length into my mouth. Longed to feel the warm weight of his balls in my hand, feel them contract and draw up as orgasm approaches, feel the spasms of his cock as he groans in ecstasy and fills my mouth with his warm spunk. Cut, uncut – doesn't matter. As long as it's clean and healthy.

I have tasted come once or twice – my own. When I was substantially more youthful I was flexible enough to suck my own cock. I'm not super-well endowed or anything like that, but I was flexible enough to get the head of my cock into my mouth. I loved to feel the slickery wetness of my pre-come and my softhard head on my tongue. I'd contort myself, my back upside-down against a wall – to help me maintain the position required to suck myself – and then stroke my cock until I erupted into my own mouth. It was *so* hot. It wasn't that I didn't have any other sexual outlets – I never went wanting for female company in my youth. I did it, well . . . because I could.

More recently, I tasted my come quite accidentally. My lovely wife, Twiddlybits, was giving me a hand-job while playing with my butthole. She did a masterful job of building the tension until I exploded with a force, the likes of which I hadn't experienced since I was 15. My orgasm was incredibly powerful and wonderful. I shot so hard that I got my face, my mouth, my hair and yes, even the wall beyond the head of the bed. *Wow*. Twiddlybits is amazing for many things, not the least of which are the feelings and physical reactions she elicits from me. I'm a happy man.:-)

The next time I tasted cock was, oh, ten or twelve years ago, now. I had spent the evening with a friend in his workshop. He was driving me home and we got to talking about our fantasies. He was a very close friend, you see, a TV like me, and a few years older than me and we had a number of common interests and likes. Well, one thing led to another and he pulled over on a quiet residential street, pulled the straps of his bodysuit off his shoulders, pushed the torso of it down, and freed his cock from where he had tucked it between his legs. I reached over and stroked it, mesmerized by the sight and feel of a cock other than my own. I couldn't wait to feel it in my mouth. I had to have it. I leaned over and sucked the head into my mouth, reveling in the feel and taste of his hard cock. It was wonderful and we were both enjoying immensely – at least until he decided he needed to play with my cock and kiss me. The playing with my cock I could have dealt with – that felt good and it could have been anyone doing it. It was the kiss that just shut me down, like flicking a switch.

At the time, I was working for a large corporation that had an amazing culture. Part of the internal resources for employees was a collection of on-line discussion forums. The forums covered subjects from integrated circuit engineering to basket weaving to gay/bi life. I was participating in one of the bi/gay forums (because there weren't enough TGs that were brave enough to join a list to create one of our own) and decided to confide to the forum about my experience and feelings. One of the members of the list replied to me that he, even though he was gay, had also had trouble with kissing another man. The sex part was easy – kissing came much harder. I took (and still take) great comfort in knowing that. Perhaps I'm not so weird.

To this day I don't know if it was his stubble, the fact that I knew I was kissing a man, the fact that he had really bad and unattractive teeth, or what – but that kiss really turned me off. Shut me down. Fast. I shriveled like a leaf tossed on a bonfire. From hero to zero in a blink of an eye.

Kissing him might have been different than sucking his cock because I could disassociate, objectify, even, his cock from him while the kiss was very obviously a kiss from a man. Dunno. It was weird. Still and all, that hasn't stopped me from lusting after cocks as sexual things. I'd still love to suck a cock to orgasm, to feel it shoot off in my mouth, to know that I could bring that level of pleasure to another person. (Side note: Even here I'm avoiding using any words that connect a hot, pulsing, silky-hard cock with a man. Interesting) I'd love to feel a real cock in my ass, filling me with its heat and bulk, touching parts of me like they've never been touched before. Stroking in and out, sometimes fast, sometimes slow, always filling me with its hardness, bringing me to orgasm. One of my favourite fantasies is to have a hard cock in my mouth, another hard cock in my ass, and my cock buried to the hilt in Twiddlybits' hot, wet, wonderful pussy. I think I'm mature enough now to deal with the feelings and emotions of samesexplay. I don't think I was when I started sucking my friend that winter's eve. I think I'm capable now of enjoying sharing my body with another man – just so long as he's not hairy. Yech. And no bad teeth or bad breath, either. Pleasant dreams, all.

10 September 2003

An Open Letter to S – or – What I Like About You
(Posted by **TwiddlyBits**)

- I loved seeing the look of sheer delight on your face when I walked into the kitchen wearing nothing but my pink camisole top and black tanga panties
- I loved the way your hands gravitated to my waist to rest on my hips and then on to the small of my back before finding their way down to my ass
- I loved the way you gently (and not-so-gently) bit me between my shoulder and neck – you seemed to know that the more aroused I was, the more not-so-gentle you could be
- I loved that you rubbed against me so I could feel your growing excitement
- I loved the way you set me onto the counter so you could lift my shirt and caress my breasts, sucking and nibbling on my nipples until I moaned
- I loved it when you almost ran to the chair in your eagerness
- I loved it when you helped me out of my panties, tossing them aside
- I loved how you threw your head back in ecstacy when I lowered my dripping wet pussy onto your very hard cock
- I loved the way you held my hips while I ground my clit along your shaft

- I loved the way you ground your hips around, too
- I really loved it when you put your finger in my ass
- I loved coming all over your cock, taking a moment to recover, then doing it again . . . and again
- I loved watching your face when you came
- I loved cuddling with you afterwards, occasionally grinding my hips into yours, rubbing my clit against you, basking in the after-shocks

3 October 2003

Labor Day, Clothing-Optional
(Posted by **TwiddlyBits**)

For Labor Day weekend, Dangly & I went to go visit our good friends A. & S. I told you about our first night there.

The next morning, we all piled into the 4WD Subaru wagon and A & S took us to some clothing-optional hot springs. We needed the 4WD because the trip included 20 miles on "unimproved road" – that 20 miles taking up approx 2 hours. A is an excellent driver and she kept the car not only on the road, but didn't bounce us around any more than necessary, either. Eventually, we pulled over at the wide part of the road and parked. We then had to hike a half mile and ford a river. There is a bridge, but you have to hike 3 miles out of your way to get to it, so we decided just to wade through the water.

That's BRISK, baby!

It was a cool mountain stream, crystal clear & not too deep this time of year. I'm told that it gets colder with snow melt in the spring and can be quite a bit higher and faster (making the bridge not unattractive, I suppose).

On the other side of the river, we continued to hike toward the caretakers' cabin, where we checked in & heard the ground rules. The hot springs are privately owned & they only let 20 people in per day. (S had made reservations for us.) We followed the path up to the springs themselves and chucked our clothes in the cabana before settling into the oh so warm and luxurious water.

The springs have been developed only to the point of making

rock pools in which visitors can lounge. Whoever did it did an excellent job because it looks really natural.

Next to the hot springs is a small, cold stream, also with a small rock pool. Both A & I went dipping in the cold water – the better to appreciate the hot spring!;-)

Anyway, when we got there, there was a nude couple probably in their mid-40s with whom we relaxed & chatted. They seemed like really nice people.

There were also some college-age kids there, including one girl who perched in the uppermost pool in a most regal manner. These kids kept their bathing suits on the entire time. Some of the guys were cute, others weren't, but at least they weren't obnoxious. They didn't chat much with us – maybe we were too old?

Another young man (mid-20s?) joined the group after the couple left. He came up to the pool and put his hands on his swim trunks as if he was going to take them off, but then he saw the college kids with their clothes on & decided to keep his on. Too bad – he was really cute and had "good vibes".

A, S, Dangly & I got out of the hot springs and went over to a big flat rock by the river – the beautiful waterfall! – where we had lunch. It was so wonderful to feel the wind kissing our skin and see the water flow by. After lunch, we headed back to the springs. The college kids had left by this time, leaving just the 4 of us and the mid-20s guy.

A & S went up into the cave portion of the springs, to the upper pool where the girl had held court previously, while Dangly & I and mid-20s guy lounged in the bottom pool. Mid-20s guy was situated such that he couldn't see A & S, but Dangly & I could. A & S started kissing and cuddling – casting amused glances down to where I was watching them with a big grin on my face – and finally A climbed onto S's lap. I watched as she ground her hips into his, riding his delicious cock while he held onto her and kissed and nibbled her ample bosom.

I rolled over onto my stomach so that I could breathe into Dangly's ear while still watching the show. Dangly slid one hand under me and began to finger my clit while asking me if I was enjoying watching them. I said yes I was and that if the mid-20s guy hadn't been *right there*, I'd've climbed onto Dangly's eager cock, too.

It doesn't take much to get me to orgasm & I shuddered several times while watching A & S and being twiddled by Dangly, all right under mid-20s guy's nose.

Of course, I have no real idea if he was aware of it or not, but he made no indication that he was.

Finally, A & S finished & returned to our pool. S's cock doesn't deflate right away after his orgasm, so he was still at half-mast which made me giggle. He put his hands on his hips (which had the effect of pointing his cock in my general direction) and said, "Are you laughing at me?" I assured him that I was, indeed, laughing at him and blew him a kiss.

By this time, it was getting late and we had a long drive back, so A, S & Dangly went to the cabana to get dressed. The cabana isn't so big, so I tarried a bit, making eyes at mid-20s guy. I eventually climbed out of the pool, making sure to give him a good view of my ass as I did it. I then walked over to the clearing by the cabana, still in full view of the pool where he was lying. I then stretched and brushed all the water off of my body in a slow, langurous, sensual way, being sure to caress my body as I did it, bending over from the waist to do my legs. As I caressed my left arm, I cast a glance back over my shoulder and saw him watching me. I smiled and continued what I was doing.

Eventually, I was dry and went into the cabana to get dressed. I had worn my tanga panties that day & so made sure to position myself in the "doorway" of the cabana so mid-20s guy could get an eyeful of them when I put them on. While I was doing that, S expressed his appreciation of them, so I wiggled my ass in his face a little, too. LOL!

Once we were all dressed, I made sure to smile & wave good-bye to mid-20s guy, who grinned back at me most delightfully. We headed down the trial to the caretakers' cabin and took our leave. When we got back to the river, S & Dangly had a mini pissing contest in which they were trying to find a way across the river without getting wet. While they were both trying to impress each other with their rock-hopping abilities, I found a closer, easier way across & made it to the other side first, high & dry. A decided to ford the river again as she wasn't comfortable jumping from rock to rock. We all piled back into the car and headed home.

22 November 2003

Stream of consciousness
(Posted by **TwiddlyBits**)

I love the reverse missionary position.

The way his shaft presses against my clit makes me feel like I'm riding the crest of a tsunami, surfing to ever greater heights of ecstasy as I thrust. I thrust, I thrust my hips over and over again, feeling the waves build, feeling the pressure build, feeling the wonder of being just one giant bundle of nerve endings, my clit growing and pulsing, my clit swelling and I become my clit, my clit surfs the waves, my clit tingles; my clit feels the pressure, the swelling waves, the pounding of the water, the rising of the tide as it builds higher and higher, his shaft pushing harder; I thrust, I thrust, I feel his breath, I feel his heartbeat, I feel his fingers grasp my ass, his legs wrapped around my waist, his breathing becoming more ragged, my breathing coming faster and faster, I thrust, I thrust, I feel the pulsating waves of his orgasm as he holds me tight while he shudders and moans, his pulsing shaft forcing me off my surfboard and into the tidal wave as it breaks on the shore; all is chaos and roiling sea and moans of ecstasy as I clutch at him, holding onto him as if he is the rock that will save me from the pressure of the waves.

Finally I surface and breathe and look at him. He is breathing too. We smile at each other as I slowly thrust my hips a few more times, enjoying the aftershocks the smaller waves that follow the massive one, the ones which kiss the shore gently and easily; we kiss, we kiss, we cuddle, we love.

30 December 2003

Catching up
(Posted by **TwiddlyBits**)

I've been slowly catching up with my blog reading. I had been remiss since nigh about the beginning of December when I got so busy that I started almost literally living in my car. I have updated my Blogroll – removing those blogs which haven't been updated in more than a month & adding some new ones which I hope will turn out to be regular reads for me.

Dangly also pointed out that I have been remiss in another way – I haven't written about our own sexual doings recently. My entry about our interpreter/guide in Asia never mentions it & so it sounds like the entire tour was sexless for us.

Not so!

Dangly & I enjoyed quite a few nights of sexual fun – damn, but those Japanese know how to build hotel room beds, don't they? Not a one of them went *bang, bang, bang,* they were all solidly fastened to the wall! And, can I just say *ooooooohhhhh* about Japanese bathtubs? I love taking baths anyway, but when the tub is actually long enough for my legs and deep enough to cover me all the way up, I simply want to moan in orgasmic delight. Combine that with a loving husband, and I discovered that I wanted to stay away for another week!

Things have not been quiet since we returned, either. Let me tell you about Friday night. Dangly had scored some really good seats at a hockey game (being Canadian, he likes that sort of thing, eh?) so he treated me to my first one! It was fun and enlightening (let's just say that I have a new-found respect for football, and leave it at that, OK?), but afterwards we walked over to Dangly's office because the building was scheduled to have the power shut off on Saturday afternoon & Dangly needed to turn off all the computers and office equipment before that happened.

So, he disappeared into the computer room while I entertained myself by wandering the halls, looking at artwork. Not being a very patient sort, I got bored and went to the back to see how Dangly was doing. Turns out he was just finishing up. It was cold in there, so we cuddled a bit, which turned into a make-out session, which turned into a petting session and, before too long, I was on my knees with his lovely cock in my mouth, trying not to touch him with my cold hands (and yet sneaking touches in just to play with the contrasting sensations of hot mouth & cold fingers). Along the way, my shirt was lifted and Dangly's roaming fingers found my braless nipples. I paused for a moment to lament the fact that I hadn't worn a skirt that day. A little while later, I paused again to tell him that I was trying to make a decision. He asked me what the decision was & I replied that I was trying to decide whether to pull my pants down & bend over so he could fuck me right there or if I wanted to wait until we got home so we could do all the other things

I wanted to do, too. After all, I do carry lube with me and there is a handy shower room across the hall from his office . . .

I made my decision – we would wait until we got home to go any further because there were things we just couldn't do in the office that we could do at home. Reluctantly, yet expectantly, we buttoned up and headed out into the night.

Upon arriving home, Dangly undressed me slowly, just the way I like it, then went and got a straight-backed chair to put in front of the bedroom full-length mirror. I got out the lube while he fetched a towel, which he positioned on the chair before sitting down. I lubed up his rockhard shaft while he caressed my breasts and twiddled my nipples. Then I turned around, bent over and applied the lube to my ass, while seductively waving it in Dangly's face. He obliged by grabbing my cheeks and planting several adoring kisses on them. Finally, I slowly lowered my ass onto his cock, savoring the sight of his face in the mirror as I did so.

It had been a while since we have done any anal play, so it took a little bit of time before I was relaxed enough to let him pull my hips down and bury himself full-length in my ass. I planted my feet firmly on the ground between his and put my hands on my knees while moving my ass up and down on his pole, really making sure he got a good show and could see how much I was enjoying myself.

Next, it was time to add toys to the equation! I spread my legs so my feet were now on the outside of Dangly's, then took my waterproof Nubby G vibe on medium vibration and slowly rubbed it along my labia, touching my clit and peeking its head into my cunt until I had had a couple of small orgasms, then I buried it all the way in and turned the vibe up to full strength, stroking it in and out of my vag in time to my gyrations on Dangly's cock.

With it buried deep in my bijou, I reached for my waterproof G Candy vibe (full strength!) and held that onto my clit as I almost literally saw stars from coming so hard. I'm sure I made noise, too; I know I was trembling when I came down.

Exhausted, I told Dangly that I didn't have the strength to continue in this position, so, still coupled, we moved to the corner of the bed and he proceeded to fuck me like nobody's business until he had a shuddering orgasm which caused me to come again, too.

After cuddling for a little while, we hopped into the shower and cleaned up before snuggling up together in bed.

postscript: There is one advantage to jetlag's effect of keeping you awake at odd hours and that is this – Saturday night, we found ouselves unable to sleep. While spooning, I wiggled my butt into Dangly's lap and sighed happily. I thanked him again for the fun we had Friday night & felt his cock start to grow as he ground into me. Not being one to waste an opportunity like this, I positioned myself to guide his shaft into my pussy and we fucked for a while in spoon position before switching over to reverse-missionary (which we both love!) and finally into standard missionary before we both came and then were finally able to get to sleep.

3 February 2004

[insert pithy title here]
(Posted by **TwiddlyBits**)

I'm on my period again this week, so y'all know what that means, right? *It's Anal Sex time! Yaaaay!* Long-time readers of this blog will remember that, while anal sex is not limited to when I'm menstruating, Dangly & I are both happy to explore this avenue of sexual pleasure a bit more during that time. Last night was no exception.

We started out in the office, Dangly at his computer & me at mine, reading email, visiting web sites, engaging in just general surfing. I was naked because I had been working with bleach earlier & didn't want to get any on my clothing *like I need an excuse to be naked?*. I turned to Dangly & asked if I could sit on him. He turned his chair to give me access & I straddled him. We held each other tightly and his warm hands caressed my skin as I held his head to my chest.

His lips found one of my nipples and my head fell back as I softly moaned in pleasure. He held me with one arm while his other hand played with my other nipple. I writhed in his lap, rubbing my cunt along his pants, and found his nipples through his shirt. He gasped as I squeezed them between my fingers. I grinned as we kissed passionately and he moved his hand from my nipple to my slit from behind. I stood up to give him better access and pulled his mouth to my breast. I don't know exactly what it is he does with his teeth and tongue, but I do know that it makes my pussy tingle. Combine that with him touching me there and I'm a puddle.

This went on for several minutes as our hands and mouths roamed over each other's bodies. Finally, I bade him stand up & lowered his pants and panties, then had him sit again. I positioned myself between his knees and took his cock into my mouth, my hands moving up his chest to fondle his nipples. As my tongue swirled around his glans and up and down his shaft, I pinched his nipples hard as he moaned, gasped and brought his hands to my head to run his fingers through my hair. I put one hand onto his shaft to hold back his foreskin so I could have unfettered access to his crown and frenulum, my tongue dancing this way and that. My nails scampered over his skin as I brought my other hand down to cradle his balls and play with his perineum.

I raised myself up to kiss him on the mouth, stopping at his chest to nibble for a bit – he pantingly asked me to suck his nipple HARD, which I did as he held my head to him. We kissed for a while longer, then I went and got a towel while he brought the chair into the bedroom & placed it facing the mirror.

He went over to the Toy Box to get the lube and our "Mr Ripple" toy. He squeezed some lube out onto his hand and smeared it all over the toy and his own asshole, then bent slightly forward as he maneuvered it into his ass, the ripples sliding in one at a time, bump-de-bump, and I held his face and kissed him, nibbling on his lips. Once it was in, he wiped the lube off his hands and sat in the chair. Now it was my turn to lube. I slathered it into and around my asshole, then onto his cock. I turned around so that my back was to Dangly & I was facing the mirror. I put my legs over his, my feet on the outside, to give myself some support as I lowered myself onto his shaft. As his cockhead entered my ass, I raised up a little to slide it back out, then in again a little more, then back out, until it was in far enough that I could stop and let myself relax.

As my hole relaxed, I lowered myself completely onto his pole, wrapped my feet around his legs and levered myself up and down. His hands came around and played with my breasts and nipples while my own hands were busy with my labia and clit. My eyes, half-open, watched it all in the mirror – I could see Dangly with his eyes closed, his head back, a look of pure enjoyment on his face, while my own face showed a similar expression of ecstasy. I smiled to see us so passionate. I laughed as well, when I saw my body reflected in the mirror and thought to myself, *Damn! I'm looking GOOD!*

Then orgasm overtook Dangly and he squeezed my tight, holding me onto his shaft as he convulsed. I rubbed my cunt and crested my own wave, then we sat there, still joined, enjoying the afterglow until his cock came out of me on its own. Then we showered and cleaned up and got ready for bed.

5 February 2004

Hump Day Fun
(Posted by **TwiddlyBits**)

After sitting here reading sex blogs all day yesterday, I was pretty damn horny by the time Dangly got home from work. I had already played once during the day – using my G Candy vibe on my clit (batteries were running low; I've since put new ones in) and my Pink Pal ex-vibe-now-a-dildo in my ass – but had worked myself up into a pretty good lather again by early evening.

When I met Dangly at the door, I was wearing my new black microfiber & lace thong with a new tight, TIGHT sweater-style shirt over a black bra that matches the thong. The top was unbuttoned down to just below my breasts and, when you stand to my left, you see just the perfect amount of skin. Combined with a bold necklace and matching earrings, it's quite a fetching *ensemble*.

I smiled and stood in front of Dangly as he put down his briefcase and took off his jacket. He smiled at me and commented, "You look very sleek today!" "Do I?" "Yes, indeed," then he held out his arms and I stepped into them and rubbed my sleek self over his still-clothed body while he cupped my ass in his hands. I stepped back and handed him the keys to the mailbox & he dutifully went out to retrieve the day's post. When he got back, he was subjected to an even warmer greeting from me. He took off his shoes & went to go get cleaned up while I attended to dinner. After seeing that it was proceeding nicely, I went back to the bedroom to chat with him while he changed clothes. I hugged him & he picked me up and threw me onto the bed, then buried his face in my crotch and pretended to gnaw on me through my undies. Then, he turned away to continue getting dressed!

"Tease!" I accused and lightly kicked his ass with my foot. He laughed! I rolled off the bed & stomped my foot. He turned around, genuinely surprised. "What's wrong?" I protested, "I'm about to crawl out of my skin & you're teasing me!" He laughed again & sat down on the bed, drawing me in to stand between his knees. "Aw, has my wife been reading porn all day and now she's horny?" "Yes," I pouted while he rubbed his face between my breasts and ran his hands over my hips, thighs and ass. "Well, maybe we can do something about that after supper," he soothed. "I sure hope so!" I replied before leaving to go finish dinner.

After dinner, I got the towel out so that Dangly could shave me. He got the electric razor, blotted me dry with a tissue (otherwise the razor "sticks" to my skin), then shaved me so ultra smooth – I really love that freshly shaved feeling. Along the way, the vibrations of the razor were having an effect on me – much more than they usually do – and I had a few small orgasms. He reversed the razor, putting the handle on my clit & I just about hit the ceiling. His eyes opened wide with surprise – I had never reacted quite so, well, "violently" before. When he was done, he held my labia apart with his fingers and concentrated his tongue and teeth on my clit until I was shuddering. Then he sent me to the shower to rinse off. After rinsing, he inspected his work and pronounced it good.

A little while later, I was sitting on his lap kissing him and he asked, "Do you want me to nibble on your pussy for a while?" I enthusiastically replied, "Yes!" and he carried me back to the bedroom and laid me gently on the bed, then kneeled down between my legs and took my bijou in his mouth.

I have to tell you, this was one of the best episodes of oral sex that I've ever had – and Dangly's provided a number of stellar performances! I was moaning and writhing and bucking my cunt against his face – you could almost say I was fucking his face, holding his head closer, closer and tighter to me. Finally, his tongue was dancing on my magic spot and I was desperately holding him tight, begging him not to stop, ordering him not to dare stop what he was doing and I didn't sail, I *rocketed* over the edge of the abyss, all circuits firing, fireworks exploding in my head.

As I collapsed back onto the bed, he lapped at my clit a few more times, slow long strokes with his tongue. He got no reaction from me because my circuit breakers had tripped and he could have done anything to me at all and I probably wouldn't have felt it at all, not until the breakers had had a chance to reset anyway. He knows this and continues the long slow strokes until he *does* get a reaction; that's when he knows that it's OK to proceed.

He crawled up my body to kiss my lips. I hungrily licked my juices from his chin, cheeks and lips. We smiled at each other & I thanked him for the wonderful orgasm. He stood up again and showed me his huge erection, pushing against his sweat pants. "Mmm, impressive," I said as I reached out to stroke it.

He took off his shirt & pants and I took his cock into my mouth, pulling back the foreskin to run my tongue over his reddening-to-purple glans. He moaned when I started fingering one of his nipples and used the other hand to grip his shaft, pumping up and down in time with my mouth, while my tongue danced around his crown.

After a little while of this, my jaw was tiring (Alex is right, a large cock like Dangly's can be tiring to suck for any length of time – not that I don't enjoy trying!), so I told him, "Stay right there," and got up to get some lube so I could finish with a hand job. I had just pumped a portion of Slippery Stuff into my hand and was turning around to return when Dangly said, "Why don't you get out the harness?" I stopped & looked at him, my hand full of lube. He grinned and said, "Well, then why don't *I* get out the harness?" He came around to the Toy Box and found the harness and selected the Kozmo vibe. I asked him to use the waterproof bullet vibe in it – not only are the vibrations nice, but the Kozmo's cavity needs to be filled with something or else it bends too easily for what we were going to do.

He inserted the bullet vibe and selected an appropriately sized sized O ring and assembled the harness. Not wanting my handful of lube to go to waste, I took hold of his cock and started stroking it, "Just to keep you interested," I said. "Uh-huh," he answered as he tried to concentrate on the task at hand. At one point, he winced and said, "If you keep doing that, I won't be able to finish this." His cock head was *very* purple, the foreskin was very tight and his balls were drawn up all the way to the base of his shaft. I could see that he was quite aroused and very close to the edge.

I let go of his cock and wiped my hand off on the towel (still there from shaving). He held out the harness for me to step into and we adjusted the straps to fit around my hips and waist. He built up a small platform with pillows and laid on his back on the bed, his legs drawn up. I turned on the vibe, then got some more lube and applied it to the Kozmo's head and shaft, then got some more and applied that to Dangly's asshole. I used my thumb to work some in and gently rubbed the whole perineal area to help relax him.

I got into position on my knees between his legs and pressed the head of my "cock" against his hole, applying gentle but firm pressure until the head went in. Dangly winced a little and I pulled it all the way back out, giving him a moment to recover. When he was ready, I repeated this, pulling it out again. The third time, once it was in, I stayed in and Dangly encouraged me to keep pushing until it was all the way in. (I have to do the same thing with his cock when I take it in the ass, too.) I took his cock and balls in my hands as I thrust my hips, pumping in and out of his ass.

He began shuddering and after just a moment asked me to stop playing with his cock and "just fuck me for a while", so I did. I leaned forward, placing my hands on either side of his chest and thrust, hoping the angle was right & that I wasn't hurting him and wouldn't flop out. Apparently I wasn't (and didn't flop out, either), as he seemed to be completely overwhelmed with pleasure, a faint smile on his face, his eyes scrinched up tight, opening occasionally to look at me.

Is this how he feels watching me when he fucks me? I thought to myself. There have been times when I've opened my eyes to see him almost studying me, then smiling when he realises I'm looking at him. It was interested to see this happen in reversed roles.

The tops of my thighs started to hurt, so I resumed my kneeling position and again started playing with his cock and balls. This time he didn't stop me and I was amazed at how *tight* his balls were; it was almost as if they'd completely disappeared and joined with his shaft. I also played with the ridge along his perineum, which he seemed to enjoy. I rubbed his cockhead and Dangly started convulsing in orgasm, shooting his load into a neat puddle on his own stomach. He flinched a little as I continued to stroke his crown and shaft, then settled down. After a few moments, I removed the dildo from his ass and wiped my hands off on the towel again.

I leaned down to kiss him, my "cock" bumping his ass, and got some of his come on my own belly. I stood up and gave him some tissue to wipe up his puddle as I wiped off the vibe before taking it out of the harness. Dangly rolled over (a backward somersault – he is *so* flexible!) off the bed and headed for the shower. I stopped at the sink to wash the dildo and then joined him.

LOL! It took a team effort to get that bullet vibe out of the Kozmo, but we eventually did it. After putting everything away, we got into our bedclothes and cuddled for a little while before going back to the office to surf for a while before bed.

This is only the 2nd time in our 3 year relationship that we've done it this way (although we've tried one or two other times). I admit that it's fascinating to watch him as I thrust – and his cock & balls are *right there* and so easy to play with while doing it! I *thoroughly* enjoy seeing him react to what's going on as I concentrate on the unfamiliar-to-me motions, even if I don't climax myself (which I didn't, although the vibrations from the bullet vibe are transmitted nicely to me via the harness as it presses on my pubic bone).

If I hadn't still been on my period, we would have used the Feeldoe double-dildo, probably with a cock ring for vibration. Maybe next time?

5 March 2004

Cunnilingus . . .
(Posted by **TwiddlyBits**)

. . . having a box lunch at the Y, canyon yodeling, carpet munching, clam diving, having dinner beneath the bridge, dipping the brush, doing it the French way, donning the beard, drinking at the fuzzy cup, eating a kipper pie, face fucking, practicing the French arts, having a fur burger with a side of thighs, indulging in gamahuche, going way down South in Dixie, growling at the badger, kneeling at the altar, performing labial titillation, licking the beaver, making mouth music, muff diving, mumbling in the moss, ocean pinking, parting the fuzz, playing in the sandbox, pug noshing, pussy-nibbling, shrimping, speaking in tongues, talking to the canoe driver, tipping the velvet, whistling in the dark, worshipping at the altar, or yodeling up the valley, *whatever* you want to call it, *I LOVE IT*!!!

Last night, as it was time to retire, Dangly sat on the edge of the bed to undress me, as is our regular custom. *Honestly, you can't expect a pampered princess like me to undress herself, can you?* I had worn a pair of tanga panties because he recently told me that he thinks they're sexier than thongs – something about the way the fabric hugs the curve of my ass. I gave him a good show while wearing them, rubbing my ass along his chest and down onto his crotch, his hands caressing my bottom, never staying still. I knew I was sopping wet when he removed my panties, so I sat in his lap, facing away from him and encouraged his hands to wander.

His fingers dipped into the well and spread my dew around, his other hand toying with my nipple while he gently breathed in my ear. I was shuddering in orgasmic delight in no time, bucking against his body.

I stood up and turned around to face him, straddling him, kneeling on the bed. I grabbed his head and thrust my nipple into his mouth. He obliged by gently biting and sucking it, one arm wrapping around my body to reach my cunt, the other hand pinching my other nipple while I whimpered and gasped.

Eventually, he ended up with his face between my legs, earnestly tonguing my clit, holding on for dear life as my hips gyrated beneath him. I don't know what the hell it is he does down there, but if his technique could be bottled, there'd be lots of happy women out there, lost in the bliss of orolabial stimulation. He should teach classes which all men should be required to attend.

Needless to say, I ended the night happily exhausted, my circuit breakers tripped, barely able to speak coherently enough to say "thank you".

I am a happy woman indeed.

5 April 2004

*Details . . . details! (a very long entry about my very first
DP experience)*
(Posted by **TwiddlyBits**)

Where do I even begin to tell you about Saturday night??

After I posted my **A little nervous . . .** entry, I had a beer to help calm my nerves.

TwiddlyBits' intoxication level: mild

F arrived pretty near the time he said he would and the 3 of us sat down for dinner – grilled T-Bone steaks topped with mushrooms sautéed in butter with garlic and a Caprisi-style salad of fresh Roma tomatoes with Mozzarella Fresca, homemade pesto and a touch of balsamic vinegar. Served with some BV Coastal Merlot that F brought with him, it was a fine feast. *(Nobody can say I don't feed my men well, eh?)*

TwiddlyBits' intoxication level: medium

After dinner, we debated going to sit in the hot tub, but decided against it because the high chlorine content would necessitate a shower and our shower's not big enough for 3. No prob. We took the 2nd bottle of wine into the living room & sat down to chat a bit, me snuggling up on the couch next to F. F asked a few questions about Dangly's cross-dressing and then the conversation turned to our first meeting a couple of weeks ago. F asked, "So what happens on the 2nd meeting?" I replied, "Anything we want!" He then asked, "Are we talking about double penetration?" I blushed and said, "Yeah. It's something I've wanted to do for a long time." Dangly & F chatted a bit about who goes where – my contribution being pretty much limited to "But where do you put your legs?" – and after some more talk of logistics, F said, "Great! Let's go do it!" and we all tromped off into the bedroom, me carrying the bottle of wine.

TwiddlyBits' intoxication level: medium-high

F is 27 years old, about my height, with short dark hair and intense eyes. He has smooth, warm skin, soft lips and a gentle touch. His enthusiasm and forthrightness were both a little surprising (to me) and quite contagious.

Once in the bedroom, Dangly & F stripped down to their undies & I removed my jeans, leaving me in just the camisole I had been wearing and matching tanga panties. I removed my big dangly earrings so they wouldn't get caught in anything and stretched across the bed. Seeing my 16 oz. bottle of Slippery Stuff on the nightstand, F asked, "Wow. You get that at Costco or something?" LOL!

He laid on the bed across my legs and I rubbed his back a bit while nibbling on his arms and shoulders (which are *quite* nicely formed, I might add – I'm definitely an arm-and-shoulder girl!) and Dangly, naked, laid down where he could caress my legs. F got up to remove his underwear and then reached to remove my tangas and camisole. I laid back down and Dangly took one nipple in his mouth, flicking it with his tongue and gently nibbling. I gasped in pleasure as F laid down and first kissed me, then began sucking my other nipple, his hand wandering down to my pussy. He dipped a finger into my wetness – and it was not "moist" or "damp" but downright WET – and he raised his head to exclaim, "It's pierced!" I laughed and said, "Yes, pierced and shaved . . ." but that's all I managed to say before he touched my clit again and I was clenching in several small introductory orgasms. F quipped, "I don't think you really need the lube, you know." I countered with, "Well, personal dryness has never been a problem of mine. But the lube is useful for other things." He nodded his agreement with that.

F raised up onto his knees and said, "Can I put a condom on now?" I said, "Most certainly!" and reached over and got a polyurethane (non-latex – I'm allergic) condom out of the box, opened the packet and gently unrolled it down his shaft, following my hand with my mouth, caressing his cock head with my tongue.

[Aside: Dangly & I did some experimentation this past week with the polyurethane condoms. He said that oral sex with the condom on is still good – he feels the warmth, the pressure and the suction – but the texture of my tongue, lips and mouth is missing. I'd be interested to hear other people's experiences with condom use in oral sex, so please comment!]

F lay down on his back and gently pulled me over to him. I straddled him and we gently guided his eager cock into my drenched pussy. He reached under my arms and grabbed my shoulders, thrusting up into me a few times while I hovered over him. I laughed and gently chided him, "You're not waiting for Dangly!" He said, breathlessly, "I am! I am waiting! Oh, you're *so* wet!" Dangly, meanwhile, had gotten a handful of lube and had slathered it all over his own cock and on my ass. He straddled F's legs and gently prodded at my back door, slipping his cockhead gently in. F asked, "Is he in? What's he doing?" I said, "He's putting it in now." As Dangly's cock slid into me, I gasped and my asshole clenched. Dangly took his cock back out. They both asked me, "Are you OK?" "Yes, I'm OK, it's OK, put it back in!", I answered as my ass relaxed. Dangly put his cock back in me and . . .

. . . and the next few moments are a blur. I have a rush of images that flicker through my mind, but no coherent time-line. I remember an incredible feeling of fullness, the sensation of both cocks sliding in and out, the wonderful friction, smoothed by my pussy's copious juices, the feeling of F's hands on my shoulders while Dangly's hands were on my hips, both holding me while they thrust. I remember my own thrusting, driving myself onto their cocks, impaling myself on them, feeling as if I just couldn't get enough, that this feeling should never end, it was so wonderful. I grunted and squealed and screamed in pleasure, incoherent, beyond words, overwhelmed as the sensations washed over me, drowning me in a flood of orgasmic delight.

Dangly withdrew his cock. F asked, "Are you coming?" Dangly replied, "No, I'm just exhausted," from holding that position. F and I continued fucking like this for a little bit while I reached over and caressed Dangly's hip. He took one of my nipples in his fingers and pinched it lightly. By this time, my own hips were beginning to tire so I asked F if we could switch positions. He agreed and I held his shoulders with my hands and his hips with my knees as we scooted, then rolled over so that he was on top. He growled as he continued his thrusting and I laughed with pleasure at his enthusiasm. I reached over and held Dangly's hand as the ever more powerful orgasms gripped me, making me scream, my legs in the air, my hips convulsing, my pussy clenching. After a particularly large orgasm on my part, F thrust into me one last time, gasping and grunting as he came.

F withdrew and settled back on his knees. I removed his condom and threw it away, then reached for some tissues to wipe off his cock. He lay back down on top of me, exhausted, but happy. He grinned at Dangly and they both agreed that that was pretty hot and a whole helluva lot of fun! I thanked him and he thanked us. We laughingly chatted a bit more, caught up in the post-orgasmic feelings of bliss. Eventually, F said he had to leave, so he put his clothes back on and I escorted him to the door. More hugs and kisses ensued and he headed off into the night.

I turned and nearly leapt into Dangly's arms, holding him tightly, thanking him for the wonderful gift he had given me. He held me tightly, kissed me and said, "C'mon, let's go shower." He turned the shower on & then went back into the bedroom to remove his own jewelry. I poured more wine into my glass, drank it and sighed with happiness. What a great night this was turning out to be!

We went into the bathroom & got into the shower. My legs were really shaky, so my main job seemed to be holding up the shower walls. Dangly washed us and dried us as we got out of the tub. I hugged him, kissed him deeply, then took his hand and led him back into the bedroom.

TwiddlyBits' intoxication level: high

My fire was really lit by this time & I was *exceedingly* horny! What follows is an account of my fiendishness – I'm always a sex fiend, but not quite always this extreme.

I laid down on the bed, pulling Dangly on top of me. His stiff cock found its way into my waiting pussy and we made love until he shuddered and came. After washing up again, Dangly decided to change the sheets on the bed (miscellaneous stains from the evening's activities) and while he did that, I leaned against the wall and masturbated frantically, crying out with each orgasm. Dangly grabbed my G Candy vibe and tossed it over to me then went back to changing out the pillowcases. As he took the sheets to the laundry room & put them in the washer, I got on the bed and decided that one vibe wasn't enough. I got out my water-proof Nubbly G vibe and held the Candy onto my clit while clenching the Nubbly in my pussy. Dangly came back to the bedroom to put some clothes on so he could go put the cover back on the grill. While he did that, I slipped the Nubbly into my ass and the Candy into my pussy and molested my clit with my fingers. When he came back, he looked at me and said, "Where have you got those?" I spread my legs to show him & he came around the side of the bed to kiss me. I pleaded, "Pinch my nipples!" and he complied, holding me as I orgasmed again and again. Eventually, the madness passed and I settled back into the afterglow. After a bit, I got up to wash myself and my toys.

TwiddlyBits' intoxication level: very high

Dangly & I got into bed, snuggled a little bit & turned off the light. I kissed him and thanked him again and rubbed my clit against his leg, which started me off again. I climbed on top of him and put his cock in me, riding up and down in a frenzy. We got into the reverse missionary position but my intoxication conspired against me and my coordination was such that I just couldn't make it work. We rolled over and Dangly plunged his cock into my pussy again and again until I had another loud screaming orgasm. He collapsed on me, both of us exhausted and we fell asleep.

So there you have it. Not only did it not hurt, but it was so incredibly good that I passed into a sexual frenzy the likes of which I have rarely experienced. I am still having aftershock orgasms thinking about it all as I write this. I think I might have to go play.

I have to change my **AFF** profile from "DP is a big fantasy of mine" to "DP is one of my all-time favorite activities!" I definitely want to do that as often as possible.

I expected to be sore the next day. I expected the skin between my vag and asshole to be irritated. Nope, neither of those happened. Not only am I not sore, but I feel great! (I was a wee bit hung over yesterday.) Dangly did say that next time, I should try it without the alcohol. He said, "While you're never a bad lay, you're better when you're sober." That's probably true and I will heed his advice, but I was awfully nervous that night!

I told F that I really hoped that didn't turn into a one-night stand. He's a nice guy, very funny, a very good lover and I think we have great chemistry together. I'm perfectly happy to be on his booty-call list – he can call me any time he wants!

25 June 2004

Tell Me Again . . . ?
(Posted by **TwiddlyBits**)

"I'm coming in to sit on you, so get ready!" I called.

I discarded my jeans and T-shirt in the bedroom and wandered into the study where DanglyBits was working on his computer. Per my request, he had pushed in his keyboard tray and pushed out his chair a bit so that I had access to his lap. He smiled as I straddled him, rubbing myself against the crotch of his jeans. He sighed happily as he buried his face between my breasts and cupped my ass in his hands.

I reached behind my back to unfasten my bra then dropped it over the back of the chair. I stood up just a little to give his mouth access to my nipples which were already nearly painfully hard with anticipation. His hands found my pussy as his teeth & tongue flicked over those "pretty pink spigots".

Taking his head in my hands, I kissed him passionately. I stood up and took his hand in mine. "Come with me," I said, leading him to the bedroom.

I leaned over lasciviously, my butt thrust into the air, to take off my panties. Dangly moaned and caressed me. I turned around and helped him take off his pants and panties, then kneeled in front of him, taking his beautiful cock into my mouth and molesting it with my tongue. He groaned in pleasure and gently touched my head, running his fingers through my hair.

With his dick still firmly entrenched in my mouth, I steered him over to sit on the bed, positioning myself between his thighs and rubbing my breasts on his upper legs. "I love having you all warm and wiggly between my legs," he whispered as I continued my ministrations.

I climbed up onto the bed and positioned my cunt over his shaft, then impaled myself upon it. His face telegraphed his enjoyment of the sensations as I planted my hands on either side of his head, pushed my knees a bit back and proceeded to ride him like a cowgirl on a bucking bronco. I had to stop periodically to let the orgasms wash over me, clenching his cock in my pussy and crying out my pleasure. I tired, so he rolled me over, taking the lead and pounding into me fast and furious as I clung to him, urging him on, bucking against him myself, my legs high in the air and toes curling. After a while, my hips tired, so I lowered my legs, trapping his cock not only in my pussy, but anchored between my thighs as well. His tempo slowed to draw out the sensation of his shaft rubbing full-length across my swollen clit, in and out, drawing moans and gasps from me as I writhed beneath him.

After several orgasms, a stitch developed in my side and I told him to roll over as I reached for a handful of lube. I took his cock in my hands and rubbed it, holding his foreskin down out of the way with one hand while the other swirled about his nearly purple glans. He convulsed and twitched and groaned, grasping at my waist. Two more applications of lube before he drew his knees up almost to his chest and I felt his cock warm and swell then pulse as it shot his hot come into my hand. "Tell me again why we don't do this every night?" he asked.

In other news, the report from my gynecologist is that all the tests came up negative, so I officially have a Pristine White Pussy.

Sweetness Follows

Mike & Michelle

http://www.no-undies.net

Monday 2 December 2002

Why I like MSN

Instant Messengers rule. They really do.

This is something Michelle and I do sometimes, her not being allowed to wear panties with skirts anymore, though this morning she dressed fast and didn't have a chance to get into some stockings.

Also sad is that she'll be busy with meetings most of the day, because I usually get her to come at work, skirt pulled up and fingers in her cunt, spanking her clit with a ruler every so often.

But today she's busy, so I'll tease her, and tonight it'll pay off.

And I've never met anyone as sexy and downright horny as her in my life.

Wow, this blog is gonna be the world's biggest over share.
Mike

Sunday 22 December 2002

Kids, Wal-Mart has beads!

Well, right now she's lying on the bed, sort of sore, more along the lines of well used, her tits, ass, cunt, all sore.

We spanked her, took pictures, and fucked hard, things in her ass, and beads.

Beads from Wal-Mart, Christmas decorations to be exact, tied into knots, 3 of them, and in her ass, and then pulled out.

Course first we started with a candy cane, melting and sweet tasting, one in the nether part, 4 smaller ones in her pussy, along with a bigger one, and picking random ones and fucking with them.

I love her, so so much, and I'm so lucky, and I can't stay and type, I have better things to do.

Mike

Tuesday 7 January 2003

Back from as holidays, with

Back from as holidays, with lots to tell, but hmmm . . . how much to actually tell.

Well, a highlight. Using the gear from that adventure kit, having the beads in her pussy, then the lil' vibe that fits into the ribbed anal thingy in there too (wrapped in a bunch of saran wrap so we could pull it out afterward), and her big wand vibrator up over her clit, and the small pocket rocket looking rig on her clit, both vibes rubbing. T'was a bit intense. Then there's us doing DP both ways, once with that green anal vibe in her bum, with my cock in her, then me fucking her ass, slowly and with about half, then her dildo inside her . . . golly golly golly.

But my favorite moment, that was tonight. Music playing, something soft and slow, and me behind her and just holding her close, swaying to the music, then touching her, the whole thing is slow motion, eventually tasting her, then her toy in her, fucking her slower while I licked her, pussy spread wide. Then just making love, tender and normal and so sweet.

We're both well, we like it all, and some nights we need to be kinky and crazy, and other nights we keep it simple, and simply wallow in the pleasure we give each other.

And yes, I love her, and I say it a lot, but it feels so good.

My last relationship ended badly, with me being cheated on for a while, and finding out through other people. We'd gotten to a point where condoms didn't seem necessary, and after there was the hurt and the betrayal, and the fear of being infected.

So, really, I wasn't feeling very dateable, and was quite happy to be single for awhile. And then Michelle came along, and with no warning kicked down all the doors, and is just . . . I don't know, I could degenerate further into cliché I guess. I just love her so much, in a time when I thought love would not be part of my life for quite some time.

OK, done for now, need to sleep.

Goodnight possums.

Mike

Tuesday 28 January 2003

Arts and Crafts

We're not at summer camp, boys and girls . . .

I haven't actually been to the site Mike's talking about, simply for the fact that I haven't had much time. In my mind, Mike is giving me everything that I need, and anyway, I don't have much time now, either. Last night was me getting out my hot glue gun, and glueing two clothespins together end to end. So that the clampy part of one faced one way, and the other faced the other way. If this makes any sense whatsoever, you have a better imagination than I do, or I have a better word sense than I thought.

I had no clue what it was for, until he had me stand in front of him, lift up my shirt, and clamp one end onto one nipple, push my tits together, and clamp the other one onto the other nipple. It HURT . . . but we're discovering that pain can dance on the knife edge with pleasure and most of the time they're whirling together so quickly that you can't tell where one begins and the other one ends.

He did spank me for a long time last night . . . so much so that I'm still walking a bit stiffly today and there were still a few marks on me this morning. Funny how I like that.

Welts . . . like reminders of last night. Mmmmm.

Michelle

Wednesday 29 January 2003

Where did Martha Stewart go?

I am a very stubborn girl. Just very stubborn. I love what Mike and I do together. I love it. But I'm also kind of frightened of it sometimes. Overwhelmed. I am a very independent person. I want to be me. I don't want my personality taken over. I don't want to give myself up just to become Slave. And I think deep down I've been fearing all that. Losing myself. Not being able to make decisions for myself. At the same time He knows what I need. He knows what is too much. I trust him completely. And it's all consensual. It's all safe. It's because we love each other so much that we can do this without freaking out all the time. I have so much responsibility at work. I have so many people I need to be in charge of all day long. It is nice to have someone take charge of me once in a while.

Last night, he decided that limits were going to be pushed. And boy were they. At first I asked if we could just be gentle and non-kink and everything. That's both of our favorite as much as we talk about being all dominant/submissive whatever; we both love just making love. Slowly and with no boundaries, no limitations, no titles. Before we started he said you know if you need anything, just ask if you all of a sudden want to be dominated, call me Master, and I'll know. Other than that, we're just making love, baby, and that's perfect do what you want, come when you want, I won't tell you what to do or anything beyond normal. It was wonderful. Intense.

But something funny: I love knowing that he wants me to come. Usually he says something like Come for me, baby whether or not we're being D/s y. Actually when he's being my Master he doesn't, he just says Come slave but you know what I mean. Last night, he wasn't saying it. And I guess subconsciously I was waiting. And I kept asking him Please, Mike Baby, you don't need to ask. Do what you want. I want to come. Well, why aren't you coming? You didn't need to ask about it. Got very frustrated and finally came out with I need you to be my Master! Well, then, come, my little slave, let your slutty little pussy come. I screamed so loudly, I'd been holding back so long, I bet the neighbors are ready to have us evicted.

After that it was time for me to be punished, because I hadn't let my Master know what I needed, so I was keeping him from doing his job. Was spanked, extremely hard. And had to count them off generally when he's spanking me, it's not SO hard. He knows how to make it hurt, but feel good. And when I count them off, when they're not punishment, I say one, sir, two, sir etc. Last night, because it was punishment and because I was a bad little slut, I was to say One, Master, two, master. Managed to get to about 9 before I slipped up and said sir instead of Master. That meant starting back at one. He got in about thirty really hard smacks on my ass and pussy before I couldn't stand it anymore and asked him to stop. Please Mike, no more. Slap. Mike, I mean it. I can't do this anymore. Slap. I think I like testing him. I'm like a little kid. In the past when I've said those things he has stopped, and that's fine. We've never had to use our safe word. Last night, there was no way he was stopping, until I finally screamed it, until I finally broke down and did what I was supposed to and said the word that could make him stop.

And that's how it's supposed to be. Afterward we made love and it was gentle and loving and good and this morning I was woken up with caresses and kisses and BREAKFAST IN BED, and I love this man so much, I can't imagine what things were like before him. Michelle

Friday 31 January 2003

Last night . . .

Last night was a bit on the surprising side to say the least. As Michelle said, she isn't so forward like that. T'was a wonderful surprise.

It helped with how horny she was – just insanely horny. I licked her and she sucked me, we used her toys on her, and we fucked and fucked and fucked.

And then she surprised me again.

"I want my dildo in my ass."

We've been working up to that, getting her ready to be fucked, and have an anal toy with a vibe and bumps. But well, she craves more.

The problem with the dildo is that it's bumpy. It's a nice silicone dildo for fucking her slutty lil' pussy with, but for her ass . . . nope, not going to work.

So, in lieu of an actual toy, we used a nicely shaped carrot, and ended up having it 4 inches in her ass with no discomfort, and fucked it at a nice pace.

Then, well, we fucked with that still in her ass, for a kinda DP. Her comment was that it felt "full".

We'll take it further, no doubt about that.

And now I'm annoyed, because she's at home, lying on our bed, playing with her clit, in the bra and panties I picked out for her this morning, getting them all wet . . .

Is it 5 yet?

Mike

Thursday 6 February 2003

Whine whine whine

. . . That is a silly subject line but one of my co-workers is doing that right now and it's getting on my nerves . . . these people can be so very juvenile. Oh, she went away. That is a good thing.

Last night. We got home, and kissed and touched, and then he had to leave. Sneaky man, got me just to that point, on the precipice of coming, just from kissing and fondling me, and then he gave me a big grin and said, "OK, baby . . . I have to go." He left, went to his meeting. I geeked out and did a bunch of work things, then cooked pad thai (mmm . . . Love that stuff and we haven't had it in a while), phoned my mother, took a bit of a nap (I mean a bit . . . probably about 15 minutes, and then someone in the apartment next door started making the most horrible noises so I woke up), and started watching one of my favorite movies, *The Princess Bride* (Fred Savage was so cuuute! I had the biggest crush on him as a child. It's funny, because he and I are the same age, approximately, but because he's been captured on film, I always feel a bit surprised when I see now-Fred, as opposed to say, *Wonder Years* Fred). Then I decided to take a bath; I usually shower, but I love just soaking in the tub now and then. It's very relaxing. Candles, bubbles, soothing music . . . my choice last night was a mix CD I'd made full of sappy love songs so I got all relaxed.

Mike came home at around 11, and ate (I assume . . . Heard him fiddling around with the microwave, so that's my assumption). Then he came into the bathroom to tell me all about his meeting. My baby did so well last night! I am so proud of him. He is so good, and has such a positive impact on so many people. He sat on the edge of the tub, and washed my back while he told me about everything that was accomplished in those three hours and I just have to repeat that I am SO PROUD of him. Then he smiled at me, said, "Come on," helped me out of the tub and wrapped me in a towel, then led me to our bedroom. I have to admit that by this point I wasn't really in the mood for the hard, kinky stuff we'd been promising each other earlier, but love is compromise and I was willing to if he really wanted it. But then he had me lay down, and took out our massage oils and told me that his mood had changed, did I mind? We are very in sync on these things; it's just odd to me. Very rarely is one of us in the mood for something and the other isn't.

Anyway . . . he just slowly, slowly rubbed my back, all lightly, and eventually moved down further, to the cleft of my ass, then my pussy . . . had me roll over and just . . . massaged me there. Lightly, and slowly, and gently, until I came to these total-body-shuddering orgasms, all the while licking my nipples and kissing my mouth, sucking on my tongue. Was so very good. Then he finally just slooooowly entered me . . . was very slick, what with the oils and things, plus my natural lubrication. And he was so hard, and I knew that he could have just pounded into me, but he held back, slow, slow, making it sooooo good for me. I think it was good for him, too, because he came so hard after awhile of making love like that.

Then we just held each other, and fell asleep . . . eventually though I woke up (I'm having trouble with insomnia lately) and he sensed it so he woke up too. Just grabbed me, pounded into me, and ohhhh, it made me scream. The neighbors were literally knocking on the wall . . . will probably get in trouble today. I came so hard. And then he pulled out, and told me to rub my clit, and he put his cock back in me and fucked me, touching my G-spot, and I was so full . . . I knew it was coming and I'm still reluctant to do it because it's all new to me, so I told him that it was going to happen if he didn't stop, and he didn't stop. It made him hornier, I guess . . . he started pounding my G-spot harder, and I couldn't stand it, and couldn't hold back, and he told me to let it go, and all this fluid came out of me, I squirted all over his cock, and then he came inside me again, and pulled out while he was coming, so it was inside me, and on me, and uhm . . . a very large wet spot on the bed last night, on his side of the bed too, but we decided to camp out. Set up cushions in the living room, and it was like a pillow fort from when we were kids, only we were naked and kissing most of the night.

I love that man so much.

Michelle

Tuesday 11 February 2003

Silly internet

This is Michelle, posting for Mike again, because his work net STILL isn't up and last night we were both too exhausted to really write much aside from what I wrote . . . he just sent me this via messenger though to put up, so here we go. Enjoy.

So, this weekend, I put clothespins on her pussy, and then got tape, and taped them to her thighs, and had her open her thighs. It kept her spread like I knew it would, and pinched and stung a bit like I knew it would, but there was an added side effect – her clit was incredibly exposed – it was swollen and hard as usual, and all the way out. I put the vibrator on her there, and she came in less than a minute. After that we used the vibes, and then I licked her, and then we fucked, and she came soooooooooo hard – it was incredible . . .

Course, afterward her cootchie had wee little dents all over it, which went away but looked interesting.

That was Saturday.

Sunday it was tender, and slow, and intense, and sweet. We just stayed in bed for half the day, and spent the other half on the couch, mostly naked, licking and kissing, and drawing out orgasms till we were half mad with the need to come.

Michelle is the best lover possible. Period. Also the sweetest girl, and my heart and my love. But also such a wonderful lover.

So, yesterday she got home before me (I worked a l'l late) and she phoned me, all horny and impatient. She had been thinking about one of our kinkier fantasies, and I took that, and told her how I thought it would go, and it turned into phone sex, with her getting wet and horny and scared (good thing for this fantasy).

If Michelle wants to tell you what the fantasy is she can – though I'm hoping to write it and post it here later in the week when I get a chance.

So, once I got home we played a bit rough, and she knelt, and I fingered her ass while she rubbed her clit, and then she was spanked, and then fucked hard for ages, and licked and nibbled on, and soon and so forth. And then we cuddled.

And then she blogged, and while she was gone I got horny again.

Actually I got horny looking at her bare bottom as she went to blog, and was hard when she got back.

And now I'm horny again – what a surprise. I always need Michelle, always, if only to touch her, and kiss her, and let her know how much I love her and need her, and are so complete with her in my life.

OK, done babbling, back to work.

Mike

Michelle

Monday 3 March 2003

Sure sure, laugh at my pain . . .

He just HAD to tell everyone about that, didn't he? It *was* funny though . . . A word to the wise: LEG CRAMPS SUCK! He just laid there on the bed laughing and watching my boobies jiggle around. Then of course, he was really nice, and massaged my calves for me, which led to rubbing my bum, which led to rubbing my back, which led to my shoulders, which led to . . . well to be perfectly honest, me falling asleep. Which was not fair to HIM, because he had had practically NO action yet, but I woke him up on Friday morning in a nice way: I saw this in Cosmo or something, probably. Hey, I get hints wherever I can find 'em.

He was still sleeping, and I snuck out of bed and went and made a cup of tea. Brought it back to bed with me, got in, took a sip, and my hands were really warm from the mug so I put them right on his cock . . . woke him up a little. Then used my mouth, which was all hot, and then, because I get thirsty in the night we keep a pitcher of ice water by the bed. The ice had melted by 6 a.m., but it was still cold. So I had a big drink of that, my hot hands still on his cock, and put my cold mouth on him. 15 or so minutes of that, and he was coming in my mouth . . . I love the taste of him. I love sliding my tongue around under his foreskin.

It just feels good to me, and tastes good . . . **sigh** I shall never get enough. I'm incorrigible.

Friday night I got home from work a few minutes later than him, and he was waiting for me with a big smile on his face. As soon as I walked in it was like, "Kiss me, Michelle!" So of course I did, I love kissing him. And next thing I know, I'm naked, and he's kind of dragging me to the bedroom, where he looks into my eyes and says that I'm going to be busy for quite a while.

Mike has long hair, and usually wears bandannas just to keep it out of his eyes. One of them came out of the drawer, and he blindfolded me as we stood at the bedroom door. Then he led me in the direction of the bed, and he told me to lie down, so I did. What I assume were 2 more bandannas came along, and tied my wrists to the headboard. Not really tightly or anything, I could still move around. He just knows I like that sort of thing, where he takes control . . . Then he stacked pillows under my bum, and next thing I know I'm getting some nice little "love taps" on my pussy . . . this wasn't full out BDSM-type thing, mind you. I love when he does this . . . It just makes my whole body more sensitive to any touch. Little bites all up and down my sides, nibbling on my ribcage, the insides of my thighs . . . finally moving up my tummy to my breasts, where he spent a LOT of time. No one but him has ever done this before, but he will lick my breasts ALL OVER, not just the nipples. And make the whole thing all wet . . . it's an incredible turn on. Of course there was sucking and licking and biting my nipples. And blowing on my tits, giving me goose bumps . . .

We have these Kama Sutra oil things. Not massage oils, but the kind that heat up when you blow on them or rub them on. I didn't realize it until just when it happened but he had them nearby . . . and poured a dollop right on my clit . . . We'd never done this before; we'd always just used them on each other's backs, like massage oils, which is silly because they're edible and why didn't we think of this sooner? But there's a first time I guess, for everything . . . and boy, what a first time. Within seconds I was begging him to fuck me because the oil made my clit so hot and so sensitive and I was so close to coming, and he was still licking and rubbing me, then he put just the tip of his cock inside me for a second . . . and pulled out. And I was like "What? Get back in there, you!".

He didn't say anything, just grabbed me by the hips and flipped me over (now understand, I am not a tiny little ballerina here. My baby is brawny), so that I was flat on my stomach, hands still tied above my head (guess that's why he didn't have them tied all that tightly) and he just rammed his cock into me . . . it was amazing. And wonderful.

And the second it went in me, I started coming, and next thing I know there's that vibrating anal toy being slipped into my ass (very gently; even in moments of madness he has his wits about him) and turned on, and I'm screeching, and he's coming, and wow, what a good Friday before-supper type thing to do!

Our weekend has been eventful, too. Aside from sex we went to see friends on Saturday, and out to see my ex-roommate's band play Saturday night. Slept in today, I made pancakes and we got all full of syrup because I can't aim at my mouth . . .

I just got really really good news from a family member, so I'm all excited and am having a hard time being really serious today, but uhm . . . yes. That was it.

Hope everyone else's weekend rocked the Kasbah.
Michelle

Monday 17 March 2003

Weekend update

Well, Michelle is in the bathtub soaking, and she's all tired, so I'm blogging for us.

So, last night Michelle dug out her old school uniform, which I'd never seen before. Apparently I have that thing where a tartan skirt makes my cock go Sproing! So, we figured beh, why not and role-played a bit, and she ended up tied up and all innocent-seeming, and I went down on her, and we fucked.

That was fun.

Today we had a quickie when we got up, and we lazed around the apartment for a while. Had nothing planned, so it was a day of rest. We were watching *Superman 2* (side note, General Zod rules!) and she just took me and kissed me lightly, and from there we made out (and yes, I know that sounds goofy), and we started fooling around and got naked, and we ended up in on the bed, fucking very frantically. So, she came, and I came, and I got her vibe and asked her to play with herself while I watched. So she rubbed and rubbed, and I got her dildo and fucked her pussy a bit, deep for a bit, sometimes right on her G-spot, and sometimes just leaving it inside for her to squeeze on.

I licked her for a while, and fingered her, and watched her use her fingers, and licked her fingers as they darted in and out of that sweet l'il hole, and she came and came and came. Think we did that for over an hour, and lord knows how many times she came during all that. Then we fucked again, and I pounded her from behind, spanking her ass while she fucked back hard on my cock, and once that was done I went down on her again, licking my cum from her cunt and kissing her.

A pretty good afternoon methinks.

So now she's all tired, and I'm kinda tired, and tomorrow starts another crazy work week, but well . . . She'll be in a towel in a few minutes, and wet and smelling nice, and soooooo beautiful, and I think maybe I'm not so tired after all.

Later,
Mike

Friday 28 March 2003

Today is *his turn*

Don't know what came over me last night. Of course Mike forgot to mention the part where he was on top of me and I was on my back, and he pushed my legs back and had me cross them at my ankles . . . I really like how that feels, and I think he does too. That was between me grabbing him at the door and me riding him . . . was very nice. I overuse that word, "nice", but I don't want to go around saying "explosive" and "supremely excellent" and things like that . . .

So at 11.30 or whenever it was, Mike came to bed. I rolled over to kiss him but THAT IS ALL. We were both exhausted and knew there would be no more of the crazy sex action . . . Seriously, it's been starting to get warm here where we live and we were both so sweaty and exhausted you'd have thought we'd run a marathon or something . . . plus I'd been asleep for an hour and everyone knows you don't disturb Michelle when she's sleeping or she might bite you really hard.

So I kissed him, and we talked a little bit, and he told me that he'd blogged while I was snoring away (he didn't say snoring, but I just think I snore). Talked about some other things, and I was all restless, moving around in the bed, and he said "Baby, do you need to come again before you can fall asleep?" I know it's weird, but that is a really good way for me to fall asleep . . . since I was a little girl, like three, four years old, I've masturbated before going to sleep pretty much every night. He knows this. So I kind of blushed and nodded, and he smiled at me, and kissed me, and just gently, gently played with my clit (there was no way we were putting anything inside me – well, the very tip of his finger, but that was it) until I had the softest little orgasm, which was exactly what I needed. And then it was midnight, and he said while I was falling asleep, "It's tomorrow, baby . . . remember? You're mine now."

I smiled.

So today I'm at work wearing a skirt and no panties, with ben-wa balls inside me, orders to make myself come here at work as many times as he tells me to over IM, and later, before I go home, I'm going to be inserting my anal toy and walking out of the building with it in, and then when I get out to my car it's up to me to take it out of my ass before I get in because obviously I can't sit in my car with that in . . . lucky I leave a bit later than most people here most days so there won't be much traffic in the parking lot because I'm thinking I'll have to lift up my skirt in the parking lot and take it out.

And again I just must confirm that I love Mike with all my heart, that he is the best person in my entire life, that I want to just be with him forever, and that I feel so lucky that we found each other. Sometimes you feel as though you're going to be Alone Forever, or that there's no one out there that fits you . . . I had always felt like something was missing from me, and now, I'm all finished, because he's here.

The End

Michelle

Sunday 13 April 2003

Weekend Update

So, yesterday I came home and told Michelle I had a meeting later that night, an emergency kinda thing. We usually get naked as soon as we get home and fuck, because well, yes, we are that horny.

So, because of my meeting we decided that we'd wait until later when we could really enjoy ourselves and take our time with things.

So, we're on the couch watching BBC World News, and I decide to pull up her top, because, well, she's not wearing a bra and I love looking at her tits. Looking is nice, but well, touching is good too. Really good in fact. So I'm sitting closer, and running my fingers idly around her nipples, and licking her earlobe and whispering all manner of filthy things in her ear.

Course then I get all curious and ask her if she thinks her clit is poking out – and yes, it is – Michelle is a very horny girl and her clit swells nicely when she's aroused. I pull her underwear and pants away from her body and have her lick one finger, and then with her pussy spread so her clit's totally out run her finger around it once.

Such a moan. So very very good.

We do this for about half an hour, and she's trying to be all cool, because well, we're waiting for tonight, but she's breathing so hard and her cheeks are flushed . . .

So I lean over, tell her I need her now, and get her pants down in like 5 seconds, and we fuck hard, and her legs wrap around me and she comes in about 30 seconds, and she keeps coming, hard and fast, and it's so intense she can't talk at all.

So, so good.

Of course there was no meeting.

evil grin

And tonight, she's getting tied up, and pictures taken, and being come on and in, and things written on her, and well, all the horrible little things we do out of love, that we enjoy and make us come so hard.

OK, kids, see you later.

Mike

Wednesday 23 April 2003

Easter Easter Easter Easter

Easter meant spending four days at Mike's parents, which meant a long drive on Friday morning, staying up really late and hanging round until we were too exhausted to do anything on Friday night . . . Saturday morning someone woke up early – and hard – and we risked squeaky bedsprings for an hour or so.

That's how it was all weekend – very quietly making love, half the time I'd have to grab blankets and bite down on them to keep from screaming and frightening the dog. We **did** get a bit of time to ourselves on Saturday afternoon, when we went for a walk, but it was pretty much just PG-13, seeing as 1) it was cold out and 2) there were other people out for walks as well.

And all the pent-up . . . whatever . . . was released full-force last night. Monday we were tired from the long ride back, plus Mike had a meeting on Monday evening. So we did make love, and it was really good to not have to hold our breath and everything. Tuesday night we had our energy back and WOW. WOW WOW WOW.

After supper he came up to me, kissed me, and told me that he was going to the kitchen and when he got back he hoped I would have my clothes off. I did . . . and he brought me to the bedroom. Mmmmm, spankings . . . pussy, ass, tits . . . really nice. Then he just fucked me SO hard, and had me suck his cock, then put it back inside me and I was screaming SO loud . . . luckily it was only 5.30 in the afternoon so we weren't breaking any noise bylaws . When he came he was kissing me so hard and I was moaning into his mouth and it was WONDERFUL.

Then we watched TV for a while, lying there, and we read to each other, and just didn't leave the bed. Oh, except at one point he got a phone call and left the bedroom to take it, and when he was on his way out he said, "Amuse yourself" (not in a snotty kind of way, in a "I'll be right back, have fun while I'm gone" kind of way) . . . Well, after about 20 minutes I got really bored, so I just started masturbating, and when he came back in my eyes were closed, and I didn't realize until I felt him start to suck on my nipple. Mmm. I kind of stopped, because well . . . you know. But he asked me to please keep going, because he wanted to see. And he got to see. Usually I'm fairly shy about things like that (go figure!) but he kept telling me how much he liked watching, and how pretty my pussy was with my fingers opening it up like that, and then I asked him to put his finger inside me while I rubbed my clit . . . After a while he asked if he could lick my pussy while I played with my clit . . . and I just kept coming, and making his mouth all wet. Soon his fingers weren't enough and I was so very happy that his cock was hard and he could come up over me and get inside me.

And now, writing about it, I'm all wet again.

Michelle

Wednesday 21 May 2003

Punishment

Now you KNOW that I'm an intelligent, adult woman. I am not a brainless, simpering idiot. Mike in no way thinks of me as being lesser, nor do I think of myself that way. *This is all consensual* and, if it weren't, it wouldn't be happening.

Clear on that? Good.

Sunday night – Victoria Day barbecue out at my friend's house. Of course, she and her husband just had a baby, the whole thing will probably be over by seven, right? Wrong. Got there, and a gathering that I thought would be the three of us plus baby turned out to be a huge bash. At least twenty people there. Tried calling Mike to let him know that I might be later than I'd originally thought, but by then he had left for **his** thing . . .

So there was wine. Lots and lots of wine. And I haven't had a drink in so long (at least since New Year's), and I'd been so sick the rest of the weekend, that after three drinks I was pretty sure I shouldn't be driving. And as Mike said, I got very sleepy very quickly, and just didn't manage to call him.

When I got home, we made out, and everything . . . we're happy to see each other. Made love. Snuggled. Then I brought it up. *I brought it up.* "Baby . . . I'm really sorry about last night . . . I don't blame you if you're angry." "No, no, I'm not angry." "Ummm . . . but I didn't come home! And I didn't call!" "Well, you couldn't call, the phones were all busy, and you were sleepy, I understand . . ." "But ummm . . . aren't you a little bit angry?" "No, my baby, not at all" (by this time I was about ready to poke

him in the eye and say it, but I was trying to be a bit more subtle)
"SHOULDN'T you be angry?" . . . Then he got it. "Michelle, do
you feel like you need to be punished for this?" "Yes . . . I ruined
our plans by not coming home." Then we talked, long, and in great
detail, him assuring me that we didn't have to, and me assuring him
that I wanted to.

Why do I want this? Again, I think it's a control thing. My job,
my life, is very . . . I am in control of a huge team of people. I can
never just let someone else take over. That's in real life. With Mike,
when I need to, he can be totally in charge, and I can just let him
have control. It's an amazing feeling, to trust someone so much that
you will let them do pretty much anything with you. We have
guidelines, we're still sort of new to all this, but so far, it just seems
right. I know he loves me, he knows I love him, and it's all very very
good.

So later last night, after I'd napped and taken about seventeen
thousand Tylenol, he had me take off my clothes and stand in front
of him. He asked me where I'd been. I told him. He asked me what
I'd been doing. I told him. The entire time he was rubbing his
leather belt against my pussy. He asked me if I realized that I had
ruined our plans by not coming home. I kind of acted a bit whiny
and told him it wasn't my fault, I hadn't meant to get drunk, and I
had tried to call, but he wasn't home, and then the phones were all
in use, and I fell asleep, and really, I was sorry, but it wasn't my
fault . . . I love playing the whiny game. He just looked at me and
said, "That just earned you five." Five more smacks for trying to
get out of trouble.

He then had me stand in front of him with my hands by my side
while he told me exactly what I'd done wrong, and how he was
going to punish me. And then it started. He made my breasts SO
red by spanking them. When I thought I couldn't handle any more
he went and got some ice, and iced them down (mmmmm) all the
while using his other hand to spank me right on my wet pussy. That
got iced down too, as he went back to spanking my tits. My tummy.
The insides of my thighs. Then he had me lie flat on my stomach on
the floor with my legs parted while he used his belt to spank my ass
. . . of course he'd miss now and then and my poor pussy would get
it . . .

Then he had me kneel. He put his hand on the back of my head, I put out my tongue, and he rubbed his balls and his cock all over my face and tongue. I begged him to let me suck it, but he said no, I didn't deserve to, I'd been bad. Then he had me start playing with my pussy, and let me get just to the point of coming, and had me stop. He did this, over and over again, until he pushed me down flat on my stomach and fucked me that way . . . I was about to come when he pulled out and had me suck his cock. He came in my mouth, and on my face, and my tits . . . and told me to lie down on the bed, where he tied my hands to the headboard, and walked out. And left me there, for at least an hour . . . He'd come in every now and then to make sure I was OK, see if I needed a drink, pinch my nipples, put ice on my pussy . . . but he wouldn't let me come. Now and then he would rub me or start licking me, but just as I started to really get into it he would stop and leave again . . .

all tingly
Michelle

Thursday 7 August 2003

The sting

Some of you know what it feels like, that hot sting you get from flesh slapping flesh over and over again. Last night my hand was stinging for what seemed like an eternity. It turned kinky. Well, kinkier, if anal is kinky. We've been playing with her ass, fucking it with fingers. She's had a few times where she's come, her vibe on her clit and a finger or two in her ass, fucking nice and fast near climax.

Last night was like that, after a while.

I had her strip, and get on all 4s on our bed. She was out of the shower, nice and soft and clean, and so I did the natural thing – I licked her asshole. Licked it, played with it, pushed it in a little bit. She was very clean and she smelled very nice, and she squirmed very nicely as well.

She squirmed, and I licked, and smacked her ass a few times. I was feeling it, and the sounds she made with each spank said the same for her.

I sat up behind her, rubbed her pussy with my palm. Heard her moan more.

Put a hand on her ass, started talking dirty to her, and slapped her pussy. That got a gasp, which made me smile. So I spanked her there again, and again, and on we went. Stopped, and she was getting red there, could hear the bit of discomfort in her voice. Told her to spread her pussy for me, nice and wide. Usually that would mean she was going to get fucked.

Started spanking again instead.

Now this time she cried out – nice mix of the sting and dis-comfort.

After that, she spread the cheeks of her ass, and her asshole was spanked. I'm nothing if not persistent.

This went on well, a while, don't know how long. What I do know is after Michelle's voice went more animal, more about the urgent need – she wanted to get fucked – as sore as her pussy and ass were, she needed to get fucked, and was demanding my come inside her.

Eventually I relented – well, actually, gave up because my hand was sore as hell. Pushed her on her side, pushed her leg up, started fucking her, pounding her pussy the way she demanded, fingers pushed in her ass, a tidy little DP. She came so hard, half growl and half scream.
Mike

Tuesday 26 August 2003

Now I have a headache

Michelle is **sooooooooo** getting a spanking tonight.

There we were all hot and heavy on the couch, that crazy intense sex we both love, she's came and came, and I'm almost there.

Earlier I'd logged onto *Trillian*, and it was running in the background.

So the vinegar stroke hits, and I'm coming, and I've been holding it back so it's a pretty big one, and someone comes online or something on Trillian, and it makes a warble – "biddily boop!!"

Right after, Mich makes the same noise, "Biddily Boop!!", and I crack up, and I'm coming, and fuck, it's not easy to come and laugh at the same time.

Yes, a spanking is totally in order.
Mike

Saturday 30 August 2003

The Secret Entry

Mike, I'm writing this at about 4.30 in the morning (actually I'm not 100 percent sure what time it is, but that seems a good guess to me) – I just got up to "get a drink" and you kissed me and rolled over and went back to sleep.

Earlier tonight we lay in bed and talked about so many things. Past lovers, and how we'd been happy with them, but always felt like something was missing. It was good to know that I wasn't the only one who felt that way – and now that we have found each other, we need never feel that way again. It seems so strange to think that I led a happy life before you – my life is so much richer now with you in it.

Our lovemaking was so very sweet tonight – from the second your hand touched my face, to the "I love you's" as you pushed inside me, to the laughter at the end when I came (why do I laugh when I come? And more importantly . . . why doesn't it give **me** a headache?), it was all just so perfect.

I love being on top of you. I love that you like that. Leaning over and kissing you, sitting back and watching your eyes as I move above you – it's all so nice. Your hands on my hips, setting a rhythm. Your hands, your fingers, your mouth, on my breasts – SO good. When I took you in my mouth later and felt your hands on the back of my neck, heard that tremble in your voice that meant that you were so close – it felt so good, and tasted so good. And later, when we were all finished, and I asked what you were thinking about, and you said "Just you. I'm awfully glad we get to be with each other forever".

I love you, my baby. It's what I was made for.

And now I'm coming back to bed to put my cold feet on you. Oh, come on. You know you love it.

> *. . . da mi basia mille, diende centum,*
> *dein mille altera, dein secunda centum . . .*

Michelle

Monday 15 September 2003

Title? Fuck titles!

So – circa this afternoon, a bit of playtime for Chelle and I.

We were in the living room, and I had her stand and strip for me, do a little turn. Grabbed her ass, spanked it once or twice. That wasn't my intention though. Had her go over and sit in the computer chair, and I got the rope.

Her hands got bound behind the chair, and I had her scoot out to the edge of the chair and spread her legs.

Earlier I'd put together a slideshow of bondage and sex images I wanted to show her, had them spaced at 45 second intervals. Things I know we've talked about, things that would excite her, scare her a little. Something else to focus on.

Then it started. Between pictures I'd take a clothespin, and attach it. Her nipples were first, then around her areolae, then underneath her breasts, finally going to her inner thighs and outer pussy lips.

Took a while to get them all applied (20 in all), and it was hard for her. She talked a lot during, and one of the things was that she didn't want to use her word, which means it was probably on the tip of her tongue. She held on, though.

Then I untied her hands, had her tap and count each of the pins, and once we had the final tally, let her play with her pussy. One finger inside, and her thumb on her clit. She was hurting, but the moan of pleasure was something to hear once she could touch herself. I stood up, took out my cock – hard and sticky by now, and started jerking off, my prick almost in her face. Bent down, and started pulling them off. That first gasp, also something to re-member.

Had them half off when she came the first time, and I followed her a minute later, my come ending up on her tits.

The more you just clicked marked the end of the scene. Kissed her, told her how proud I was of her, and unclipped the remainder of the pins. She was still very much on the verge of crying with the intensity of it all, so she got picked up and carried to the sofa. Held her, kissed her head, made sure she knew how well she'd done.

Just showed the entry to Michelle, here's her 2 cents:

They know about the mindset I get into when we're doing things . . . I want them to know about what state of mind you get into. You know?

So, my state of mind. Well, it's a calm place. Very calm, maybe a little chilly. At the same time though, I'm excited, aroused. Also half my concentration is on what I'm doing, the other half is on what she's doing, how's she's reacting to what I'm doing. I want to push her to the limit, but I don't want it to be too much. It's no good for either of us if she has to use the safe word.

She's used it once if you were wondering. I made her do it – wanted to make sure she would actually use it if it was too much. Didn't do anything terrible, just made it a lot at once, sensory overload.

Anyhow, enough of this chatter – must go make couch burritos with my girl, finish out our weekend reading to each other.
Mike

Saturday 20 September 2003

snort

I have been working like a crazy lady lately, and it's been . . . probably a good three days since Mike and I have had any time for anything aside from a (VERY QUICK) quickie the other morning. And then starting yesterday, but mostly today, I have come down with this horrid horrid flu. So bad that this afternoon I actually came home from work early. IM'd Mike to let him know I was home, said "hi" to friends who were sending me messages, then went off for a nap. Well, a nap with a porn movie and my vibrator. Nice, nice, nice.

Mike got home and was treated to naked, congested, sneezing and coughing Michelle begging him to fuck her. I'm sure THAT was attractive, but he rallied the troops and managed a full frontal assault. I kept trying to avoid kissing him, but we're both such . . . kissers . . . that it just sort of happened. So he'll probably end up sick soon too . . . I hope not.

Plus the sound of me screaming "Oh, yeah, fug me, Bike . . ." We laughed **so** hard.

But I love laughing. I love how I can laugh with him. How we don't feel we have to be all serious and like, dramatic during sex . . .

And now, back to bed. Well, soon. *Pretty In Pink* is on TV and when I'm sick, I get to watch all the cheesy movies I want and Mike doesn't complain. Also the fact that when I'm sick I tend to give him more blow-jobs, because you can't catch the flu through your cock . . . can you?

Michelle

Monday 22 September 2003

Just a quickie . . .

I'm not really in the mood to post, as I still have the lingering effects of my flu going on (plus I've just taken some NyQuill, and want to get this typed before the Big Fuckin Q kicks in . . .), but we all know that if I don't post right away, then I forget, and we wouldn't want that, now would we?

One of the major benefits of being sick is that you get pampered. Not to say that Mike doesn't pamper me other times, oh no no. He does. But this weekend . . . – I got to watch *Pretty In Pink*. Twice. – We had soup for every meal and he didn't complain. – He kept telling me to go back to bed and sleep even when he was moving furniture around and could have used my help. – I got amazing back/foot/neck rubs without even looking like I needed them. Mmmm . . . – He brought me magazines to read in bed – When I asked him for pickles and a chocolate bar, swearing that was the only thing that would make me feel better (yeah yeah, I know . . .), he brought them, without giving me weird looks. – He went out and bought a bunch of new pillows so that it would be easier for us both to sit up in bed together – He stayed in bed with me most of the day, risking life and limb and his own health. – He brought me popsicles – He kept offering to call my boss and tell her I'm sick and won't be in tomorrow (I won't let him do this, though). Because . . .

I am feeling way better than I did yesterday and swear that I will feel 100 percent better tomorrow. Because I'm stubborn and don't like missing work. Ever. Unless I get to miss it but have fun. Fake sick days are so much better than real ones, don't you agree?

We've had some very gentle, loving sex this weekend. We've also had to be a little experimental, seeing as too much jostling wasn't such a good thing for me most of the time. He enjoyed my fevered mouth on his cock . . . and enjoyed when I would suck on a Popsicle in the middle of giving him head, then return my mouth to him . . . but it gave him ideas.

This afternoon I woke up to find that my nightie had been unbuttoned down the front (NyQuill! make Michelle deep sleeper!) and Mike was trailing a Popsicle all over me. At first I thought "ugh, cold!" . . . But I let myself relax and enjoy the shivers it sent through my body. My nipples were as hard and pointy as Milk Duds, and he took them into his hot mouth . . . mmm. Then he started running the Popsicle down between my legs. I was a bit hesitant at first because well, ever had your tongue stuck on a frozen piece of metal? Yeah, didn't want that happening with the cooch . . . but it turned out OK. It turned out more than OK . . . I ended up with my pussy spread open and the Popsicle moving in and out of me, melting pretty quickly . . . and then the shock of heat as he pushed his cock inside me. Ohhhhh, wow.

Let me say it again: Ohhhhh, wow.

Of course now I have telltale purple splotches all over me, but I think we're going to take a shower now. No worries.
Michelle

Wednesday 24 September 2003

Sniffles no more

Michelle is feeling better.

She was on the road to recovery Monday – seeming more her usual self. It's a savage little flu virus going round, and I was worried she'd be sick the entire week.

So, woke up with the alarm this morning, thumped the snooze button. Chelle was out of bed, and I figured she was in the bathroom or taking some meds. I lay there all snuggly, occasionally opening an eye and glaring at the alarm clock.

Then the unexpected happened. I was pounced on, I shit you not. Michelle bundled in the room, nose still a little stuffed, but otherwise 100 percent better, and pounced on me, trying her best to tickle me through the bed clothes. I'm very very ticklish in certain areas, a fact she took full advantage of.

I struggled a bit, and the bed clothes ended up down over the end of the bed, and she ended up on top of me, straddling me and kissing, rubbing her butt on me. She sat back up, pulled down the straps of her pj's, leaned down and kissed me again, and wiggled on me some more.

What followed was some very nice, very energetic and playful lovemaking, much needed after the weekend.

So, fast forward to tonight. We had a nice romantic meal, and Chelle is soaking, taking a nice relaxing bath. In a moment I'll join her, wash her back, and kiss her a little. Then I'll kiss her a lot.

After that, who knows what'll happen.
Mike

Friday 17 October 2003

A few hours ago

I can't remember what Chelle was doing – fiddling with something or other. I was pawing over some new EBay swag, geeking out and such. She made a funny little comment, and I told her she was going to get a spanking for it. She said something to the effect of "uh huh, right", and in that second I decided yes, she was going to be spanked. My voiced changed, and I told her I was serious, so over she came, "yes Sir" once she came over close. I sat down, undid her pants, slipped them down, followed by her underwear.

I sat back a little, patted my lap, and she leaned down, lay there. Held her snuggly to me with my left arm, and started rubbing her bare skin with the right. Pale, shapely and beautiful.

The first slap rang out loud, made her gasp and left a nice red handprint on her ass. Right after I started running my fingertips lightly and slowly over where I'd made impact, tracing outlines of where she was now sore. She started to push her bottom against me a bit, which brought me to the task at hand, and another slap, this time on the other side.

Red again, and another outline to trace.

Once we were done, her ass was quite red, quite hot to touch. She stood, and I did likewise, kissed her and hugged her.

Sitting wasn't going to be an option, so I asked her if she wanted to go lie down. She nodded, and I took her hand and we walked to the bedroom. She lay there on her tummy, still naked from the waist down, head sideways on the pillow and her eyes closed. I sat behind her, ran my hands up over the backs of her thighs, up over her stinging cheeks. They were still very warm, and to me quite beautiful. She parted her legs in turn a little, so I spread her ass – all the better to see her pussy of course. To say she was wet would be a horrible understatement.

Out came my cock, which had made a nice sticky mess in my own undies. Leaning down, parting her legs more, roped up on one elbow I ran my cock-head up and down her wetness, then slipping just the head inside. She'd been moaning since I started touching her, but she redoubled her efforts with that. Moved very slowly and shallowly, as gentle as I could, kissing her shoulders and neck, whispering that I loved her, all the little things. We didn't last long like that – it had been a day since we'd made love, our morning ending up a rush thanks to us sleeping through the alarm clock. Still, neither of us complained. We cuddled, and she fell asleep with her head on my chest. I let her sleep for an hour, and when she woke, I made sure she came, teasing her with my tongue for as long as she could stand it.

Mike

MODEL MISBEHAVIOR

Kris Madison

http://www.krismadison.com/blog

Wednesday 31 July

A Day in the Life of a Web Girl

9.00 a.m. – My alarm goes off. I groggily stumble towards the chatter coming from my dresser & hit every button until it shuts off. I return to my cozy bed.

10.00 a.m. – I'm awake now but pretending I'm still sleeping. I have so many things I need to do today. I really should get out of bed. Piggy needs to be walked. I have to hit the gym before it closes for cleaning. I should really get up.

10.30 a.m. – I finally drag myself out of bed & head towards my computer. I check my email & add more things on my growing to-do list that never gets any smaller.

11.00 a.m. – I take Piggy for a run instead of going to the gym. I'll get in a work out & then I don't have to walk him later. It's already scorchingly hot though. Piggy, my little black Pug, is not the best motivator for getting me moving. He finds a shady spot & lays down, refusing to budge. I sit down for a bit & stretch, then carry him most of the way home.

12.00 p.m. – After showering, I grab a bowl of cereal & settle in to read my webmaster boards. Junk mostly, but since I'm in an industry that I can't really discuss with my friends & family, these on-line personalities have become the closest thing to real friends I have in my business. Sometimes there is great information & new ideas about marketing or improving your web site. Sometimes it's just a lot of gossip & bickering. Either way, it's entertaining & is a daily habit of mine.

12.30 p.m. – I really need to do some work. I make a new to-do list & add simple things like "shower" & "pay credit card bill". Now I can cross a couple of items off & relieve my procrastinating conscience a little.

1.00 p.m. – Check my web site stats to see if I've gotten any new sign ups. Nope. Damn. I remember that I haven't turned on my voyeur cam & if I'm going to be working all day, I might as well give my members something to look at. Oh yeah, and I'm naked.

1.30 p.m. – I have a phone sex appointment scheduled for 2.00 p.m. He's already paid in advance for a 20-minute phone call. I put on some music & pull my pink jelly vibrator out, just in case. I figure I have a little time before my call, so I set up a new shoe auction on an adult version of EBay. Not really sure what the bidders do with my high heels once they receive them, but they are very sweet guys & I'm happy to Feng Shui my closet for cash.

1.37 p.m. – I get a nasty email from the phone sex guy saying, "So are we doing this or what? Who's calling who? Don't I need a number?" A little annoyed, I email him back with my number & say that I'm available to start earlier, if he likes.

1.39 p.m. – Nasty email number two from phone sex guy. When he set up the phone sex time, he said, "2.00 p.m. your time". Fine. Sounds good. Turns out he thought I was one hour behind instead of two hours – a problem that could have been easily solved if he had let me do the time conversion myself.

1.42 p.m. – My phone rings & we start talking. I'm already a little annoyed but I lie down on the couch & try to get comfortable. Then he starts coughing. "Sorry, I'm just getting over a cold. I really wanted to talk to you though & didn't (cough, cough) want to wait any longer." Uh, OK. So I start into my little phone sex fantasy since he didn't really have any input & just wanted to listen. I start off with him rubbing my neck, nibbling my ear lobes . . . arch my back & press ag (cough, cough) . . . press against you. I can feel your (cough, cough). Sigh.

He takes a break from coughing to let me know what he's wearing – panties! Yay! A little flustered, I try to cover up my surprise. "That's hot baby. I bet they feel tight around your . . ." (cough, cough).

1.16 p.m. – I hang up the phone & head to the kitchen to fill up my trusty water bottle that is always by my side. Shaking my head, I decide that after only 4 sessions, I'm finished with phone sex. It can be lots of fun if you get to talk to someone you click with, but when the onus is on me to do all the talking . . . well, I'm just too shy. I'm not exactly a writer for *Penthouse Forum* & it's surprisingly difficult to come up with new & interesting ways to describe riding cock. Maybe I should run a contest – come up with new ways to describe my pussy. So far I've got pink, wet, hot, tight, sweet, a little salty . . . did I say wet? Damn. Good thing I'm retired.

1.30 p.m. – My boyfriend comes home & I tell him about the phone sex call that belongs on the bloopers reel of my life. He laughs but seems uninterested. Although he's never said anything, I don't think he likes me talking to other guys on the phone – unless he's at home & listening, of course. The second call I had he listened the entire time & ended up masturbating with me while I was still talking. I don't think the caller had any idea he was having a threesome.

2.00 p.m. – It's a beautiful day so we head out in search of somewhere to take photos. The parkade of my apartment building has a nice view & we stop to do a few shots of me leaning over the railing. Some guys are sitting on their balcony in the building across the street & they notice us taking pictures. I flash my boobs for a couple of shots & right after, the guys go into their apartment. Thinking the coast is clear, I hike up my dress a little bit to reveal a flash of pink panties & we keep snapping pics. The guys return to their balcony, however, binoculars in hand! We quickly take a few more pics & then head for the elevator, worrying that we may get in trouble with the security guard in my building. The guys start yelling across the street at me, "Is the show over???" I give a quick wave & laugh all the way to the car.

2.30 p.m. – We've been driving around for half an hour & finally find a decent spot to take some photos. I lie down on a blanket in the grass & slowly strip while the camera flashes away. We're in an open clearing in the woods which isn't very isolated, but I figure if anyone comes walking down the path, I should be able to spot them in time to throw on some clothes.

2.47 p.m. – My body is contorted into an awkward position that accentuates my curvy hips while disguising my less camera worthy features. A mosquito is biting my thigh but John says the pose looks so good that I must hold it until he can get a picture. The stupid digital camera is still "processing" so I have to wait . . .

2.49 p.m. – He gets the picture & then I run around, yelling at the damn mosquitoes. He snaps a pic of me running, much to my annoyance.

2.56 p.m. – After a few more shots with my ass in the air, John's shorts are developing a noticeable wet spot. He's had enough & wants to get wild in the middle of the wilderness. He tries to toss the camera aside, but I won't let him. Instead I make him lie down on the grass & climb on top, camera poised for action. We take a bunch of cool photos creating our own nature special, all from our own perspective rather than that of a smarmy porn producer. They turn out quite well, despite the 23 mosquito bites I endured.

3.17 p.m. – I'm just pulling my shorts on when a car drives by not 10 feet away from us. Somehow, we had completely missed the gravel road that is the entrance to the camp sites. Thanking our lucky stars, we decide it's time to pack up & head home.

4.00 p.m. – I check my stats again & am delighted to have gotten a new member. Hurrah!

4.05 p.m. – I start building a new photo gallery of my outdoor adventure & upload it to my web site.

5.00 p.m. – I pick a few of my favorite shots & send them in to an amateur picture post site where people send in pics of their girlfriends & wives. They provide a link back to my website plus my email address, so it's a fantastic way to meet new members. I dig through all the pics until I find the last ones I sent in & browse the comments left for me. Here are a few highlights:

> *I'd like to apply as your personal photographer. I'm ready to start at your bottom and slowly ascend your corporate leg.*

> *wow. beautiful lady. I showed my sister your pics and well we both masturbated looking at them.:) :) cool. thank you sexy. :)*

> *Always try to show yourself from head to & including your feet & toes. You did a great job & I know its difficult shooting yourself. I shoot women nude & always show full body whether lying down or standing & always in heels or on tip toes.*

Everyone's a critic.

7.30 p.m. – John & I get cleaned up so we can go out for dinner. We're meeting another local web girl & her husband who have been in the industry for a few years. I'm very nervous because I'm terrible at meeting new people, but I am looking forward to knowing someone in real life who can relate to the craziness of what I do. I'm also hoping that there will be a spark between us so we can do a girlie shoot together. Yum!

9.30 p.m. – Several margaritas later, we're having a great time laughing & relaying stories about the oddest requests we've ever gotten from surfers. Mine? A guy emailed me who had seen my pics but couldn't afford to join my web site & wanted to know if I would mind sending him some of my pubic hair the next time I shaved. Surprisingly, I decided to pass on his offer. At least my friend's strangest request was willing to pay her for accommodating his weirdness. He requested a 20-minute custom video of her sneezing over & over again. She kept snorting pepper & sticking q-tips in her nose to make herself sneeze. Crazy, but she made $200 for 20 minutes of work – if you can call sneezing work!

11.00 p.m. – We get home just in time to watch *Sex in the City*, one of my favorite shows. Shocked?

11.30 p.m. – Check my stats again to see if I have any new sign ups & then hit the blog of one of my favorite web girls, Tasty Trixie. Despite condemning myself to desperate loser status, I'll admit that I have an on-line crush. She is so unbelievably open with her emotions that it's addicting. If she's having a bad day, I worry about her. I almost sent her flowers when she broke up with her boyfriend! Fortunately, I realized how weird that was before it was too late. It's bizarre how you can feel close to someone you've never met & who has no idea who you are. I suppose this must be how some of my members feel too.

12.00 a.m. – I get ready for bed & try to fall asleep early. I promise myself that I will get up early tomorrow & get some work done. My boss is a real bitch, you know? Better not get fired!

Tuesday 5 August

Downtown Living

You know you've lived downtown for too long when it doesn't even faze you to check the park for folks sleeping before you unleash your dogs. I forgot to check behind the lone structure in my dog park this morning & had to drag the dogs away from a sleeping couple & their belongings. Looks like the park dude nabbed himself a lady.

In other urban living news, I just returned from a lovely walk to Second Cup with a yummy cup of chai. Fortunately for me, there's a coffee shop within two blocks of my place. I say fortunate because my last attempt at making my own chai almost set my house on fire. Those little paper tabs at the end of tea bag? They're flammable. Just so ya know.

Thursday 7 August

BAHAHAHAHA!

For me, the best thing about DVD porn is the preview clips. I hate dialogue & story lines in porn, despite being a woman. I'm not sure who decided that women want substance with their porn but they definitely didn't interview me before creating that little factoid.

If I want to see a movie with a plot & character development, I'll go see a real movie. If I want to jack off, I'll pop in a porno. Why would I ever want to combine the two? I don't want to be entertained by my porn. I want to be turned on. Hell, if I have to listen to what the porn stars have to say, I might as well just fuck my boyfriend.

Anyways, in one of the horribly edited preview clips there was a big circle jerk scene with a woman in the middle, sucking each guy off. The guys were coming on the back of the woman's head for some reason (she wanted the extra protein for her hair maybe?). As one guy started spurting his load onto the top of the smut starlet's head, the current suckee jumped out of the way as if he'd been shot, leaping dramatically to the side & safely out of sperm's way. On second thought, I think he may have actually moved *faster* than if a loaded gun had been fired at him.

Which makes me wonder – how does one so afraid of come land himself in a 5-to-1 cock ratio movie? Chalk it up to one of those scenarios that sounds appealing when you read the script scrawled on the back of a Busty Ranch Saloon napkin & know your rent is past due, but turns out a little icky in real life, literally. I wonder how he fared for the rest of the flick. Almost makes me want to rent it.

Sunday 10 August

3.19 a.m. – Finally Something Interesting on my Spycam

After months of watching me typing away on my computer in pajama pants & zit cream, I'm finally doing something interesting & no one is up to watch! My girlfriend, Sabby, & her husband are over for a few drinks & we're playing strip poker. Surprise, surprise – John still has all his clothes on! I suspect he's been dealing from the bottom of the deck.

Whoops. I've been corrected. He had to lose his socks. Sabby & I are both buck naked. Missed the straight again. Doh!

2.11 p.m. – Panda Puffs Never Tasted So Good

Up at the crack of two, I'm devouring a bowl of cereal (organic, World Wildlife Fund supporting & gluten free, brought to my attention by Houseboy, my favorite hippy) & poring over the snapshots I grabbed last night. If the round of strip poker wasn't surreal enough, I had to get photographic evidence of the naked guest sitting a little too close to John for his comfort. Sabby's mantoy kept leaning closer to John while he kept trying to lean further away. It was hysterical. And then a funny thing happened . . .

I'm not a natural exhibitionist. I've never flashed my tatas at a party. I've never felt comfortable doing cam shows. I don't wear skimpy clothes when I go out to try & attract attention. I do like taking pictures & knowing people are seeing them on the net, but it's in a very controlled manner, from which images right down to the context in which they're presented.

On the flip side, a true exhibitionist, a born cam girl, was never displayed in such raw form as my friend Sabby. The minute I pulled out the camera, she started performing. I had it hooked up to the TV so she could see what the snapshots looked like & she responded instantly, hopping on John to give him a lap dance, bouncing her bubbly boobs around. It was like firing up the lightning bolt to Frankenstein's monster, only with double Ds & no bolts jutting out of her neck.

Like everybody else, Sabby can sit around ranting about work over a couple of beers, but she loves her job. She works harder than any cam girl I know & she's very successful at it. I originally attributed her success to her smarts, being a bright, fluffy business-woman. Her looks don't hurt either, reminiscent of Heather Lock-lear (of Melrose Porn Place). But it's her born to perform quality, that sparkle of life even a Hollywood surgeon can't provide, that's the true key.

It doesn't take my high school career aptitude counselor to note fundamental differences here. It's not news to me that I'm not physically built for the porn world, but I celebrate that, proud of the fact that I'm offering a different face on what's considered sexy. I've always had wide hips & a generous ass. At 5'5" I was constantly reminded that I looked nothing like the girls smiling on the pages of the glossy magazines I grew up with. But when technology made it possible for any housewife with a digital camera & a copy of FrontPage to toss up some nude pics of herself, it became clear that it's only fashion designers who subscribe to that one standard of beauty. Amateur porn revolutionized the net & earned so much money that even mainstream porn producers took notice, launching their own brands of amateur porn in unheard of categories like "mature" & "BBW – Big Beautiful Women".

However, being devoid of a personality that thrives on attention, preferring to curl up under the covers than perform for an audience is a bit more of a pickle.

I've been thinking a lot lately about where I want my site to go. I haven't come up with any conclusions yet, but last night's antics confirm my gut instinct to forget trying to compete with the status quo. And yes, there is one even in the on-line porn world. If I were to try & keep up with the Joneses of Porn, I'd be wearing a cheerleader uniform & taking three cocks in my ass while blowing up a balloon. Not gonna happen.

I think my site will gradually become more & more about my life, as un-sexy as it may be. Having your work all encompassed by one aspect of your life, not even the most prominent aspect of **my** life, feels (not surprisingly) unbalanced. I love posing for the camera, from choosing new outfits & dreaming up role-playing fantasies to the satisfaction of sitting down in front of my computer to go over the images I snapped using the self-timer, knowing that I created this, all by myself. There are certain niches that get my juices flowing, creative & otherwise. I adore traditional nylon stockings with garter belts & heels. I love painting my toenails different shades & shooting in the grass where they remind me of glittering jewels between the blades. Though I don't get to as often as I'd like, posing with another model is a blast, bringing a totally new energy to the scene. But trotting around in a saddle because pony play is a hot selling new market? That's turning my sex life into work.

Unfortunately, I think I've let that "Well, everybody else is doing it" attitude erode some of my personal boundaries. Even the computer savvy naked housewife loses her amateur status when she starts charging for memberships. It's a tough path to walk between running & marketing a business effectively & doing what you love while earning some money for it. Periodic gut checks like this one are a great way to remind myself that I'll never be able to make every pervert happy, so why not satisfy my own pervy desires? I may never have as many fans as a cam girl of all trades like Sabby, but the ones I do have I'll have a much better chance of really connecting with on a more personal level.

And who knows? Maybe when the pressure to be sexy all the time is lifted, my inner horndog will grunt its way to the surface. John can only hope.

Thursday 4 September

Shaving Accident

Did I mention that I'm incapable of shaving without causing major damage to my body? I was trimming my little patch yesterday & whoops! Took a big chunk out of one side. I kept trying to balance it out until finally it looked so ridiculous I was forced to shave the whole thing off.

My kitty is completely bald & smooth now, looking so foreign to me. It *feels* weird too, like I'm touching someone else.

I'm all for variety & do like to mix things up. Sometimes I'll let my patch grow, loving the feeling of a gentle tug on the long curls. Sometimes I like to trim it into a triangle with nothing down below. But completely bare? Not my style.

Each time I glance down between my legs (which is pretty often since it's been much too hot to wear clothes around the house the last couple of days), I'm treated to a little surprise, remembering again that my patch of hair is gone.

I like the feel of the smooth transition; running my hand along the soft skin of my belly, then down further, suddenly caressing my clitoris long before I was expecting to reach it. That little tuft of curls, though seemingly insignificant, is like a road sign declaring, "Turn here. You're almost there!"

I think some further experimenting is in order. More thoughts later.

Saturday 29 September

Best Investment Ever

The best purchase I've ever made, if you don't count the computer I use to whore myself on the 'net, has to be adopting my two dogs. For pure entertainment value alone, they are worth their weight in gold. Yesterday at the park, for example, Piggy, my black Pug with the most embarrassing name at the dog park, was running around in the leaves like a little boy. He was up to his bulging eyeballs in one big pile of leaves, a big grin plastered across the face that only a mother could love! He looked hilarious & I was kicking myself for not having my camera with me.

FYI: "Piggy" was not a name I picked, lest you think I'm one of those daft Paris Hilton-types who forces her dogs to wear ridiculous outfits or throws birthday parties for her cats. He actually had a name when I adopted him, but with his constant snorting, curly tail & the squeals he'd let out as a puppy when I tried to pick him up, I kept exclaiming, "What a little piggy!" as he wriggled out of my arms. The name, unfortunately, stuck.

Kiero, on the other hand, is one freaky little chick. She's a Chihuahua crossed with a Jack Russell terrier that I rescued from the SPCA. She was actually my least favorite dog at the pound, but was the only apartment-sized dog that didn't try to bite Piggy's face off at first contact. With her ribs sticking out & a steady shake, I figured she was the dog most in need of rescue. She's adjusted quite well to her new home & quickly became the dominant dog, humping her brother right off the couch some days. She's fixed. He's neutered. She's the boss. But that's not why she's freaky.

They were both sniffing around the same spot at the leash-free park yesterday. Piggy lifts his leg to mark it & what does my little girl do? Runs right in to sniff what's going on. Yup, my Mexican rat is into golden showers. Piggy peed on her head! I dragged her home (after laughing my ass off) & tossed in her into the tub.

Today was more canine comedy. I figured I would soak up some Indian summer sun & read a book while they ran around. Would they leave my side to explore the park? Nope. Such momma's dogs! They were so close to me the entire time that I have paw prints all over my book. At one point, I was lying on my tummy, trying to read, while Piggy was standing on my bum watching people walk by & Kiero was standing in between me & my book with my chin resting on her back. I couldn't stop giggling. Hell of a lot better value than the last Adam Sandler shitbomb I went to see!

Monday 5 October

Keeping In Touch

Between the nagging guilt that is my inbox overflowing with 1619 messages & a recent blog entry by a fellow webwhore, I've been pondering – how long is too long to reply to an email?

It's not that I don't like receiving emails, quite the opposite. I adore the little bursts onto my screen, effortlessly filling me in on the details of what's going on in a friend's life or letting me know that someone enjoyed my recent photo shoot. I check my email a gazillion times a day & read every one. But I rarely respond right away. I usually let them pile up until I feel too guilty to get any work done & then I fire through them. If an email is older than a month, I usually just delete it without responding. A month is a long time & whether it was my sister or an on-line friend, it's probably been so long that they don't remember writing the email anyways. If it was someone just passing by my website, they probably don't remember **me** at all.

Like my webwhore counterpart, I do feel guilty about not giving more of myself, especially to my fans. But let's face it – a big part of why my chosen profession involves sitting at home alone in front of my computer for 12 hours a day is the simple fact that I'm an introvert. Interacting with other people exhausts me.

If I didn't have a scheduled standing Girls Night, I wouldn't see my friends more than once every 4 or 6 weeks, when I finally got lonely enough to pick up the phone. It's no accident that my family lives two provinces away. I don't keep in touch with any of my friends from school other than tidbits that filter through my mom. My voyeur cam watchers can probably attest to my anti-social nature by the number of times they've heard my phone ring, watched me check the call display & then promptly not answer it.

Though I'm two cans of Lysol away from building my own Spruce Moose, most people would never guess it. Once I'm out,

I'm talkative & always make people laugh. I've often been told I'm the life of the party, even before I've had a drink or twelve. But the effort it takes me to get there is tantamount to running a marathon. A less sweaty marathon filled with giggles & sex talk.

At the end of the night I'm always glad that I went & promise to get out more, but I'm also relieved to come home to a quiet apartment & the furry companions who rarely expect me to be witty & entertaining. A bowl of kibble? I can handle that.

Grabbing my Gatorade & hitting the inbox.

Wednesday 8 October

Blonde Afternoon

After wandering around my apartment complex looking for my car, calling John three times with no answer & then calling the towing companies to see if it had been towed, I finally found it hiding in the very last stall of visitor parking, only visible from three feet away.

I drove for almost half an hour to get to my soccer game late. Surprise! No one was there. The field was completely empty. Half an hour of cursing later, I stomped back into my apartment & re-checked the email I received about our make-up game. Lo & behold – the game is NEXT Thursday. There goes an hour of driving for no fecking reason.

Grabbed the dogs & threw them into the car, headed to the off-leash. It was a beautiful day & I figured they deserved some exercise, even if their Mom wasn't going to get any that night. But my lovely plan was foiled! A stupid woman with her stupid Weimaraner was at *my* leash free park. And since Kiero, all 8 pounds of her, likes to go for the throat of large dogs, she had to stay on her leash.

I walked my dogs up & down the field, waited for the stupid woman to leave & did some more cursing. How dare she? How dare she ruin the evening I was attempting to salvage?

Finally the bitches departed & Kiero was free to run. She ran the length of 10 soccer fields before she finally slowed down. Not a dog designed for apartments, clearly.

Piggy took notice of some white plastic wiffle balls a grandfather

& his little ones were playing baseball with. When I say "took notice", I mean he stole them & ran away. Fortunately, the kids & granddad all thought this was hilarious, so for the next half an hour, I sat in the grass while the kids threw the balls for the dogs. The smiles & giggles from those two little rugrats were adorable. Even notoriously snotty Kiero got in on the fun, batting about the lightweight balls with her paws & chasing them all over the park.

It turned out to be one of the nicest evenings I've spent in a long time, in the company of strangers.

Wednesday 15 October

Why Porn (a.k.a Did She Just Say That???)

I love pornography. For as long as I can remember, I've been intrigued, excited & aroused by pornographic imagery. Not very many people will say that out loud – even fewer women. On top of the social silence, there are scads of women who would have you believe that enjoying sexual imagery that isn't disguised as art means you couldn't possibly be a feminist. That's just stupid.

Having sex, feeling desire, being titillated by erotic imagery – these are all completely natural emotions. We are sexual beings. Regardless of whatever political agenda you may be marching sexual desire pulses through your veins at one time or another. So how could celebrating the imagery of sex be such a bad thing?

Fundamental feminists will try to tell you that pornography degrades women. That nude photos and XXX videos promote the view of women as sexual objects. I've got a news flash for ya, sisters – women ARE sexual objects! So are men. At some point in your life, you will see someone, be it a man in a Calvin Klein ad dripping wet with only a thin cotton T-shirt covering his rippling muscles or a woman on the bus wearing stockings with seams drawing a line up beyond the hem of her skirt and guess what? Your thoughts will immediately jump to sex. That's OK. That does not mean you're a pig. That does not mean you're a bad person. It just means you are alive!

Whether you're attracted to men, women, cross dressers or the transgendered, there is going to be at least one "type" of person in the grab bag bag of folks we call humanity that is going to do it for you. That little twitch in your pants, a sudden blush to the cheek, a raging fucking hard-on, whatever – the look of that special someone will illicit a reaction from you. Being attracted to someone because of their looks is perfectly natural & it doesn't automatically indicate that you wouldn't be interested in getting to know that sexy someone on a more intellectual level. It doesn't mean that you wouldn't value him or her as a complete person once you got to know him/her. It just means that you're alive & human. And that's A-OK in my book.

How does pornography come into all of this? Blame MTV. We just don't have very good imaginations anymore.

If it were socially acceptable, when you spotted someone on the bus on the way home from work that really turned your crank, you could just whip it out right there & jack off. However, that would land your sorry ass in jail, and rightly so. The saucy bus tart may be coming home from a long day at work & is probably not attracted to you. She likely wants nothing to do with your little fantasy, if she did, she'd probably be sitting beside you & actually talking to you instead of facing the other way. Hell, if you'd gotten up & given her your seat, she might have actually chatted with you, providing a perfect opportunity to ask her out, you lazy fuck. But I digress.

Folks with lively imaginations have no need for pornography. That man on the bus could've dragged his Sum 41 sticker-covered knapsack home with his female fantasy on the brain & added her to his mental collection. With hot water streaming down his back in the shower, his mystery bus lady would appear, roll off her stockings & climb onto his small crooked member. Safe from the eyes of the bus babe, as well as law enforcement, our masturbator is free to choke the chicken without anyone being degraded or getting come in their eye. Unfortunately, too many years of watching *My Mom Off the Island So I Can Marry a Millionaire!* have killed that mental function. Combine this with the overwhelming political correctness that teaches men not to think of the women they encounter in day to day life as sexual beings, they turn to fantasy where neither the scenarios nor the women resemble reality.

And that's why porn is here to stay.

The porn magazines don't make us horny – we're already horny people. The magazines just give something to focus our sexual energy on for the minutes it takes us to get that release. Sure we could do it on our own, using our own imagination or the bus ladies of the world for fodder. But the fact is that would take a lot longer. And who wants to promote more water consumption? Don't care about the environment???

Friday 1 November

Steal This Webpage

I went to log into my site today to check something & started getting whacked with pop ups. Huh? I don't have pop ups on my site. I soon realized it was my host's version of a 404 page. Naturally, I freaked. Where the fuck did my members' area go???

I tried:

- logging into a couple of other pages I have bookmarked in my members area. Same problem.
- FTPing to the members' area to see if all my files had somehow been erased. Nope . . . all looked good.
- checking the .htaccess. Seemed fine.
- checking my password files to see if some weird redirect had been added. Un-uh.

Everything seemed fine except that my members' area was still missing!!!

After a panicky call to my host, I discovered that my members' area was perfectly intact to everyone except me. It turns out that my personal password was somehow leaked. My host's security program detected too many logins by my username & blocked me, redirecting me to the pop up pages rather than my members' area. I blame the snotmonkeys at Globalbill, my ex-billing provider that closed up in the middle of the night, completely unannounced.

Needless to say, the rest of the afternoon was spent furiously changing every password I have on every site I have a password to. That's a whole lotta passwords. It got me thinking about on-line security & the identity theft stories the local news are always so fond of ~~promoting~~ reporting.

I'm generally a pretty trusting person. Living pretty much my entire life on cam, I'd have to be. But how much do I really trust the trained seals they have doing "tech support" over at my domain registrar? Those guys don't even bother changing out of their pizza delivery uniforms before they slap on their headset & settle into their Strongbad-plastered cubicle for the night.

What exactly does Ted the tech guy have access to? Let's see . . . my full name, address, phone number, credit card number & the password I use on that site. It wouldn't take too many nights delivering medium peps before his girlfriend starts ragging on him that his 1984 Honda Accord with the "FUCK YOU & YOUR ONLINE JOURNAL" bumper sticker stinks like a pile of day old 'za. "*You know, Ted. There's a good chance that Kristy has used that password before. Let's see what else we can find . . .*"

Good thing I have no money.

Drat! Ted is foiled again! Muahahahahaha! I win by poverty default.

Tuesday 17 November

Reverend Kristy Rantsalot

Thanks for the words of support, guys. My friend is absolutely fine & it turns out it wasn't a heart attack. She has very high blood pressure from being the official worrywart of her entire family & this attack was just a case of stress-induced angina.

The concept of creating so much stress in your life that it actually makes you physically sick is a serious one though. I am grateful that I realized at a young age life truly is what you make of it. When you surround yourself with negative energy, your life is negative. I apologize for the hippy-speak, but it's true.

I was absolutely miserable when I worked my corporate tech support job, even though I was making a ton of money for a 19-year-old. I bought into the idea of climbing the corporate ladder & "networking" with people I had no respect for. I spent all day listening to people yell at me because they couldn't get their email (*Um . . . you're on dial up. Did you connect to the Internet first?*) or because the evil Internet had *somehow* put a sex site into their history file that there was *no* way someone in their household could've *visited* (*It's only you, your husband & your 16-year-old son that use the computer? Gosh, I have no idea how Tremendous-TittedTarts.com could've gotten in your history file.).*

Then I'd have to hear one of my eight managers, none of whom knew anything about computers, reprimand me for forgetting to say "Thank you for calling HyperMegaGlobalCorp" at the end of my nineteenth call with the password problem lady who always had her caps lock key on.

"Oh & by the way, Kristy, your Calls Per Hour is down to 8 & we need that up to at least 9.2, so can you try to teach these people how to use their computers quicker? That'd be great. Thanks!"

Everyone I worked with was a zombie. There wasn't a single person at that company that actually enjoyed his job &, over the course of the two years I was there, I watched tech after tech go on sick leave or start taking anti-depressants. The rest lived for the few moments after work & on their breaks when they could get high. After a long, boring shift, we'd head out to a local pub & drown our sorrows. I can't remember ever having a conversation that didn't revolve around how much we hated our jobs.

But for most of them, the money was enough of a pull to keep them there. They worked just hard enough to not get fired. And the company paid them just enough so they wouldn't quit. Fortunately, I escaped.

I had my light bulb moment while watching the movie *Fight Club*. If you never caught that one, just the first half of the movie is enough. The Ikea-ed condo scene was like the hand of God coming out of the celluloid & smacking me across the ass. That was the sum of my life. I went to a job I hated every day. I spent my weekends at Ikea, picking out new items to decorate my condo with. I lived with a boyfriend who wasn't even someone I was in love with, just someone that I didn't ever fight with. It was a Prozac life – no extreme lows, just a steady monotone hum without any crescendos.

At that point, John & I had already met but were both in other relationships, so we hadn't acted on the spark between us. We became good friends & I helped him set up his new apartment when he finally did split up with his ex. But I wasn't quite ready to take the plunge & leave my rock steady life until that night watching *Fight Club*. I got up from that movie theatre, phoned him & told him I loved him. I moved out a couple of weeks after that, quit my job & created a new life with him. And I've never been happier.

Granted, a lot of it is still the mindset. The friend I mentioned earlier, for example, has nothing to stress over. She has a healthy, happy family. She has financial security. She has a husband that loves her. But she's always searching for something, somewhere that is wrong & she fixates on it. So instead of seeing how lucky she is, her life is filled with stress.

She wouldn't be able to get out of bed in the morning if she lived my life. I have zero financial stability &, being self-employed, I have a very feast or famine lifestyle. By working in the sex industry, I also run the risk of burning my bridges in the mainstream world so, should I ever need to get another "real" job, it may be very difficult for me. But ultimately, if I decide to be happy, I will be. I can focus on my lack of security or the freedom my job affords me. I can become consumed by the number of people I offend by posing nude or be grateful for the amazing friends I've met in this industry. It's entirely up to me.

Allright . . . now it's just about 4 a.m. & Reverend Kristy has probably ranted enough. But I do hope that somebody will stumble across this entry & maybe hear something they needed to hear. And to everybody else, make it a wonderful day! It's entirely up to you. How cool is that?!

Friday 30 November

Are People From L.A. Really That Fucked? (a.k.a If You're Appearing On Reality TV, Make Sure Your Underwear Is Clean)

After two very long work days for which I earned virtually no money (seriously . . . I made more money when I was 18 & working at a coffee shop), I treated myself to pizza & some pay-per-view. Decided to skip the sweaty man-on-man love, also known as UFC, & went straight for the boobfest of Blind Date Uncensored. Good gawd! There are some fucked-up people on the dating scene.

The hero of the evening was a 25ish, fairly attractive guy who seemed like a pretty good date throughout his clips. His date was into the bad boy type so he intuitively tried to step it up a notch. Apparently his efforts didn't go unnoticed as they ended up back at his apartment, stripped down to their skivvies. The chick was still playing hard to get, but c'mon now – when you're half naked & about to give an equally half naked guy who you just met a few hours ago & whose last name you don't even know a massage, you're not exactly the Donna Martin of dating.

Yes, I did just make a Beverly Hills 90210 reference. So sue me! I haven't had my morning chai yet & the analogy well has run dry.

Fuck. I think I just plagiarized Dennis Miller.

Back to the date from hell . . . as I'm-Really-Not-A-Slutbag hops onto the bed to massage her suitor, she & the millions of trashy reality TV viewers, including myself, are made painfully aware that the dude has shit his pants. His underwear had huge nasty stains on the seat! And not just skid marks, 'cause this was on the outside.

I laughed & cringed so hard I actually fell off the couch. Well worth the $3.99, thank you very much.

Wednesday 9 December

Beautiful Snowfall

Yesterday evening I was watching the snowflakes twinkle as they floated to the earth across the black night sky. It looked so peaceful & beautiful, a fresh coat of perfect white blanketing the grit & concrete of downtown. I bundled myself & the dogs up in our winter gear & headed outside. They bounded across the fluffy white snow into the quiet night, broken only a few seconds later as I started cursing like a truck driver.

"Hurry the fuck up & pee! It's motherfucking cold out here!"

Ah, Canada.

Monday 21 December

Birthday Blues

As the end of year draws to a close, like any good consumer who's bought into the idea of having a house, car, family & secure job, I'm reflecting on the year behind me. The bonus pressure of adding another digit to my age, magnified by an industry where anything over 21 is considered "mature", is the straw that broke this webwhore's spirit. That's right. I'm in a birthday funk.

Technically I do have a condo, a car, a boyfriend & a job that doesn't appear to be down-sizing me any time soon. I've even lost weight this year, a goal usually at the top of everyone's New Year's resolutions. But those nagging "shouldas" keep getting to me.

- I shoulda earned more money this year.
- I shoulda saved some money this year (like money to pay my taxes with, for example).
- I shoulda learned how to put the motherfucking baseboards on (4th year running & still sitting in a dusty pile).
- I shoulda figured out how to discuss issues without yelling by now.
- I shoulda at least *decided* if I want to have children or not.
- I shoulda started brushing my dogs' teeth regularly.
- I shoulda dropped off the Goodwill box that's been sitting in my front hallway for two months.
- I shoulda learned to quit boring my blog readers with the minutiae of my life.

Is there a certain age when you feel like a grown-up? I really thought that by now, I'd have my shit together. I'd be one of those fully-functioning women with a swanky condo & perfect nails who's always throwing dinner parties for her fascinating group of friends. A snapshot of my real life is more likely to reveal a pony-tailed, Sketchers-wearing girl in a disaster of a living room typing away on her computer with chipped sparkly pink nails & still calling her parents' house two provinces away "home".

I'm glad I'm leaving tomorrow to visit my family for the holidays. I think I just need a hug from my mom.

Monday 4 January

Plane Is Still Grounded, But My Mind Left Days Ago

Technically I'm not on holidays yet. My plane doesn't depart until later tonight. But my mind left days ago.

Let's run a quick tally on what I was supposed to have completed before leaving:

TASK: 25 reviews for new client.
RESULT: 0 reviews completed.

TASK: Photo shoot & update.
RESULT: Charged the camera batteries.

TASK: Marketing work so my projects won't lose all traffic while I'm gone.
RESULT: Refer to exhibit A – rolling tumbleweeds.

I've somehow managed to consume mass amounts of time doing absolutely nothing. My grand accomplishments for yesterday included doing the laundry & packing. Full stop.

I do, however, look & feel fabulous. I got my pre-holiday fake tan working & am floored at what a difference it makes. My tummy looks flat & muscular. My blue eyes pop out instead of my blemishes. My shoulders look absolutely kissable. I'm hooked!

For people who can tan all summer long, this probably comes as no surprise. But for someone who either freckles or turns lobster pink, this is heaven. Being a complete narcissist doesn't hurt either.

While I should be working madly since I have huge bills to pay upon holiday return (taxes, anyone?), I don't feel one bit guilty. This is a change of phenomenal proportions. I feel relaxed, happy & completely free of the stressful *chicken-without-its-head* hysteria that usually precedes leaving for holiday. I'm usually up until 4 or 5 a.m. the night before a trip, feverishly attempting to get everything finished. Of course, this makes the first day or so of holiday tense as it takes a while to unwind & shake that "what did I forget?" or "I can't believe I didn't finish _____!" feeling.

I didn't finish any of it. I forgot most of it. And I couldn't care less.

I'm going to Vegas, baby! Here's to warm weather, cold beer & plenty o' trashy hotel room snapshots.;)

Saturday 11 January

Things I Learned In Vegas

1. **Treasure Island rocks!** The hotel rooms were large, beautiful & cheap. It wasn't a 5-mile hike through a maze

of jangling slot machines to get to the elevators. It was probably just as fast to walk from Treasure Island to the conference space in the Venetian as it was to walk from the actual rooms in the monolithic Venetian itself.

2. **Chicken Venetian is to die for.** The yummiest meal I had in Vegas & a recipe I am going on a no-holds-barred search for.

3. **Four days is too short.** The last day we were there was the only time we took to kind of relax & do the touristy stuff. But it would have been nice to have had that day to wander around, catch a movie, hit a buffet & then get up the next morning to return to "convention mode". I had some great photo shoots & met kick ass people at the parties, but after four days I was burned out & needed a break from the small talk & constant, "Yes, I'm really a webmaster, not a porn star" clarifications.

4. **Vegas is therapy.** The trip was literally worth the money for the simple fact that I was able to overcome my fear of meeting new people. Usually in situations where I don't know anyone & I'm forced to mingle & make small talk, I get phobic. My mom was like that too & absolutely dreaded going to my dad's stupid corporate parties & whatnot. I've always been the same way, except in the company of friends. In Vegas, I didn't know anyone although I had chatted with some folks through email. Surprisingly, I had no problem at all! I had a blast & wasn't shy about introducing myself to new people once I got on a roll. Suck on that, Dr. Phil!

5. **I heart Seska.** I've had a crush on this Montreal amateur model for ages, so getting the chance to hang out with her & do a shoot together was great. I was very nervous & it likely didn't go as well as it could have, but I'm hoping we'll get to meet again. I'm not sure what it is about Seska that girls love so much, but I am just one member of her popular fan club. Trixie & I are already planning a video where we get to take turns wearing a black wig. "It's my turn to be Seska!" "No, I want to be Seska now!"

6. **I belong in this industry.** I've never been quite sure if I fit in with the other amateurs & pornographers since I'm

not a swinger, I've never been a stripper & to be honest, I'm really not much of an exhibitionist. Sure, when I get drunk you might catch me dancing on the tables. I like having sex outdoors & feeling the rush of almost getting caught. But I'm not one of those girls who would just flash her tits because somebody caught my eye. Despite my unlikely porn star status, in Vegas I would say that I really clicked with 95 percent of the people I met. This never happens. In fact, John & I joke around about how we just generally don't like people. We have a hard time finding cool couples that we could see ourselves going on holidays with without wanting to bash their brains in with coconuts after day three. But in this industry, the ratio of people I've met that I really liked is insane. I have a huge list of people I would love to visit & I find myself wishing I lived somewhere more accessible to the rest of the smut peddler population.

7. **I am so glad that John came with me.** He has been completely inspired by the people he met in Vegas & is now going to get more involved in the industry. Up until now, I've run my sites 100 percent on my own. He takes photos of me sometimes, but I still have to plan the shoots, the poses & usually drag his ass behind the camera. He works very long hours, so I can't blame him, but now that he's all fired up about his own ideas, I can't wait to see what he can accomplish on his own. Plus it will make our own dinner conversation more interesting as there will be less of me droning on about who did what & who wrote this or that in her journal. OK, I'll still probably talk about that stuff, but at least he'll know who I'm talking about now!

8. **I am very bi.** Yes, I've always had some measure of attraction to other girls. Yes, I've kissed other girls & once went down on a stripper with a room full of guys watching. But considering the vodka/cran factor compounded by the "putting on a show" factor since we had an audience, the fact that I was extremely attracted to her showgirl good looks isn't rock solid evidence that I'm bisexual. Each photo shoot I did in Vegas, however, just seemed to get better & better.

Joy, a tall, tanned & toned blonde was gorgeous & very sweet with me, ensuring that I was completely comfortable each step of the way. By the end of our shoot, I just wanted to pounce on her! Seska was an absolute doll & I wish we'd had more time together. And Trixie? My on-line crush completely rocked my world. I had hoped that we would get along well since we read each other's blogs & I felt like I "knew" her before we had met. But . . . wow. I could never have anticipated how amazing we would be together. Kissing her soft lips & looking into her eyes – it felt like I was falling in love with her, as corny as that sounds. Women definitely have a stronger emotional experience in regards to sex, but I had no idea I'd get smacked upside the head like that, cartoon hearts swirling around us. Now I just have to figure out how to smuggle her up to Canada.

9. **I love my job.** This is probably the most important revelation that hit me in the desert. John & I were waiting at the airport & a group of "Wheel of Fortune" slot machines were just crossing the $1 million progressive jackpot. So while we were waiting to board, we started plugging what was left of our American change into the slots. Of course, we chatted about what we'd do should we win 1 million USD. You know what? I would still do my site. I've been getting so excited planning nylon & foot fetish shoots that if I had won the $1 million, I would absolutely still be doing my site. I would just throw way more money into hiring models & buying equipment. I bet there aren't many people who can say that if they won the lottery, they wouldn't quit their jobs. It was the first time it really hit me how happy I am with what I do.

This is going to be a really good year.

KILLBUNNIE23

http://killbunnie23.com

About Me

I was born in New Jersey and have been trying to live it down ever since. Anyone who has ever grown up in New Jersey will know exactly what I mean. I lived with my mother and her parents in a comfortable and curious home on the side of a mountain. They were kind, opinionated, very funny, and always gave me the room I needed to grow. I spent most of my childhood with my nose in a book or obsessing over horses, and I wanted to grow up to be an artist and never ever get married.

When I was 14 I discovered boys, or *a* boy, to be more specific. He was a 16-year-old rat-faced metalhead with a skateboard and, for some reason, I found him appealing. I suppose in a town that was less than 2 miles square he was about the edgiest thing going. One evening while my parents were out, he pretended he was deaf and ignored me out of my virginity; I said no about a half dozen times and he just didn't seem to hear me at all. I only mention this event because I believe that it changed me, it left me with so many questions, and I never really looked at men quite the same ever again.

I spent the remainder of my high school career snubbing my peers and slumming it in New Brunswick with bands like The Bouncing Souls. I felt stifled by the conservative environment of middle-class New Jersey and I think it's fair to say I was an overbearing pain in the ass, but what teenager isn't? I had sought out the punk rockers in hopes of liberation but found them to be

just as restrictive socially as high schoolers were. How can something that's supposed to be about anarchy have so many rules? I
was desperate to find a place where there were no rules and NYC
seemed like a safe bet. They say you should be careful what you
wish for, but I had always thought that was just a tired cliché. Little
did I know.

In 1992 I was just about to turn 18 and I left New Jersey to go to
college at the New School for Social Research in NYC. I had every
intention of being a thoughtful and serious student, but things
don't always work out as planned. The lure of NYC nightlife was
too strong and I decided to trade in classes on Hegel and Marx for
downtown raves. I was brainwashed by the bright lights, candy
colors and repetitive music (the ecstasy probably didn't hurt,
either). In the beginning the scene had this really inclusive positive
vibe going; I had never experienced anything like that before and it
was infectious. It was also short-lived. I soon noticed that at every
party at around 5 a.m. this strange group of people would show up.
They weren't like the ravers, they were more like elegant monsters;
they were the club kids. They lounged in the corners, observing
everything and talking in tight little cliques and I knew that's where
I wanted to be. I had had enough of pigtails and pacifiers; I wanted
to move on to bigger and bitchier things.

By now the school year I had not attended was over and I needed
a job and an apartment. The apartment was easy; I found a one-
bedroom to share with a Jersey skater kid. He was an ideal roommate, we were never home at the same time and I hardly saw him
the whole year. The job, it turned out, was pretty easy as well. I
browsed the back of the *Village Voice* and found an ad that said
"fantasy role-play, no nudity, no sex, no experience required", I
was savvy enough to realize that meant S&M and I thought I might
be qualified. I had some experience in boy torture and figured I
could easily learn the rest. The dungeon was really a three-bed-
room apartment on 30th street and the interview process was fairly
nonexistent. In short, I got the job and became a teenage dominatrix. This also proved to be my entrée into the world of the club
kids.

You see, to become a club kid it didn't matter where you were
from; you could be a trust fund baby like James St James or from
the suburbs of Ohio, like my friend Sacred, it never really mat-

tered. You just had to have a hook, something that made you different and special. We were all self-created creatures and I had finally found a place with no rules. The more twisted and bizarre you were, the more popular you were. Michael Alig was our ring leader and was the most twisted of all, and in time it would be his undoing.

But before we get to all that bad stuff, there was a lot of fun to be had. Every night was Halloween, a new theme, a new party and a new costume. Peter Gatien built us an oversized house of cards on the third floor of the club where we could all hold court and indulge in our favorite pleasures. He paid us to look fabulous and behave outrageously, and we did our best to live up to his expectations. My job was to dance in the Shampoo Room, on a tiny wobbly podium, to Whillyem's eclectic mix of 80s, disco, new wave and hip hop. I had to beware of records that had a skip in them since it amused him to fling them at me like a frisbee. On Fridays I held the velvet rope to the VIP area; basically, I was that bitch you had to get past to get to the good party, but fortunately for most people I was easily bribed. Saturdays I was back up on the podium, teetering in my platforms and dodging vinyl. My days continued to be filled with sweaty businessmen begging for spankings and licking my boots. The whole thing was held together by constant momentum, drugs, and eyelash glue, and it was only a matter of time before we all succumbed to our own fabulousness.

As time passed the theme of our parties became darker, and our choice of drugs more serious. We traded in Clara the Chicken and ecstasy for Blood Feast and heroin. Drugs used to be something that enhanced our experience and it degenerated into the reason we threw parties at all. Emergency Room was an excuse to dress up like doctors and hand out rohypnol, and in one of Michael's more obvious moments he threw one for the World's Largest K-Hole. He actually distributed flyers advertising this event all over NYC and then was surprised when the DEA took an interest in the Limelight. Things were taking a bad turn, but we were all too fucked up to notice or care, and besides we had always counted on Peter Gatien to take care of those details. What we didn't know was that Peter was in just as much trouble as the rest of us. Mayor Guiliani had pledged to clean up NYC and the Limelight was one of his prime targets. Too bad Peter was too busy being holed up in the Four Seasons Hotel with Michael smoking crack to do anything about it.

We had all gone off the deep end, and no one more so than Michael. He was on more drugs than all of us and if he could get his hands on yours he would do those too. In fact it was his passion for drugs that made him invite Angel, a local wannabe, to move into his apartment. Angel may have been a wannabe, but he was also a very proficient drug dealer and desperate to be in Michael's inner circle. Michael, in typical form, exploited that need for acceptance and convinced Angel to open a line of credit, which was Angel's first mistake. His second was to leave his stash at home unattended. A blizzard trapped Michael and his friend Freeze in the apartment with nothing to do for four days except consume all of Angel's product. He came home and confronted Michael and no one can be perfectly clear what happened but we do know this:

- Angel was furious, and a fight ensued.
- Michael fought back but was losing, so Freeze decided to help with the aid of a hammer, three times to the head.
- Angel was bloodied but not dead, so Michael and Freeze decide to finish the job with a pillow and some household cleaning products.
- They then move him to the bathroom and leave him for about 10 days.
- Freeze buys Michael a bundle of heroin and a set of knives and leaves him to it.
- What's left is boxed up and dropped in the river.

Unfortunately, instead of sinking as they had hoped, it floated to Long Island, where it was immediately found by the police. Now you would think that the cops would figure something like that out quick, but they don't give a shit about some gay Puerto Rican club kid drug dealer. It took 8 months before they arrested them, and then only because Michael would confess to anyone who sat still long enough to listen. He really believed that no one would turn him in, but apparently he was wrong because they sent him away for about 10 years. He managed to murder not only a human being, but a whole subculture in one drug-addled afternoon.

I left both the club scene and the S + M world in the same year.

The two were interdependent in my mind and when one collapsed so did the other; besides, I had a burgeoning heroin habit to support, and the money just wasn't good enough. A taste for heroin was part of my Limelight severance package, along with a very cute but very unemployed boyfriend, who also shared my inclination for the powder. We moved into a hotel, a place famous for being a home to various hookers, transvestites, artists, crazies and a fair number of European tourists on a budget. On any given day you were as likely to run into Madonna in the elevator on her way down from a photo shoot as you were to trip over someone OD'ing in the hall. The rooms were slightly larger than a walk-in closet, and contained no extra amenities, including a bathroom – you had to share one with the whole floor but if you were lucky you might get your own sink. There was something incredible about that place, though. I don't really know how to describe it. The building itself held so much energy and history, sometimes it felt like you were residing in a living thing. I was supporting myself and my boyfriend by stripping at the Harmony Theater, one of the most notorious strip clubs in NYC. To say it was a hole would be generous; I never quite figured out if I was working there to get heroin or if I was doing heroin because I worked there. Either way, after a year, I realized I was well on my way to becoming a cliché and I wanted out.

I left everything – the job, the drugs, the boyfriend, the hotel – everything. I took time off, I traveled, I spent some time in Dallas (hot) and some time in Miami (hot and humid), mostly sitting on my couch watching *Northern Exposure* and playing with my cat. After a year I returned north and moved to Connecticut and started over. It is a quiet place, nothing like the city. I am surrounded by trees and animals and, in the winter, I actually need the 4-wheel drive on my car. It was a tough adjustment at first; I was bored and lonely but I bought a camera and everything changed. Here was the perfect thing to fill my time, indulge my obsession for dressing up, to document life around me and to communicate it to the world, all without ever having to leave my house. I took all that time I had alone, and all those costumes I had collected from my club years, and I let my imagination play itself out for my camera. Here was the ultimate opportunity to express myself; my camera felt like a projection screen for the inside of my own head and an extension of my own hand. Some pictures were love letters, some were inside jokes to myself: all of them are a reflection of something that matters to me, something that I wanted to share with everyone here.

Monday 21 July 2003

Ok, I just had the strangest phone call.

The BigMan has all sorts of odd and annoying friends, which is why I never answer the telephone and I don't know what possessed me to do it today. This particular odd and annoying friend writes terrible lyrics to horrible musicals and likes to keep me on the phone for an excruciating amount of time making up rhymes about my name.

This, believe it or not, isn't so much the strange part.

I had forgotten that, in addition to his passion for rhyme, he harbors fantasies of dominant women tickling people till "they feel like they are going to die". I had also forgotten that he knew I was a dominatrix at one point and liked to get me to talk about my old tickling customers. All of this forgetting made me remember why I avoid him on the phone.

He called me once and sort of made a few rhymes and skirted the tickling topic and then hung up on me. Then he called back and grilled me on the tickling directly. There were strange grunting sounds in between questions and I couldn't tell if he was asthmatic or masturbating. Either way, I did what I always do in these situations, which is answer the questions as obtusely as possible. I know the answers he is looking for, and of course I refuse to give them to him. His fetish may be tickling but mine is to skirt the edge of someone's satisfaction and then deny it. He pursued it doggedly for a few more minutes before giving up and moving on to some rather personal questions about what I liked most about Miste. He didn't mean anything sexual, but it was still personal anyway, so I remained dense and unpliable. Exasperated, he eventually wrapped it up with a half-assed rhyme and hung up again.

See why I don't answer the phone?

Saturday 13 September 2003

You would think after all I have seen I would be really cynical by now, but I'm not. In fact, I still have a tendency to be an idealist and believe the best of people; that's why I was so bitterly disappointed by my experience last night.

I went into the city to go meet Mr SeriousArtist who I met at the Party Monster after party. That evening we seemed to have a good conversation and he went as far as to suggest that I might work as his assistant on his next project. I didn't get too excited about that prospect but I was vaguely interested . . . so I go and I meet him and I realized something was wrong right away, and it wasn't just the white foam collecting in the corners of his mouth making him look like a cokehead freak or that he kept whipping out his comb to run it through his vaseline-soaked hair like Fonzie. The whole thing seemed to go from feeling like a meeting to feeling like a date, and then from feeling like a date to feeling like a really bad date. He knew I was married to Mister from the first time we had met, so I am not really sure why he was expecting more, but when I wasn't down with his plan he became very rude and dismissive. My favorite part was when he told me he had enough platonic friends. What is interesting is he had spent so much time telling me how different he was from other guys, and how much he really loved women (heads up, girls: guys who say they aren't like other guys most assuredly are and men who make a point of telling you how much they love women most likely don't). The whole thing left me really depressed and with a slight case of penis envy, just because I suspect this doesn't happen to male artists quite as frequently.

Monday 6 October 2003

Conversation overheard in the ladies' room of a NYC lounge between two women sharing a mirror:

"Your nose is so cute."

"I know."

"It's so tiny and cute."

"I know, I measured it. It's a half-inch."

"It's so little."

"A half-inch exactly."
"I just love it!"
"I know, me too."

So much for the Village being full of intellectuals.

Friday 21 November 2003

I have kept a diary off and on more or less since I could write. The first one I remember having was a little red vinyl Hello Kitty book with a lock on the cover. In fact, I still have it, along with the 20 or so other books I have collected over the years. sometimes I write a lot, sometimes I don't write for months, but to me somewhere along the way I have formed the inherent opinion that existence is pointless without documentation.

However, the lesson I have learned repeatedly is that with documentation comes trouble. I have never had a diary that has not been read, the reading of which usually results in some sort of personal drama. My solution was initially to keep two diaries, one that could be left around and one I would keep hidden, but that only works as long as the second one isn't found, which of course it always is. So then that led me to keep three, one in the open, one decoy secret one, and then one really super secret one with all the good stuff. Can anyone guess what happened? of course you can . . .

So what does this have to do with life now, you might wonder (or you might not); since this diary is online and obviously public, how can it be stolen and read? The short answer is that it can't, but it has raised a whole new set of problems. When I began this page it was intended for strangers, people who I would never see, but through one means or another it is now in the hands of most of my friends, people I see or speak to on a near daily basis. On the one hand I am pleased that they can share something I have worked so hard at putting myself into. On the other hand, it can be quite frustrating. I have to constantly self-censor for fear that I may hurt or annoy someone. I have to make sure that I do not tread on toes because I have to face the fallout of it in real life. I want to be honest about the things that are going on in my life, or even the things in others' lives that inspire tangents of thought (which often leads to the creation of art) but how do you do that and not hurt feelings?

My web guy heard my whining and created an online super secret diary, just for me, but we have seen the luck I have had with those before and I am too chicken shit to actually use it. So for now I am stuck. Mentally constipated you might say . . .

Wednesday 10 December 2003

I really don't even know what to say. I am not entirely sure how the whole issue came to a head in the first place, but when it did I was ready to abandon this site, my journal, and my photography.

Mister and I were discussing an unrelated topic. Somehow the conversation managed to turn to my photos, this site and all sundry associated with it. He isn't always comfortable with certain aspects of this project, more specifically the sexual nature of some of the images and the number of people who write to me, most of which are men. I think he has a fair point; I often think if the shoe were on the other foot I might not be so casual, which of course leads me to feeling guilty for doing it myself. It's unfair, and it brought me to a whole new set of disturbing and confusing questions.

Questions about why I create and post things like this in general. It is something I take such great pleasure in but am often embarrassed to talk about in other areas of my life. My family, my in-laws and etc all know I have this hobby and it is frequently discussed in the abstract but whenever anyone wants to see anything I tend to give the runaround. It would embarrass me for them to see it. They would probably feel the same, so why do I do it. The question plagues me and I have no answer.

I panicked and started to wonder if what I was doing had any merit at all or if I should just stop. But, merit aside, I don't want to stop because it makes me feel good. This place, my blog and these photos, are the one thing I have that is all my own. I can play out all of my fears and fantasies here to whatever degree I choose, but I am having a hard time reconciling how to be a good wife and true to myself as an artist (if I can even be called that) at the same time. These two sides of me move further apart every day and I am left feeling torn.

This has registered itself in the fact that I haven't taken a new photo in three months. Oh, sure, I have projects in the works and whatnot, and I think about pictures all the time, but whenever it comes down to actually setting up and shooting, I always find some reason to put it off. I feel paralyzed, too scared to move forward, but too scared to give up what I have. All this shit has been building up for a long time and, like I said, yesterday it just all came out.

Astro and Lauren met me in the city and gave me their opinions. "Be brave," they said. "This is part of who you are and you should not give up, and don't worry, families don't stop loving you over a few photos."

Monday 15 December 2003

This isn't true of everyone, but I notice a lot of times when I meet someone new that I am interested in becoming friends with, they lose interest in being friends with me once they realize I am married. I find this incredibly depressing.

I know it's tough when you meet someone you think is cool and you are interested in them or whatever and you get disappointed when you find out that they are taken but, Jesus Christ, it makes me feel like a walking fuck-hole with some extraneous body parts attached. Is my only worth my potential as a date?

It just makes me feel real small, you know?

This is one of the reasons why I frequently hate being a female. For years I wouldn't even acknowledge it in my own head. I still prefer to think of myself as neither sex, or perhaps both, but definitely not one or the other. Sometimes I wish I could erase my genitals and the responsibility and complication that comes with them. I hardly ever get a period and I really believe that I just flat-out willed them away. I have been to tons of doctors and they can find no cause. I simply could not face the continual bloody reminder that I am a girl. How do women do it every goddamn month? 4 a year is the MOST I will tolerate.

At the same time I don't want to be a guy, although I do think I would enjoy the novelty of external plumbing for a few weeks, I just want . . . Oh, it is impossible to explain what I want.

I guess I want everyone to understand that to me my body and my gender are happenstance and are not a reflection of myself. It is just the space I occupy. In a way I almost envy my transsexual friends. They knew they were in the wrong body and they had the means to correct it. There is no third option; I am stuck here for good.

Jesus, this is not what I expected to get into when I sat down. I was just a little upset that I think a potential friendship I was really looking forward to has faded and suddenly all this crap came out . . .

Let's move on to other things . . . Right now I am up in Albany at Bryan and Sacred's house. We are supposed to be working on a new shoot but the ends seem to be fraying. It is a simple shoot; we just keep getting stuck. And now everyone is out at work and I am here in the house with nothing to do and not even any pot to keep me fuzzy. But it's not so bad, I decided to use my time alone to dress up as Bryan and take a few pics of me playing videogames like the regular guy I wish I was today. Oh, and I also made a meatloaf in the shape of a human head. That always cheers me up.

Monday 22 December 2003

The other day my horoscope told me to go plumbing through my old diaries for inspiration, and while I have said before that I only put limited stock in astrology I figure it is never a bad idea to go through old things. I didn't find much in the way of inspiration, but I did find out a whole lot of things that only make sense in hindsight. My first choice was the book that covered my time in Hotel 17, right when everything was on the verge of falling apart. I sort of know in my mind how awful things were, but it was so completely different to see it spelled out on paper. It is amazing really what the mind and time can do to one's memory; in my head it had all taken on a soft amber hue, horrible, but more like a sad movie I had seen a long time ago, *Old Yeller* in my head. While I reread my passages, I was shocked at the direness, desperation and tragedy that filled nearly every day of that year. At the same time, I was proud to see that I never gave up faith. I was always working to change; I always knew that it was temporary and there was another life for me. Looking back, I see I was just as much lucky as I was right.

Not everything I read was so heavy. I did find some amusing things. One was I realized that I hooked up with a semi-famous actor and forgot all about it. He was no one then and I am not going to tell you who he is now, but I see him on one of my favorite shows every week. In the entry I was in a nightclub (quel surpris) and I picked up a pretty boy on the way to the bathroom (yet another shocker); he said he was an actor. I feigned interest as we waited in line; he talked about his Hallmark movie of the week that was on the next night and his part in a movie that was coming out. He lied about his name (which I found out the next day, when I watched the Hallmark Special) but he told the truth about his parts. What can I say? He was fun to make out with and I forgot all about him till I read that entry. For a laugh I looked up the movie he was in on IMDB and to my surprise it was someone whose name I recognized immediately; not only that but he was in one of my all-time favorite "teen" movies which happened to be on my TV the exact moment I was looking him up! Weird, huh? He was a lot skinnier back then, which is probably why I didn't recognize him . . . or at least that is the story I am sticking with.

Tuesday 13 January 2004

Here is a typical conversation in my home. I am speaking in italic and BigMan is speaking in regular text.

I don't want to drive the black car any more.

Why not?

I think some animals have been living in it. It smells like cat food and pee.

Oh, well, that can't be too terrible. It's just a little water.

What water? I said pee.

Yeah, that water.

You think pee is water?

Well, yes, basically.

Hmmm . . . (Pause)

So if I went into the other room and peed in a glass, you would drink it?

Uhhh . . . errr . . . no.

But I thought you said it was water.

Well . . .

So you wouldn't drink it, but you want me to drive around in it?
  Realizing I may have had a point, but not wanting to concede defeat, he said, "Ehhh," and followed it with a noncommittal gesture of the shoulders. The pee car issue is currently unresolved.

Saturday 17 January 2004

Sometimes I fantasize about shooting myself in the head, just to make the noise stop. I don't really want to die or anything, I just want a little break from the constant relentless thinking.
  It never stops. Tangent builds upon tangent and there is no end. Most of the time I am pleased with this; I very rarely am ever bored. I don't even need to carry a book to the doctor's office or anything because all I have to do is disappear into my own head for a while and it's all good. I have a library and six thousand channels of satellite TV built right in. Usually I would consider this way better than real TV, but real TV comes with a remote control and more importantly an off button and my head does not.
  I just want a little vacation from my brain, or maybe I could send my brain on a vacation from me. I wonder how it would feel about two weeks in the Virgin Islands . . . or Hawaii, perhaps?

Sunday 25 January 2004

I get a pretty decent amount of mail. Most of it is full of praise and encouragement, and whoo boy I love that. Positive feedback keeps me going when I want to throw in the towel, but this morning I got an email of a sightly different variety. Not critical, not mean, but he definitely wanted me to explain a few things. His questions were relevant so I have reposted (most) of our correspondence.

  Hi
    I read your\"about me\" page and I read some of your blog.
    I'm sorry to read about your fucked-up life when you were living in NYC. I &'m glad you outta that – but I just don't get why you maintain ties with it by dressing up and having photos taken of yourself in prop clothes/heroin chic/etc.

I'm as open-minded as the next person, but if you're pleased you're out of that scene, why not cut all links with it entirely? Leave the heroin chic and the mind-fucky attitude?

I'm not implying you should do the above by means of asking questions, I'm generally unsure as to why you are like what you are like.

Anyway, whatever you do, I wish you all the best for the future.

B

My response:

Hi B

Firstly, let me thank you for writing me one of the first really interesting emails off my site ever. 99.9 percent of the mail I get is from people telling me how much they like what I do, and hey, I am certainly not complaining about that, but a little dissenting opinion is nice. It forces you to look at your work and your words with fresh eyes. Debate is good, it keeps you sharp.

Now on to the topic at hand.

Please, please, please do NOT feel sorry for me about my "fucked-up life", because I certainly am not. I cherish every experience I had; I have seen and done more in those years than some people have their entire life. I regret nothing, not even the most painful parts, and there were plenty, but there was also more than my share of fun. We are talking Studio 54-sized fun.

But I digress. You wanted to know why, if it was all so horrible, I do not just cut ties . . . The short answer is because it wasn't so horrible. And besides, there was really nothing to cut ties with. I was mind-fucky before I got to NYC so it stands to reason I would be after I left. I was born like this; you can even ask my mom. In fact, if you reread my bio, you will see that I deliberately went to NYC to find other like-mind-fucky individuals. My time there with them allowed me to experiment and develop what has become my personal vision/aesthetic. Some people go to university. I went to nightclubs. The end result is essentially the same.

I am slightly confused by your repeated reference to heroin chic. That was a real 90s look and I think I can safely say there is no evidence of that in my photos. Heroin chic is based on über-skinny hollow-eyed fashionista junkies, which I may have resembled somewhere in 1996, but as the size of my ass will attest is no longer the case. I do not promote or reflect the use of heroin in my photography; I do not wax nostalgic, it was a dark time in my life, but I report it because it happened.

I take the photos in the prop clothes because . . . well, mostly because I enjoy it. I like being able to indulge my imagination and play out little mental scenarios. It's fun. Besides, I have all these clothes and things lying around; I might as well use them. Taking photos of myself is a way to reinvent myself on a regular basis; I can be anyone I want, the bored 60s housewife waiting to meet her lover, the washed-up show girl about to get murdered, a day in the life of my ex-boyfriend . . . whatever I want. Some of the photos aren't for me; many of them are private messages to people in my life: It's a way to express humor and affection. For example, I started the pin-ups as a means of sending visual love letters to my (now) husband when we were dating long distance. My photographs can serve any purpose I wish them to; the possibilities are limitless.

So you see, I am not tied to my past. My history liberates me; it has taught me how to be free both as an artist and a person. I don't know why I am the way I am: a combination of nature and nurture, just like everyone else, I guess.

Sorry for the excessive length of this letter, but you asked some big questions, so you got some big answers. I hope this clears things up a little, but if not I am happily here for further dialog.

I wish you all the best in return Bunnie

Wednesday 4 February 2004

People who have been following this blog for a while are probably intimate with my bizarre sleeping habits by now, but for those of you new on the scene let me fill you in . . . I do all kinds of weird crap in my sleep. Most notably I get up two to five times a night and sleepwalk to the kitchen and eat all things sugar-related. This is confusing to me because during waking hours I have little interest in eating sweets. For a long time the top choice for my midnight feedings was ice cream; it got so bad I had to have a padlock put on my freezer, to which Mister holds the key. That worked; I would just run unfulfilled laps to and from the kitchen all night, but then I made the mistake of going to Costco and buying Mister a big bag of those gourmet JellyBelly jellybeans.

Who can resist a jellybean?

Not me.

It's one of the few sweeties I am tempted by during waking hours but I thought I could control the situation by getting another lock for the cabinet we keep them in. I must be a far more clever or determined little monkey than I thought because I have figured out how to slide my hand up and into the cabinet, circumventing the lock and grab tiny little fistfuls of jellybeans. I know this because I have been waking up feeling like I have been poisoned; sugar makes me feel worse than a hangover, but the real evidence is that I keep finding all of the flavors I don't like in strange places around the house. A coconut bean on the kitchen counter, a banana one on the back of the toilet, licorice under my pillow and, the final and most damning, two root beer jellybeans in the back pocket of my pajamas.

Thursday 12 February 2004

The funny thing about keeping a blog for me is that I can only do it if I pretend no one is there . . . or not really no one, but maybe more like a big faceless amorphous mass of people, which according to my stats is fairly correct. 30,000 hits from 30 different countries (wheee!). Somehow that is less scary than when I find out the guys in my webmaster's office are reading it. Then I start imagining a face to put with the name and an imaginary life to go with the face and then imaginary opinions of my blog and all starts to go horribly wrong from there. I become self-conscious and clam up. I start scrutinizing everything a little too closely and become super self-critical.

This is usually the point where I contemplate chucking the whole thing.

Happily I never quite get there; I am not sure what brings me back, but I always come back.

Writing here usually makes me feel better, whether I am communicating with someone, no one, or everyone. I get what drove Leticia off for a few days; it can be a lot of pressure to be interesting all the time. I guess the flip side is it can be a fun challenge too . . .

Sunday 15 February 2004

Ugh.

Unless you plan on having babies, and I don't, there is just no point to being a girl.

Fucking cramps are killing me.

I'd like to cut my uterus out and feed it to the vultures.

I don't use the damn thing anyway.

I would so much rather imagine that beyond my cervix was a black hole, something that threatened to suck away anything that got to close into oblivion.

Now THAT would be fun.

And come to think of it, pretty useful, too.

I could use my pussy as a giant vacuum cleaner, sucking away anything from errant dust bunnies (just imagine me scooting across the floor of my house) to undesirable elected officials.

Saturday 28 February 2004

Today has turned into an unexpectedly exceptional day. As you know from the previous entry, this morning I have had a sudden jump in hit counts. So I went out about my business, shopping and such, and I arrived home all excited because I found a pair of pants that fit me (miracle!!) and took a quick peek in on the site and was floored to find the hit count had jumped another few thousand. It jumped so many that it reset itself to zero and started all over again.

I should be happy about this, but I don't know if I am; I am too busy feeling guilty for being naked, for being perceived sexually, for the way it hurts the people close to me, for me to enjoy it. I should be happy; people are noticing me for doing something different. It's what I have always wanted since I was a little girl. So why aren't I happy?

Monday 1 March 2004

It would be tempting right now to sit back, bask in the new attention and think all sorts of nice things about myself. It would be easy to indulge the ego . . . but I think today I am going to do the opposite. I am going to spend the day scrubbing my kitchen floors, cleaning my toilet and telling everyone else how great they are for what they do and how much they mean to me. Why hoard the goodwill, right? I am also going to make a point of spending a little romantic time with my Mister; he has gotten a little bit left aside in all my excitement/exhaustion. He is kind enough to allow me to share myself with the world here, so I need to remember to share myself with him too. His support means the world to me and I am grateful to have it. Many husbands would not be so understanding . . . so I'm going to make a point of showing my appreciation at some point today.

Tuesday 2 March 2004

It seems there was no need to manufacture jobs with which to humble myself. Life has turned to shit of its own accord, literally.

Woke up this morning to find our sewer pipes backed up and the basement flooded. Nothing brings you back down to earth quite like a mini sea of poo in your home. The plumber is down there now trying to sort it all out; I am just praying it's a simple problem that can be solved today, because sooner or later I am going to have to pee and I would rather not have to do it in my yard.

Friday 12 March 2004

I am not feeling well.

I don't think it is just the head injury either, though I am sure that doesn't help.

This is a more amorphous non-body not feeling good. Some-times I feel a hole break open inside me and all sorts of things starts passing through, most of them unpleasant. Pain, fear, and deep deep sadness . . . I feel it all just pour into me, even if it has nothing to do with me, and I have no choice but to carry it around until it dissipates.

Maybe it's an over-developed sense of empathy.

It seems like most of the people close to me are going through something painful, or confusing, or depressing, and I wish I could just take them all and tuck them safely into my belly until it's all over . . . but obviously I can't.

I can't protect anyone from anything, I can't save anyone, I can't do anything but sit here while all of this collects in me and pray my seams don't burst.

Sunday 14 March 2004

I told a lie yesterday.

Barb and I were having one of our little chats and I told her that I hated people and that I wish we would all die out as a species. She looked so hurt when I said that.

I imagine in my mind sometimes that I have my finger on a button that could vaporize every human on the planet. Do I hesitate? Not in my mind I don't. So where's the lie?

The lie is that I don't really hate us all at all, it's just sometimes easier to feel that way than admit how disappointed I get. I get frustrated when I see how small we can be, how cruel, selfish, wasteful, deceitful, petty . . . well obviously I could just go on and on, so I won't. Secretly, under all this cynicism I am a closet idealist; I want to believe the best about us, that we have the capacity to be better . . . or at least kinder and slightly less fearful . . . but then I turn on my TV or take a look around and . . . well imagine it like this, like you poured your whole heart, soul and trust into someone you love, only to find out they have been fucking your best friend behind your back the whole time. A most painful betrayal.

So Barb, I am really sorry I lied; It's just sometimes I can't face the truth.

Saturday 20 March 2004

I got this email a little while ago, and I tried to respond directly but for whatever reason it kept getting bounced back to me, so I am just going to post it here.

> Yeah hey I can imagine you getting a lot of emails and whatnot from guys with all of your pictures (which I don't find appealing at all, but maybe that's just me) but I would just like to say that you are exactly the type of person I had desired to be for a long time. Relatively intelligent with sex appeal. I admire you some, I admire how you seem to not give a damn what anyone thinks and that you are able to live your own happy life the way you want to. I was just curious, however, as to why you would subject yourself to the life of a stripper and sleep around? The question is not meant to be inclusive at all and if you do not wish to answer, that's fine. Thanks. Oh, btw, how old are you? I'm 15 (if you wanted to know).
> Cheryl

Hi Cheryl, Thanks for writing to me. Sorry it took me a while to get back to you but I have been swamped under emails and I really wanted to give yours the attention it deserves. You can ask me any question you want; the ones I would find intrusive no one ever thinks to ask me anyway.

You wanted to know why I subjected myself to the life of a stripper and to sleeping around . . .

It was fun.*

My mom always said if you want you can go through life always making the safe choices, but it sure isn't going to be very interesting. I guess I really took that to heart. You are right, I live how I please and I don't care what anyone thinks. I can't think of a compelling argument to do things any other way, can you?

Hope that answers things for you. Best, Bunnie

*If that doesn't satisfy you I will address it at greater length. I never really considered stripping something I was subjecting myself to; it was something I wanted to do, even though it wasn't always pleasant, easy or fun. Sometimes it was downright awful, but I think sometimes I like awful. When I was in my late teens/ early 20s (I am 29 now) I was hungry for a diversity of experience. I wanted to walk the edge of darkness and come back to tell the tale. Most of the time while I was stripping I felt like a scientist; I wanted to observe people and that was a great place to do it. I learned more about human beings, men in particular, there than I did in all of my time in school. I guess some people might be uncomfortable with the idea of running around naked, or being viewed and handled as a sex object, and I admit sometimes I didn't like it either but mostly it didn't bother me. I guess I just don't think about things that way, to me, my body is just the space I happen to inhabit. I detach easily so it is simple for me to view it as nothing more than a tool or a prop I can use to suit my own ends, as i continue to do with my photos. If anything I always thought the joke was more on my customers than it was on me . . . They were the ones handing over all their hard-earned money and for what? A peek at my boobs? Hahahaha, morons. They would have been better off getting a hooker, at least then they would have gotten something in return. Oh you probably think I am awful now . . .

Sleeping around was a lot less complicated. I did it because I wanted to. you only get one ride on this planet and I wanted to do/ try/feel/learn everything I could. I do not want to get to the end and find myself saying "I really wish I had . . ." Fill in the blank. I don't sleep around anymore, not because I have a moral issue with it, but because after all that sex what I have learned is that it means very little to me. Despite what the media is constantly pushing us to believe, most sex isn't that exciting or even very good and so I have no compelling reason to seek it out. Looking back over my partners I would say maybe 10 were ever worth sleeping with at all, but hey maybe I am just a critic.

Monday 5 April 2004

I didn't realize until I logged on today that it is the 10-year marker of Kurt Cobain's death. Naturally AOL has to attach a stupid poll about whether or not he was a genius . . . 58 per cent said yes. I was honestly surprised he ranked even that high, considering the crowd. The poll was, as always, linked to a message board.

AOL message boards are the bane of my existence. I am irresistibly attracted to them, even though I know I will leave them infuriated and doubting the worth of human beings in general. Today was no exception. Today's posts fell into one of two categories, ones that say Kurt was a whiny drug addict loser who got what he deserved, and others blaming Courtney for killing him. To the critics who blame him I say:

People, please, have some compassion. Does taking such a hard line benefit anyone, including yourself? It's not like drawing these rigid little conclusions can protect you from anything, especially pain. We can say, "Oh he was so talented, he was rich, he was famous, what was so rough about his life?", but what do any of us know? Sometimes the things you think you want the most are actually the things you need the least. As everything on the outside grows brighter, the things on the inside grow exponentially darker, add drugs that can simultaneously alleviate and exacerbate the situation, and who knows what can happen from there?

I know, first hand. I won't bore you with the details but suffice it to say I have deep sympathy for Mr Cobain. It's almost amazing how easy it is to slip into these spiraling thought patterns. You are literally not thinking straight, and yet with each passing thought you become more certain you are seeing things clearly for the first time. You know you are really fucked when the idea doesn't even scare you anymore; you are beyond fucked when not only does it not frighten you, but it seems like a relief.

Today actually marks the 10-year anniversary of another death for me. Philly Dave, also known as Frankenberry, was a kid from (where else?) Philadelphia who broke out in the NYC rave scene in 93. He was just sweet as pie when we first all met him but that was before he turned into an overnight ecstasy kingpin. I caught him on the tail end of his sweetness, dated him for a few months and so had the vantage of watching him sour. I am not even really sure what happened . . . I remember us having a lot of fun. He had just started dealing E's and we were going to parties all over the East Coast, then he started to change. He became very successful in his chosen field and it seemed the more money he made, the meaner he got. One afternoon stands out in my mind . . . I was fishing behind my couch cushions, looking for change to eat that day (I was a very, very poor student at the time) and he comes trotting up my stairs with a big bag of McDonalds from downstairs (this was before I realized how evil they were and was just obsessed with fries). So he sees me and what I am doing and he asks me so I tell him and says, "Oh," and sits down and EATS ALL THE FOOD, right in front of me. I am talking like six cheeseburgers and a couple of large fries. And he is sitting there, looking at me, and I just KNOW if I ask for a single crumb he is going to go all batshit and say I am only dating him for his money and drugs and yada yada blah blah.

Like I would fuck this guy for ecstasy and fries. Please.

So that was what you might call a relationship-defining moment for me right there. I took it as a personal challenge and we spent the next couple of months embroiled in some pretty fucked-up power games. When all was said and done he was left out in the cold and I was stuck with a lesbian for a year, but that's another story; this one is about him.

We didn't speak for a year after our last fight. I kept tabs on him, though; I knew he was hurtling forward at a rapid pace, his appetites voracious. He consumed more than anyone I had ever met, – food, sex, drugs, money . . . everything, anything. he would think nothing of popping 18 E's and topping it off with some coke, K, rohypnol and a bottle of diet Pepsi. Did I mention he was a diabetic? not healthy . . . so one night at 5 a.m. he comes up to me, so high his eyes were rolling back in his head, jaws chattering. He says, "Bunnie, I am sooo sorry about this last year; we were so fucked to each other and I don't want to fight anymore. We were friends before anything and I want to be friends again." I was surprised; I was moved; I agreed. We hugged and we parted. I went home and four hours later I got the call that he was dead.

When I went home, he went to an after-hours in an apartment on the lower East Side. All I know is this, he went into a bathroom with freeze (the same one that later helped kill Angel Melendez) and when he came out he sat down and slowly aspirated on his own vomit. I know this because Jenny told me she sat there and watched him die, too fucked up in her heroin/K hole to help. His diabetes needles were missing and by the time an ambulance arrived so was the ten thousand dollars that he had in his bag from his evening's sales. It's fair to say I have my suspicions.

I hope he can hear me thinking about him, so he knows he wasn't forgotten. I think that is what he worried about most. It was almost like he always knew he was going to die young and so worked that much harder to leave an impression. Mission accomplished, Philly, because I am never going to forget. You really pissed me off on the regular, but I cared about you anyway.

Friday 7 May 2004

I don't know what it is lately . . . I think I am losing interest in the Internet.

Maybe it's a weather thing. Winters are so conducive to indoor amusements, it's easy to settle in front of the monitor, or behind the camera, but summer is another story entirely. All I want to do is get up early, go outside and work in my garden till I drop of exhaustion at sunset.

We have about two acres of overgrown, untended land infested with tree-killing vines. There's hardly anything growing that would be considered little more than a weed. I arm myself with the loppers and hack my way through the tangle, I rake miles of leaves, I build rock walls, I prune, I haul, I dig . . . matters are not made any easier by the fact that BigMan, the owner of the property, holds the international title for LAZIEST MAN IN THE WORLD and has used the back yard as his own personal dump for the last 25 years. I have excavated tons, literally tons, of trash from the garden behind the house. In addition we have three (three ! ! !) cars on various parts of the lawn that do not work, three that do work, and one that thinks about working sometimes. That is seven cars, people . . . Seven fucking cars. If I didn't know better, I would think we were a family from a John Waters film.

So forgive me if I am distracted, but at this point in time the day-to-day mundanities are far more interesting to me than my ephemeral life in the Net. I like digging in the dirt, I feel grounded, safe, and happy . . . but at the same time less creative. I haven't taken a new photo in months and I let the lapses in my blogging get longer and longer. I am not really sure why.

Maybe I think I have nothing interesting to talk about . . . After all, how much is there to say about working at a big tag sale and gardening? I thought maybe I should start organizing and writing up some of my favorite stories from the past, dominatrix days and club kid nights . . . Lots of good story fodder to be composted. I was ready to submit and give up one of my old favorites, completely vintage Bunnie, the kind of tale I could tell in my sleep . . . But first I consulted a friend of mine, who wrote me and said:

> A blog is the purest form of personal performance art. By its very existence, you define it, and it can be whatever you want it to be. Your hit rate alone should assure you that there's people out there who want to know what you're doing, be that gardening, making taramasalata, or rubbing peanut butter into your nipples.
>
> So if you decide that your blog is to be a gardening diary, and that the only photos you're going to take are going to be a day-by-day carrot growth chart, then that's what it is. If you lose 99.956 percent of your readers by doing that, then that's OK too – your blog isn't something that you do for other people, it's something you do for yourself.

Well, fuck me if he isn't right.

I forgot the plot, that I am not here for you, I am here for me. Maybe that is what has been hanging me up with the photos too . . . I became so distracted by thinking I had to be perfect, that I had to please my audience, I forgot what it was all about in the first place. That this is MY space . . . I can do something with it, or nothing, and since I pay for it I don't owe anyone a goddamn thing. I don't have to take a photo for a fucking year if I don't feel like it. Sure I will lose my audience, but in a way . . . so what?

I love that you all are out there, that I have communication with you, but it isn't what brought me here in the first place and it shouldn't be what keeps me here. I am here because this is the one place in the universe where I dictate all the rules. So maybe someday I will go through some of my old stories because some of them really are worth telling, but it isn't going to be because I am afraid, it is going to be because I feel like it. For now it might just have to be gardening.

Sunday 30 May 2004

I stopped by a tag sale while driving around this weekend; two items jumped out at me immediately and I grabbed them. I took my selection to the guy having the sale; he eyed my choices and said, "I think I want to go to a bar with you sometime . . ."

Can anyone guess what I had selected that would inspire that comment?

An antique riding crop and a giant bunny suit.

Friday 4 June 2004

For a while I thought that I was inviting too much in by keeping myself open; I thought if I made my world smaller I would reduce my chances of encountering anything really bad, but that just isn't true. If you care about even one person you open yourself up to tragedy.

Something has happened to someone I care about. I am not going to tell you what it is because it isn't mine to tell. All anyone needs to know is it was sufficiently awful to knock me back, jolt me out of my little cocoon and remind me just how horrible the world really can be. I am sick with disgust.

When I go out I have to shade my eyes because I am afraid that if people look into them that they will see the endless emptiness that I feel right now. I know that beyond the emptiness there is a rage unlike anything I have ever faced before. I can feel the agitated tremors of it in my bones; my cells glow with it. I want to take the human race and wring it of evil and obliviousness. I am paralyzed by my impotence, unable to do anything but use each private moment I steal to cry. It doesn't change anything or even really help, but there is nothing else I can do, no place else for all this emotion to spill over to, so it wells up from my chest and out of my eyes.

It will run out eventually, as it always does, but right now I wonder if I even care. Is there anything to even come back for? Why keep investing yourself in something that can be so gravely disappointing? All of my life I have questioned the value of our existence, but always with a reserve of idealism . . . I wonder now if that is gone.

I will be unavailable for the next few days.

Friday 11 June 2004

I listen to women talk about having, or wanting to have babies . . . they speak of it with such reverence and certainty. They actively seek out partners and deliberately work towards the day they can have families . . . I have to be honest, it confuses the living shit out of me.

That part of me, the part that could even *consider* it, just does not exist. I look around inside myself, (you know all the usual places, under the couch cushions, behind the drapes . . . misplaced things are always the last place you look) for a maternal instinct or even a base urge to reproduce and I got nothing. Zero, zip, nada, bubkas. Aside from the total absence of urge, the whole thing just seems like a raw deal. You get to relinquish your body to what essentially is a parasite, spend multiple hours in pain passing it, to get the delight of cleaning up its shit for the next few years and taking attitude for the remaining ones. Maybe I am missing some-thing, because even though I was really enjoying the company of the children at the party (they are way more fun to play with than the adults), all I could think when I saw all the pregnant ladies was, "Dear God, please don't ever let that happen to me."

Is there something wrong with me? Maybe . . . a lot of strangers/acquaintances certainly seem to think so (though not any of my friends, many of whom are parents themselves, they are way too cool to hold my non-breeding status against me). When people drop phrases into conversations like, "Someday when you have your own you will understand . . ." Or when they inquire about when Mister and I will be starting our own family (a fucking rude question to begin with), I patiently and politely inform them that I don't think it is for me . . . Usually I am met with one of two responses: a look like I just said I'd like to eat their children for breakfast, mixed with intense pity followed by a condescending, "Oh, well, I am sure you will change your mind, everyone does." Or occasionally something more hostile. One man spent the better part of an hour telling me that I was a selfish human being for not sacrificing myself on the altar of motherhood and that without children my life would be worthless.

Is that true?

I just don't believe it. If anything I wish I could be mom to the whole world. I would give it hugs all the time for no good reason and I would give it time outs when it got unruly. Why give your love away only to the people who share your DNA? I wanna give mine away to everyone.

Sunday 13 June 2004

Had a dream I ate Mister's penis. Just sat down at the table with it on a plate, looking for all the world like a kielbasa, and gobbled it right up with a knife and fork. Oddly, he didn't seem to mind.

Maybe I miss eating meat more than I previously thought.

Thursday 17 June 2004

Word to the wise: always clean your room before the cable guy comes to install a new system.

I had completely forgotten he was coming at all . . . totally slipped my mind.

Normally it wouldn't matter, aside from a few errant bits of clothing on the floor I generally keep the bedroom tidy. I am usually particularly particular about keeping certain items discreetly stored, but of course this was the one day where everything had slipped out of my grasp and out of its hiding spaces.

I let the cable guy in, thinking he will be working on the office TV or one of the ones in the upstairs rooms, and so continue on about my business, wiping crud off my kitchen counters. Then I hear a rustle in MY bedroom and run through a flash check in my mind of the room's status . . . You see, our housemate was recently away on vacation and, well, privacy is a precious commodity in this house so Mister and I wanted to make the most of the time we had with it to ourselves . . .

I tried to sort of casually slip into the room while he was working, ostensibly to you know, be helpful or something, and then started attempting to execute an elaborate series of manoeuvers to remove items from view. Usually I am pretty good at that sort of stealth, I can make objects disappear at will, but I was outmatched this time: the bedroom was a minefield of contraband.

He had already headed straight for the TV (of course) where there was a mixture of yoga DVDS and porn sitting on top of the set. He turned his back for a moment and I whisked them into the closet. When he turned the other way, I tossed a shirt over my glass piece. I thought I was on top of the situation but after my auspicious start things started to unravel.

The thing about cable guys is that they always have all this wire they want to run everywhere. Over, under, above, and behind every blessed fucking thing they can get their hands on. So, before I know it, he is running wires under the dresser, where I suddenly remember throwing some girlie magazines like two years ago. Sure enough, he starts digging around under there to feed some cable and a couple of titty mags slide out. Great. I am hoping the layer of dust covering them is thick enough to obscure the covers and try to nudge them back under with my toe. Moving on, he starts testing the TV, turning it off and on, trying to get the signal to load. I have one of those little 13-inch combo things that you buy at Costco for 89 bucks that has a VCR built in, pretty convenient, but if there is anything sitting in the VCR it ejects it when you hit the power button. Sure enough, he hits that power button and a tape pops out with a label emblazoned across the side with the inspired title, in my own handwriting, 'PORN TAPE VOL.2'.

Will the embarrassments never cease? Apparently not yet because then he started running the cable behind my bed . . . I am not even going to get into what he may have run into back there. Even I draw the line somewhere.

I suppose as a cable guy he must have this sort of thing happen all the time. When I think about it, its enough to tempt me into trying to get a job in the field, all those personal spaces to explore . . . and I guess it all didn't make such a terrible impression on him because before he left he also installed a memory card in my computer, gave me a new modem for it, and also a hug on the way out. Now that's service. Maybe I should start hiding porn under my kitchen and bathroom sinks so I can get a sweet deal when the plumber comes . . . do you think it would be too obvious if I duct taped a few DVD's to the back of the toilet?

Diary of a Nympho

http://nymphodiary.blogspot.com

6/5/03

Sexcapade

I needed sex. It had been about two weeks – too long. There's always my trusty buddy, P., when I'm in dire need and there's no other way to be satisfied. We have the greatest friends-with-benefits deal around. We're good friends, and can have straight-up sex and even hardcore fucking with no strings attached whatso-ever. Afterwards, we're both back to just relaxing and talking like nothing ever happened. It's the perfect set-up – no extraneous feelings, no awkwardness before, during or after. So when P. called yesterday while I was at work and mentioned he was experiencing the same dilemma (i.e. horny), I told him to come over after I got off work – and bring some beer. It helps me loosen up, and I love a cold beer after work.

He came, lay on my bed with his shoes off while I played on the computer at my desk – we chatted. Very casual. The subject turned to sex – always does. I can't help myself – even if I'm around someone I don't want to have sex with. We started looking up dirty pictures on the Internet. I lit a cigarette and he started massaging my back – standing behind my desk chair. I took a big swig of beer as he made his way to my neck – my most sensitive part. I sat up straighter, arching my back – decided to put on some mood music. Which playlist? "The Fuck List"? No – not into that soft porn music today – I wanted hardcore. The "Hard" playlist. Godsmack blared from the speakers, he's biting my neck, licking my chin all the way up to my mouth. He slipped his tongue in my mouth, grabbing my face and chin in both hands and angling it towards him. It was wet, urgent, rough. P. isn't the best kisser. He doesn't move his lips, rather holds your mouth open against his own and duels tongues. It's not bad – not at all – just not my style. But it seemed to fit the mood. I didn't want to kiss him, and turned away to take a drag of my cigarette and a swig of beer. He was licking my chin, my neck, and found my mouth again. He pulled my shirt off and freed a breast from my bra – stroking it, bending over and sucking the hard nipple. The same treatment was given to the other. After a few moments, my hand found his hard cock and I began massaging it through his shorts. Those came off and I continued to stroke him through the soft fabric of his cotton boxers. I pulled away from him and pulled his cock out. I took a swig of beer, to make my mouth cool and I licked at the head. He shuddered. I took him into my mouth. He was quickly moaning and stroking my hair, moving his hips with my rhythm. He wanted to get on the bed – tease my pussy with his dick. I told him OK, but I didn't feel like actually having sex – some of that and we both get off on oral. He said that was fine with him (that's how we usually do it). I climbed on the bed, pulling off my bra and shorts. He climbed on top of me, slapping his cock against my pussy-lips lightly. Seeing I needed some work, he scooted down on the bed and lightly flicked my clit with his tongue. I love to be teased – and the light, feathery caresses of his tongue got me immediately wet. I moaned, pushing my hips towards him, and he began to lick a little harder, going deep in and dragging his tongue the length of my pussy. Then he would go back to teasing my burning clit. I was whimpering, and getting more turned on than I'd thought at first possible in this casual tryst.

"Put your dick in me," I said in a pleading voice. He grinned at me – excited that I'd changed my mind from just oral gratification. He got up on his knees and rubbed his cock on me. I moaned, loving the anticipation. He slid just the head in – sliding in and out slowly – then pulling out and rubbing my clit again with it. This went on for a while, with his going a little deeper every time, and I was being worked into a frenzy. Suddenly, as he was sliding in a little more, I grabbed his hips and pulled him into me. He grunted and I let out a long moan. He started to fuck me just like I liked –

slow, long and hard. I grabbed hold of him, so turned on I only wanted to get off – and started grinding into him at my own pace. He matched it and I felt myself coming to a loud orgasm. I screamed, my pussy contracting around his dick, and I clawed at his back. After my orgasm, he held my legs up and began fucking me hard. I put my hands above my head to steady myself against the wall, and he pounded into me. I felt my breasts swinging heavily with the force – I turned my head towards my arm and screamed and yelped. It didn't take much of this before I heard him groan that he was going to come. He pulled out and I sat up, trying to catch his throbbing cock in my mouth. He just missed – shooting a warm glop of come on my cheek before I sucked him into my mouth and finished him off. He ran to get me a towel and I lit another cigarette.

Afterwards, I was back at the computer and he was back lying on the bed – this time clad only in his boxers. "My legs are still shaking," he said, and I laughed. I told him he wasn't so bad himself. "You're just so intense," he said. "And I love how much noise you make – porno noise." I smiled at that. I'd always been loud – hell, I want the neighbors to know I'm getting fucked. Porno noise. Had to keep that one in my catalog of self-descriptions and positive points.

27/5/03

Sexcapade

P. was over visiting, actually half-snoozing on the bed. I was on the phone with J. – the one I want but can't have. He lives far away. J. and I were talking about sex – we're always talking about sex. "I want to hear you," he said. I just giggled. "Tell him to fuck you and let me listen," he said; he was laughing but he wasn't joking. I glanced over at P. "He wants to listen to us fuck," I told him, taking a big swig of beer (P. always brings beer when he comes to visit – I think he knows what the amber liquid does to me).

P. just smiled and strolled on over to me, leaning over me where I sat in my desk chair. I moaned slightly as he brushed his lips over my neck – it's so sensitive there. "What's he doing?" J. asked.

"Kissing my neck," I said, softly. I leaned my head forward to give him better access and pointed to the back of my neck. P. knew the drill and sank his teeth into the nape of my neck. My back arched and I gave an excited and tortured little moan. "Harder," I breathed. "He's biting the back of my neck," I said to J., who also knew what that particular act did to me. I downed the rest of my beer – it helped me get over my stage fright. I have to admit, I was a little nervous about someone listening to me during the act. I'm VERY vocal.

"Get on the bed," P. said, pulling at my arm.

I crawled over onto the bed next to me, explaining to J. what I was doing. "Where's P. at?" he asked me.

"Between my legs," I giggled, and then moaned softly. "He's flicking his tongue over my clit." It felt so good and I was immediately wet. J. moaned a bit, too, then and told me he had his own cock out and was stroking it as he listened to me.

Soon P. was on top of me, running his dick along the length of my pussy – which I love. "He's teasing me," I told J., giving P. a wicked grin. In answer, he slid himself inside me, slowly. I let out a loud cry and bucked my hips towards him. He started pumping into me pretty hard, but I grabbed his hips and pulled him into me even deeper and made him slow his rhythm down to match my own. Soon I was at my regular ecstatic staccato moaning and crying out. J. was loving it, and kept whispering dirty things into the phone. I was making so much noise myself I couldn't make out what he was saying, but it didn't matter. He's got such a sexy voice it was all I needed. Even with all of this extra help, I couldn't come. I have the same problem when someone is watching me masturbate. I love an audience – but it makes me try too hard (which is the surest way to stop-up an orgasm!).

Finally, P. was tiring out and I told him to go and get my vibrator out of the bathroom. He did so, and within seconds was sliding it into my steaming cunt while simultaneously flicking my swollen clit with his tongue. He turned the vibrator on high, and it felt soo good. I wanted to buck my hips against him and make the vibrator go even deeper, but I couldn't even move. Moans turned into screams of "Oh, God" and "Fuck" while J. was telling me to come for him in that seductive voice. "I'm gonna come with you," he told me, and I could tell he was just as close as I.

It only took a few more seconds of all of that for me to start to peak, "I'm gonna come!" I screamed out and felt P. speed up just a little while J. cried out and moaned right along with me. It took me a few minutes to calm down after that – I just lay there panting and trying to calm my racing heart. Finally I got my voice back enough to get out, "Fuck, I need a cigarette."

I went to the bathroom while J. raved over my performance.

"I told you I made porno noise," I told him, giggling.

24/6/03

Memoirs

I lost my virginity at a Motel 6 in the summer of 1996. It didn't start out especially pleasant. We'd rented the room, along with another couple, to do just that. However, just previous to the renting of the room, my best friend and I had gotten our belly-buttons pierced – and liquored ourselves up with a bottle of vodka between us to calm our nerves (it was my first extraneous piercing). I vaguely remember some heavy making-out before I passed out. The next thing I remember was hanging over the toilet bowl with my first mate holding my hair. Rather than take advantage of me, he took care of me. We went back to bed after I expelled the evil fluids from my body – and awoke in the early morning hours. He looked at me and said, "Let's take a shower together."

We took turns soaping each other up, washing each other's hair and spent a great deal of time caressing each other's wet, slick body parts. We kissed under the pounding water and he lifted me up and tried to enter me. I was so tight; we had problems. We got out of the shower and commenced on a towel we'd spread out on the bathroom floor, and then somehow ended up with me sitting on the counter near the sink. I'm sure this tight pussy he seemed to be having trouble getting into was frustrating, but he didn't show it. He smiled at me, grabbed a bottle of conditioner and slathered it all over his cock – then rubbed some on me. He slid into me, slowly, in one fluid motion and my life was changed forever. I'll never forget that initial sensation of having a hard cock sink deep inside of me. That first moan – a mixture of sudden, intense pleasure and mild, pleasant surprise. A fiend was born.

25/6/03

Memoirs

I like to call this one "A Tale of Two Dicks".

I thought it was going to be yet another typical and terrible Monday, but midway through the workday I received a phone call from a male friend of mine I'd been casually seeing. It was always a treat hanging out with him because even though we'd never officially done the deed, we talked about it a great deal. The air around us was always crackling with sexual tension! He was going out of town for a few days and wanted to spend a few hours with me before his flight left. He picked me up from work, and we went back to my place. We were doing our usual, talking about sex and getting all hot and bothered with the mere mention of past dirty deeds and torrid trysts. I asked him to tell me about his dick . . . to tell me what it looked like. He seemed to get very turned on by the idea of describing his cock for me, from the look of the large bulge that began growing in his pants. A little shy at first, he soon got into it, and began getting very explicit. I could no longer control myself and begged him to let me see this magnificent cock he was describing for me. Gladly, he pulled his smooth, hard dick out of his pants and I found myself going in for a much closer look. Quickly, I had him in my hand and was slowly licking around the head and along the length of his shaft. He moaned and begged me to suck him. I slowly slid my lips over the head, sucking it, and went down and took all of him inside of my mouth. I fell into my own rhythm, running my tongue along the underside of his dick as I came up. Soon, he put his hand on my head and pushed me up and down on his dick, as I struggled to keep up with the pace he desired.

"I'm going to come," he cried out, but I knew this already. I latched on and sucked even harder as loads of his hot, sticky come shot into my mouth. I continued sucking, slowly, milking every last drop out of his throbbing cock as he shuddered. I pulled away with one long, last suck and swallowed every drop he had pumped into my mouth. I gave him a sexy grin, and swiped at my mouth with back of my hand. There wasn't much time to do anything else, so I got him a towel and he cleaned himself up. He had only ten minutes now to make it to the airport, and he gave me a quick, appreciative hug and was out the door.

All worked up myself, I sauntered into the bathroom and quickly climbed in the tub: my favorite place to masturbate. A few moments of rubbing myself was all it took to bring on my own thundering orgasm. I got out, and started making dinner when the phone rang. It was a male friend of mine I hadn't seen in almost a month. The last time we had got together had been hot, and I was so excited just to hear his voice on the phone asking if he could come over. An hour later, he was knocking on the door and soon after that we were all over each other on the couch. My hand snaked down his pants before I realized what I was doing. He moved off me to give me easier access, and I soon had his hard cock out and in my hand. I quickly went down, licking his balls all the way up to the head teasingly. "Put it in your mouth," he said in a husky voice, but I felt he needed a little more teasing first. I slid my lips softly over the head, barely caressing it and flicking my tongue over his hole before pulling back again. I ran my tongue along his impressive length a few times, before returning to lightly tease the head. He was moaning and asked me again to take him in my mouth. I swirled my tongue a few more times around the head, before suddenly taking his entire cock in my mouth. He groaned and grabbed my hair. I started off very slowly, going all the way down and pausing – sucking him deep into my throat – then moving back up while sliding my tongue along the underside of his cock.

Apparently it felt good – too good. His hands tightened in my hair, pulling it, and he began pushing me down on him, forcing me to speed up. Always happy to comply, I accelerated my rhythm, adding my hand to the base of his cock and matching my stroking with my sucking. It was but a few seconds of this when I heard a low, "Oh, God," and I felt the first stream of hot come pouring into my mouth. He came so much, he almost choked me, but I didn't stop swallowing and milking the last drops from him. I sat back on my heels and watched him trying to catch his breath. Whoever thought a Monday could be so enjoyable?

8/7/03

Memoirs

Want to learn how to ensure you never get a repeat performance with me beneath the sheets? Read on.

It was the first guy I'd been with since my ex of four years had left me. No, I wasn't some vulnerable, sobbing mass of emotions that could easily be taken advantage of. I was a hot and horny nympho who was having to adjust to a life without a regular supply of sex. It wasn't an easy adjustment.

We wound up on the couch and I straddled him. He was a pretty good kisser and I found myself grinding my crotch into his. I was enjoying myself, so I slid off him and undid his pants. He had a nice cock and I hungrily started sucking it. He didn't let that go on for too long – said it felt too good. Next thing I knew he was on top of me and sliding his dick inside me. I moaned, and started to swivel my hips to match his quick thrusts.

A little too quick – there was one, two, three thrusts and he blurted out, "I'm going to come." To which I responded, "Already?" He didn't even make it through the fourth. But, that's not what banned him from my list of potential fuck buddies forever. I'm not that shallow; shit happens. He apologized, saying he hadn't had sex in about three months. Fine, cool, whatever. *Then* he said, "Well, I gotta go." He stood, put on his clothes, kissed me on top of the head and left – while I sat there in stunned silence. Come too quick, we can work on that. Not so outstanding a performance, I love to train. Sex-jitters that make you keep losing your hard, not a problem, I'm patient. Get off and don't even *attempt* to get *me* off – arrivederci, asshole. And you won't ever get a second chance.

23/7/03

Memoirs

I'm not a fan of big dicks. Size never really mattered much to me. There were a few reasons for this: 1. My first was just average and he was *amazing* in bed. We were wild, and had lots of threesomes, and I got to experiment with bigger cocks but I wasn't impressed. I truly believed that any size was just useless equipment if you didn't know how to use it. 2. I'm only 4'10" – there's not a lot of wiggle room there, if you know what I mean. Big cocks just hurt me. I also find it harder to give a good blow-job when said member is so damn long you can't get much past the head down your throat without having it tickle your intestines.

So, everyday-size cocks were A-OK with me. That is, until I met Really Big, Gorgeous Cock Guy. RBGCG was this very sexy and very sexual man I'd met online. After talking so for months, we went out to a club together. I really wasn't expecting to get with him – but he had me so turned on by the time we got home that I was all over him. Imagine my dismay when I pulled him from his pants to give him a good suck. I know, I know – most women would've been drooling over this massive prize I held in my hands. It was definitely the largest I'd ever seen and all I could think was, "I'm not going to be able to enjoy this because it's going to feel like he's splitting me open." Still, ever the trooper, I dutifully sucked away (as well as I could around that thing).

Soon after we'd rearranged ourselves and I was lying on my back, awaiting the impalement and hoping he would come quickly and not hurt me too much. Imagine my shock – and complete and utter delight – when he slid that massive cock inside me *and it felt like fucking heaven*. This was new. A few good minutes into this, I was leading him over to the couch – I had to ride this one.

He later admitted he was a bit skeptical at first of letting me straddle him on the couch – claiming most women didn't know "how to move" that well in said position. Little did he know he was with a trained and masterful nympho! I climbed on top of him, enjoying every single inch of that cock as I came down on it – then began fucking the shit out of him. I couldn't believe how good it felt and how much it *didn't* hurt. Never had I experienced this sensation of being completely filled up. I was nearing my orgasm when he cried out that he was going to come – so I rode him faster, hoping to beat him to it, or, at least, come with him. I missed – he scored. He apologized – saying he wasn't used to a woman knowing how to ride him like that.

Still, being the sexy gentleman he'd been all evening, he got me off with his skilled fingers. Though I still had an amazing, explosive orgasm, I do regret not getting to come all over that really big, gorgeous cock of his.

25/8/03

Sexual Blather

I promised details – and I always deliver.

Friday night arrived in a cacophony of mayhem – I had to work late and was, therefore, running late. I'd had possibly the most stressful work week of my life and was ready to kick back, relax, have a drink and view some new sex toys.

Oddly enough, my two friends and I arrived just on time. There were about ten women there, most of whom I knew vaguely, and we all sat in a big circle in the living room around what, at first, appeared to be an altar to Aphrodite. It was covered in assorted bottles of oils and lotions and creams, and various other sexual playthings. The toys weren't out yet, but there was underwear and lingerie laid out as well.

The spiel was lightning quick and, before the first twenty minutes were done, my hands and arms were covered in lotions and oils that served varying purposes, and my chest was aglow with glitter. We got to sample just about everything. I had the strangest taste in my mouth, since all of it was edible and I'd mixed it with my beer. There are oils and lotions for *everything* you can dream up. "Like A Virgin" was an oil that made your pussy tighten up for a tighter fit; there was one that numbed the back of your throat to kill your gag reflex, and even one that loosened up your asshole for anal penetration. I can't even remember half of what I saw, there was such an assortment. It was a rich nympho's dream and a poor nympho like me's utter frustration. We took a short break as she picked up the bottles and laid out the real stars of the night – the toys.

I've never seen so many dildoes, vibrators, clit-suckers, butt plugs and weighted balls in all my life. I wanted one of everything. Of course, my meager paycheck does not allow for many sexually oriented splurges, so I really had to get *just* what I desired the most.

Let me take the time now to introduce you all to my new friend who is as-yet-unnamed. His given name is the Jelly-Gyrating-Beaver and he's as fun as he sounds. I honestly wasn't going to buy a new vibrator. As I said, the one I have works just fine and is new. Yet as I sat there looking at the ones in front of me, I remembered that when I'm using a vibrator (outside of the tub) I always wished for something to also be vibrating on my clit. This is one of those deals you see with the little beaver on the top of the vibrator that stimulates your clit whilst the other part is fucking you. I was in a mad rush to find batteries Saturday morning as soon as I woke up, and let me just say this about my new friend . . . *wow*. I really wasn't expecting it to be quite as good as it was. I'm sure you'll be hearing more about this new toy in posts to come.

The next purchase, that I'm equally as satisfied with, is a cream called Nympho Niagra. This was gotten on recommendation from the hostess of the party, a good friend and fellow-nympho-Scorpio. She raved about it, and I remembered another nympho-Scorpio friend telling me the same thing about the cream. I had to try this. As opposed to those warming-to-make-you-tingle lotions (which I'm not fond of) this is a cooling one. I will admit that I spent the better part of Saturday just rubbing this stuff on my clit and pussy while I went about doing my everyday chores. As soon as it would wear off, I'd dab on some more. It's listed as an "arousal stimulator" and I can say that I certainly was more aroused than even usual (which is really saying something). When P. dropped by to see my new toys and help me try them out, we were both amazed at just how much I came afterwards. I wasn't wet, I was *sopping*. So, if you can get some of this, **do**.

Not much else to report at this point. I've been playing with both of my purchases all weekend long, and as soon as money permits, intend to contact the saleslady and order a few more things. I promise to divulge any new and exciting exploits involving these new things . . . and you know, I always deliver.

9/9/03

Sexcapade

I can't leave my loyal readers high and dry for too long. Time to get everyone all wet again with a juicy, recent exploit.

I think my favorite sex is wake-up sex. There's just something utterly delicious about coming out of sleep right into some groggy groping, leading to a few yawning moans, flowing into some slow, stretching grinding and ending in an orgasm that makes a morning caffeine jolt pale in comparison.

The alarm pulled me rudely out of my slumber. It went off for a few moments, and even though he was closer, he didn't move to turn it off. I leaned over him and swatted around the top of the clock until my fingers hit the right button. Snooze. I scooted my body closer to his, he was warm and the a/c had, overnight, turned the apartment into the equivalent of a meat locker. I tucked my head into the crook of neck and shoulder and felt his hand in my hair. I hadn't even realized he was awake. He started stroking my hair, playing with it, sometimes running his hand down the back of my neck. In that premorning haze I perked up just a bit – could he be horny? B. isn't usually known for his sexual enthusiasm and I always hold onto the glimmer of hope that a little push from the Morning Wood Fairy will up the odds in my favor. Could this be one of those mornings? I decided to be a little brazen, and kissed his neck softly (coming on to B. is the equivalent of sneaking up on an alert deer – you never know when he'll turn and run the other way). His gentle answering moan was all the confirmation I needed. I let my hand snake down between his legs to find the fairy had, indeed, blessed us this early morning. I stroked his bulge through his underwear and felt his caressing go down my arms, to my belly and thighs. Rolling on my back to give him better access, I felt a finger slip over my pussy-lips – already moist – teasing me with slow, long strokes along the length of it. I moaned, trying to concentrate on still stroking him, but enjoying the feeling of his sliding fingers almost too much. This didn't go on long, the teasing and stroking and moaning, before I uttered that I wanted him inside me.

I turned over on my side in what is known as the "spooning" position. It's one of my favorites, as it allows ample opportunity for him to rub my clit while I gyrate in my own, preferred rhythm. He scooted up against me, pulling me even closer to him and I raised my leg up as he stroked me with the head of his cock. I squirmed a little, trying to get just the right angle for him to penetrate me, and finally felt him slide all the way inside. He collapsed against me with a little moan and his fingers quickly found their way to my clit. I swirled my hips and thrust back against him as he simultaneously pumped back into me. With his fingers strumming my clit, this couldn't last too long.

I came in a matter of minutes, crying out and bucking up against him. He held me tight while I cursed and shuddered and, as soon as mine ended, began pumping into me with fervor. Within seconds, he was coming too and his cries of pleasure were as pleasurable to my ears as my own orgasm had been.

Can I say, there is simply no better way to start off the day.

12/11/03

Sexcapade

Oh, it's been *way* too long!

It had been a lazy day all around. The golden autumn afternoon had been filled with honeyed talk and the light amber cool of cheap Chardonnay. We wandered outside to enjoy the fading light and the growing chill to the air, our eyes heavy and drooping as the setting sun.

I wandered back inside. It was darker inside; the only light was a washed-out pale gray shining through the slats in the blinds. I lay down right there on the floor, the new carpet thick and lush underneath me. I soon felt him lie down beside me, wrapping an arm around and pulling me closer to him. His warm breath on my neck made butterflies flutter in my stomach. I soon heard his rhythmic breathing and knew that he had dozed off. I found myself lulled into a light slumber as well as the light around us grew dimmer.

I slept only for a few minutes, but when I opened my eyes the room was darker. Some light still came in, but dusk was approaching. My movements awoke him and I felt the soft, wet of his lips on the back of my neck. I moaned, stretching my body and inching it even closer to his. His hand slipped under my shirt and I gasped as his fingers closed around my nipple, pinching it roughly. I pushed my ass back against him, feeling the hardness of his cock through his boxers. His moan drove me on, and I began rubbing my ass against him as he bit down harder on my neck.

Soon his hands had a new duty in mind, and I felt him pulling his boxers down with an urgency that made me even wetter. I rolled around to my other side so that I was facing him and scooted down so that his hard cock was right in front of my face.

"Oh, God," he moaned as I slid my lips over his cock and flicked my tongue over the head. That delicious little wine buzz I'd been experiencing all afternoon kicked into overdrive, and I found myself suckling and licking him with a fervor and intensity that had him crying out and pulling at my hair. It wasn't long before he was begging me to stop, afraid he would spill his seed before we had a chance to actually have sex.

I couldn't stop. I pushed him over on his back and went at it from a different angle, knowing this would slow down the rise to orgasm for him; for a few moments anyway. I climbed on top of him, running my hands up under his shirt and clawing at his chest. I was struck with a sudden urgency – I had to have him inside me.

I slid up his body, licking his lips and moving down to nibble on his neck. I felt his hand down there, guiding his throbbing cock towards my pussy. "I want you inside me," I purred in his ear. As I felt the head of his dick graze my lips, I quickly pushed and slid down on it – eliciting a long moan from the both of us.

Oh, there's nothing I like better than riding a man. Or perhaps, it's just that I love being in control. Either way, it was evident that neither of us was going to last long in this position. I started swiveling my hips and sliding up and down his dick with obvious delight. He grabbed my ass and quickly matched my movements. The room was almost completely dark now and the only sounds were our low whimpers and noisy moans.

Every few moments we'd pause; he was having trouble keeping himself from going over the edge. Finally, I felt the rise begin inside of me and my movements fell into a deep and deliberate dance.

"I can't . . . stop . . . if you keep doing that," he panted, but I barely heard him. I was on a mission and my own orgasm was my goal. I knew that he would come when I did. I cried out, picking up speed as I felt the first wave hit me – waves that rode up, each higher than the first, cresting into the next surge. I screamed – and then I felt him coming. This was all I needed to hit my peak. I could just barely feel him digging into my back, and his screams and cries seemed to match my own. But it was hazy – as if I was hearing it from some distant place somewhere above us.

And then it was over . . . as suddenly as it began. I found myself back in my sweaty body, lying on top of him – both of us panting and trying to calm our breathing and slow our hearts. I looked down at him and he gave me a smile. "Let's go take a bath together."

What better way to end a perfect sexual romp?

10/1/04

Sexcapade

Even though the setting was public and over-crowded, it seemed we were the only two people in the world. Had I inched any closer to his warm body, I'd have been in his lap. Our heads were bowed down and together, talking low and whispering indecent things into one another's ear. We had finished eating and it seemed that both of our minds were now on one thing only. The table offered no covering to hide any indecorous act we might wish to engage in, but my J. can be ingeniously surreptitious.

His breath was hot against my neck and his wet tongue so deft in my ear that I thought I might come from the simple contemplation of such skill being employed elsewhere. Suddenly he took my hand and began to guide it towards that warm and hard spot between his legs. I pulled away, giving him an astonished look. How could we, my eyes asked, with all these people around? Even though we sat in a corner of the room, there were crowded tables around us on two sides. The room was full of eyes that could turn our way and perceive our indecency at any given moment. "Trust me," he responded without ever speaking as I watched him rearrange his jacket as to make his nether region less visible.

He slowly undid his pants, watching my expression and glancing around to make sure we were not noticed all at once. I caught my breath as he pulled his magnificent cock into view. I am a cock connoisseur and it was pure delight to see one so fetching. My first instinct was to take that hard, smooth member and put it into my mouth – it begged to be bathed by my tongue and suckled with ardor. I could not, naturally, as hiding my head bobbing in his lap would have been ultimately impossible. Instead he took my hand again and led it back between his legs. I heard his soft moan as I wrapped my cool hand around his warm, throbbing cock. I began to stroke him, twisting only my wrist so that the obvious movements of my arm would not give us away.

What if we were caught – what if someone sees us? The thoughts raced through my head as I stroked him. I felt worried, but the wetness in my pants indicated what the situation was truly doing to me.

"Wait," he told me suddenly. He took my hand, and cupping it, spat into it. I smiled, and when I placed my hand and went to work once more, I knew he wasn't far away from coming. I was able to work my magic much better with the lubrication.

"I'm about to come," he told me, leaning forward and crushing my lips with a passionate kiss. I could feel his mounting climax in his uncontrolled kiss and my hand picked up its speed. He moaned around our dueling tongues and I could feel his cock throbbing with his orgasm. Hot jizz dribbled over my fingers as I squeezed the last drops from him.

I pulled my shaking hand away, grabbing napkins from the table, and glancing around furtively – suddenly once more aware of my surroundings. I handed him a napkin so he could clean himself, but I doubted there was any way to wipe the grin from his face.

17/2/04

Lascivious

Letter to My Beloved,

Why I Did Not Give You That Quickie In-Public-&-Under-the-Table Hand-job the Other Day

I hope you don't think I was ignoring him or that I was simply refusing to give him any attention whatsoever. Both of you must think I dislike him, but nothing could be further from the truth. You must know that I am completely mesmerized by him!

You may just think that I'm reticent and apprehensive about doing it in public during our short visits – but it is much more than that! My first impulse is *always* to get my hands on him as soon as he makes an appearance. You have no idea. You see, he is simply god-like in my mind. It seems almost sacrilegious to go at him with anything but reverence and respect. To simply have quick and non-meticulous contact with him is akin to eating a communion wafer and wine as a snack with no pre-ritual! It is feeding caviar to your dog or pouring Dom Perignon out on the ground as soon as the cork is popped. It is taking something that should be sacred and revered and making it base and mundane. I don't feel *right* skimming over something I feel should be savored, studied, worshipped, and handled with respect.

When I see him, I am drawn to him like a moth to a light. I want to trace every contour of his being with my finger and then my tongue. I want to memorize every mark, every movement, every curve and twist of his body. I want to learn everything that pleases him, and to what degree he enjoys each of my endeavors. I want to *know* him; every nuance of his existence. So much so that I desire the time and ability to do just that – and to interact with him on any level less seems down right blasphemous.

You must never think that I like to ignore him or that I enjoy teasing him. I want only to treat him as he truly deserves, and as I really want.

Always,
Bendis

10/3/04

Sexual Blather

My best friend once said of me, "You're the only person I know who proudly displays their vibrator in their soap dish."

I really believe this had more to do with the fact that I'm rather lazy than anything related to my unquenchable thirst for all things sexual. Still, while it may not be evidence that I am a true nympho (but am a slovenly housekeeper), it certainly is an indication of my sacred bathtime ritual.

When I was a young teen, I spent many hours masturbating – more than once a day, too. I often daydreamed of when I'd be a grown woman and how I would have the most amazing collection of sex toys; especially vibrators. I was fascinated with vibrators even though I'd never seen an actual one outside of the local Spencer's. I loved the idea of being able to have something that hummed and quaked that I could stick inside me. Now grown, I own only three vibrators and I never use two of them. I found, once I finally began having sex, that having something that hummed and quaked inside me couldn't even compare to the soft warm hardness of male flesh.

That said, while I may not have the vast sex toy assortment I hoped for as a teen, I have all I need, all any woman needs, to keep me happy. My hand-held shower massager. It's not just for showering anymore. Trust me.

Now I can't see a woman alive *not* enjoying the thundering rain of water pounding against her clit, but I believe masturbation via water holds an even more erotic feeling for me. My first ever experience with masturbating was in a swimming pool – lined up perfectly with the pump jets. I didn't know what I was doing, but I knew it felt good; damn good. I've been obsessed with "water sports" (no, not *that* kind) ever since.

So it was with much delight that I finally ordered a slim waterproof vibrator for my tubtime fun – and yes, Bubbles sits in my bathtub's soap dish. The combination of humming vibrator and pounding-water-on-clit is a sureproof come-within-seconds orgasm for me. It has become a bath time ritual for me. Shave – bathe – wash hair – masturbate. I come out feeling *completely* cleansed.

I usually bathe with bubble bath and plenty of candles in the room. Sometimes I'll have a glass of wine or champagne, or just a beer. The entire time I'm in the tub, while I'm doing all of my other "cleaning duties", I'm thinking about sex. Hot, dirty, nasty, wet sex – whatever scenario fits my mood at the time. By time I get to the last part, I'm more than ready.

I turn the massager on jet-spray, the high-powered one, and tease myself with it for long moments at a time. Moving from my clit down the length of my pussy. There isn't an inch of it that doesn't love the feel of that jetstream. When I've gotten myself completely aroused and ready, I take Bubbles, turn him on, and gently slide him just inside myself. I hold him there, barely pushing, and let the massager work its magic on my clit – the more aroused I get, the more I open up, and the more the vibrator slowly slides inside. It really doesn't take long, once that's slid in, for me to have the most amazing orgasm.

It almost beats the warm flesh of an actual cock.

Almost.

22/3/04

Sexual Blather

My first boyfriend and I lived together for four years and had the wildest sex life I've had with anyone to date. We were both nymphos, and kinky ones at that, with an open approach to sex that was as healthy as it was fun. We'd try just about anything once, and neither of us had any hang-ups about experiencing pleasure in whatever form it could be found. In other words, we were/are both bisexual.

For those that don't know it, there is something absolutely amazing about bisexual men, and women who think it's too un-masculine or consider it an unattractive thought are truly missing out. Perhaps it's that I've always been so comfortable with my own sexuality, knowing I was attracted to women long before I was ever attracted to men, and accepting it without much thought or worry. I jokingly referred to myself as a "dyke who likes dick" for some time. Whatever the case, I have always been drawn to bisexual or effeminate men. This became clear to me only after a guy I had the hots for, a close friend of my boyfriend and mine, turned out to be a cross-dresser. We, being regular and full-time freaks, were the first people this man had ever confessed his secret to and we joyfully helped him go out shopping after that for dresses and wigs; it was fun. I've heard that today he lives somewhere out in California as a full-time Dominatrix; and as a woman. That was the first time I noticed a pattern in the men I was attracted to.

My current boyfriend is the only straight man I've ever dated – and, while he's all man, he still falls somewhere in the middle; probably more metrosexual than anything though I hate to use the term because it's been so over-used. I had hoped he'd turn out, after all, to be into men – but he's as straight as an arrow. Hey, you can't win all the time.

Most of my female friends are confused by my love of bisexual men. They can't imagine dating a man who is into other men – who's, basically, half or almost gay. The idea they have in their heads, I'm sure, is of some foppish, flaming individual who is a total bottom. Nothing could be further from the truth. To me, a bisexual man is a true hedonist – a man so into carnal bliss and the heights of pleasure that he is open and willing to experience it in *any* form – whether it be making love to a female or another male. A man so comfortable in his sexuality that he can love and fuck *either* sex without sending his own mind into a state of turmoil is an exceptional individual – especially in the society we live in today where's it's just becoming "slightly" OK to be gay and completely looked down upon by almost *everyone* to be male and bisexual (from straight to gay people). I can't think of a single thing more erotic than seeing my man, my normally strong and manly man, succumbing to the taboo pleasure of another man's touch.

The men I've dated that are bisexual have been amazing lovers. Never will you find a straight man (my present one included) so in touch with feminine desires and needs. I've never met a straight man that was as sensual as the bisexual lovers I have had (and I've had my share of both). I'm not saying there are not totally straight men out there that are in touch with their feminine sides and are sensual and adept lovers; just that the majority of the ones I've come across were not. There is something intriguing about a man that can be attracted to other men – something dark and mysterious and erotic; to know they are so into sex, such lovers of pure pleasure that they would seek it out in any form. That is a man this nympho can get into.

25/3/04

Sexcapade

This nympho's sex life has been something akin to the Sahara Desert lately, folks – as you might have been able to tell from the lack of actual sex posts lately. So it brings me immense pleasure to bring you all a long awaited (by you and I) Sexcapade:

He popped open a bottle of red wine moments after we both walked in the door. It'd been a long day for me – work, leaving early for a doctor's appointment, going to the DMV, going to the pharmacy, pre-rush hour traffic. I was grateful for the warm, bittersweet liquid as it trickled down my throat. We sat at our computer desks – exactly opposite one another – idly chatting, sipping and surfing as we did most afternoons.

"I need to go and take a bath," I said casually, as he poured me a second glass.

"I want to take a bath with you," he said, cocking a playful eyebrow up at me.

I was surprised. B., as previously noted here, is not known for his sex drive – if he even has one. Though in recent talks he has agreed that he needs to be more giving with the cock. So far, he's been living up to this goal nicely.

Delighted, I went and poured us a hot bubble bath, lighting the small bathroom up with candles and giving it a lovely, warm glow. He came in as I was undressing and playfully gave my nipple a little tweak, grinning at me affectionately. He climbed in and leaned back as I followed, lying back against him. We talked and giggled as he idly stroked my body, sometimes finding his way down to my clit. I leaned back further, turning my head and he met me in a hot and wet kiss. His finger was making delightful circles around my clit and I moaned around his tongue as I felt his cock growing hard against my backside.

Suddenly he broke away. "My God, baby," he said, "I can feel your wetness – even under the water."

I grinned, handing him my poof after I'd drizzled it with lavender-scented bath gel. He bathed me slowly and teasingly, spending extra time on my most sensitive areas. After that we grabbed my best friend, the hand-held shower nozzle, and he washed my hair – giving me a luxurious scalp massage. I was feeling good all over and could no longer control myself when he began nibbling on my most sensitive part – my neck.

I grabbed both sides of the tub and hauled myself up while he quickly slid directly under me. Slowly, I lowered myself down onto his waiting cock – my aching pussy literally quivering with desire. Both of us moaned as he slid in and I began with slow, circular movements that ground myself into him.

Realizing the shower nozzle was still going strong, I excitedly grabbed it and shot it straight on my clit.

"Can you feel that?" I asked, my own voice almost cracking from the intensity.

"No," he said, "But keep it on there if it feels good for you."

I have never had the chance before to combine my two favorite things – my hand-held shower massager and actual sex. I began riding him faster, the water lapping up just almost over the lip of the tub with a rhythmic whoosh as the massager pulsated a heavy stream of warm water right onto my clit. The effect was dizzying and I came almost immediately – crying out and almost losing my balance in the midst of it all. He pulled out of me and said he wanted to wait – and go at it again soon.

We ended up having company, and I went to bed early. But as I awoke in the a.m., I decided to try my luck a second time. I scooted closer to his warm body and kissed him lightly on the cheek. He smiled, though he kept his eyes closed.

"Baby," I whispered in my husky, just-woke-up voice. "Make love to me."

He moaned, and stretched out a hand that found my breast – nipple already hard. He breathed down my neck and nibbled on my ear as his hands caressed my body – always coming just inches from my pussy. This slow and deliberate teasing always gets me so worked up. Finally his mouth found my own and his fingers found my clit with the fast and sure skill that I love about him. I was moaning and suddenly begged him to be inside me. I couldn't take this anymore.

He rolled on top of me and I wondered briefly when he'd had the time to take his boxers off. Without a moment's hesitation he was sliding inside me. I cried out in utter delight, wrapping my legs around him and pulling him down fully on top of me. We began our dance and he slid his hands under my ass, lifting me up so that he could slide even deeper inside.

With such a good work-up beforehand, it didn't take me long – I felt it first as a warm tingling in my thighs, that spread up and over my stomach and turned into a heat all throughout my body. I screamed and clutched at him as it rose, throwing my mind into that realm of confusion and intense pleasure, and rode the wave out – it ebbed slowly and he finished himself off as I recovered from my own.

I think he's making up for lost time; and I have to say he's doing a damn good job of it.

CAPTIVE HEART

Katy and her Master

http://www.captiveheart.us/blog

These posts took place over 17 months' time. When it began, we were in a long distance (and international) relationship, visiting whenever time and money allowed. He came to visit me at Christmas 2003, then moved in with me in May 2004. I've noted on the posts whether we were apart or together at the time of the writing.

9 March 2003 (long distance)

Why this blog? by Katy

Why air intimate details of our relationship to strangers? Part of it is altruistic: there is a lot about BDSM on the web, and quite a lot of it is either scary as hell or completely unbelievable to someone new to the scene. We thought the experiences of a real life couple (yes, we *are* real!), one of us the experienced mentor, the other the eager student, might be educational. Part of it is explorational: it's a tool for us to explore our own feelings as we work out the day to day details of our life together. And I will admit, quite a lot of it is exhibitionist. We don't get to be Out to most of the people we encounter daily. This blog is a place for us to be Us.

Master and I have been together for either a few months or forever – we haven't decided which. I suspected that I might be kinky and Master (of course, he wasn't Master then) agreed to answer my questions and guide me as I explored my submissiveness. He wanted me to be careful and wanted to be sure I didn't get into a bad situation by trusting someone I shouldn't. The friendship evolved from mentoring to active lust to formal submission to passionate love. Perhaps that phrasing is wrong, because we didn't stop being any of those things, we just grew and claimed more and more of each other's souls.

Loneliness hurts like hell. I was romantic enough to ache for a soulmate and pragmatic enough to doubt that such a thing existed. So I locked up my heart to keep it safe. Defenses to rival any fortress kept me from loving anyone enough to get hurt. And then my Dark Knight found me. He swam the moats, climbed the walls, and slayed the demons that had gathered like vultures. He set my heart free and claimed it for his own. Though my heart is his captive, my soul has been freed.

He is my Master, my owner, my lover, my father figure. He cares for me and meets all my needs. All he asks in return is my obedience, which I am happy to give. I am his willing slave who lives to please him. "Slave" is such a strange word, though, for he does so much for me. Little things, like brushing my hair, or bringing me a cup of tea, or rubbing my neck. I am less a slave than a goddess, pampered and cherished and spoiled. And loved. Always loved. Love beyond measure, beyond words, beyond fear.

Master, you are my whole world.

8 July 2003 (long distance)

Loving Master's Cock by Katy

To be on my knees before Master is bliss. I feel complete. I feel enveloped in his love and support and dominance. I feel *myself*, the me that was locked up in a virtual chastity belt for so long. Not only am I doing what *I* want and need to do without shame or guilt or fear, I am doing it with someone who wants me. I once thought that I would be happy just to have someone who would pay attention to me for half an hour a day. With Master, I always have his attention, whether I am on my knees, caressing his cock with my hair, or when we are both at work, an ocean apart.

Obviously I prefer the former.

For this telling, I will imagine that Master has given me permission to make love to him in any way I choose. There are other times when he grabs my hair, pulls me to my knees, and fucks my mouth.

And other times when he orders me to clean his cock after sex. There are so many ways of loving his cock with my mouth that I can write about this for years. And will.

I am at Master's feet, nuzzling his cock with my face and hair. We often sit like this, perhaps with the television on. Perhaps with one of us reading to the other. Just being together requires nudity. We could no more keep barriers between us than fly. And whenever possible, some part of me is touching his cock.

I love Master's cock. It is beautiful. It is very thick and long and intact. His pubic hair is thick and dark, and I often burrow my nose into it and inhale. I enjoy licking and kissing the shaft of his cock. He says he can barely feel it. My hair is soft and fine, and I love to drag it over Master's body, his legs and cock and balls. I am growing it long as a gift to Master. By the end of the year, I may be able to wrap his cock in my hair.

Master, how does it feel when I lick around the circumference of your cock near the base? When the ends of my hair brush against your skin? When my wet lips trail kisses from the base of your cock towards the head?

8 July 2003 (long distance)

Master's response by Master

To say that my pretty slavegirl likes to worship my cock, would be something of an understatement. For me, having my submissive at my feet reinforces everything I am: dominant, sadist, etc. It doesn't actually matter whether my cock is in her mouth. Having her leaning against me, arms around my waist, head resting in my groin, while my hands are in her hair, is emotionally very powerful for both of us. This is one of my favourite positions to collar her in.

Katy is misremembering one thing – I have not said I can barely feel it when she kisses and licks my shaft. I have explained that most of the nerve endings are in the head, and also the foreskin, and that stimulation anywhere else is not as effective. That doesn't mean I don't like it!

My last two partners both had TMJ severely – Katy has it mildly. One of them also had an aversion to bodily fluids, and even preferred the taste of latex to the taste of my cock. (It wasn't a hygiene issue –

Katy will tell you how fastidious about keeping myself clean.) I was mildly offended by this, although I tried to hide it.

It is difficult for me to describe how powerful are the emotions caused by having a slavegirl who actually *wants* to worship my cock; who actually enjoys it and loves to swallow. I have very intense orgasms during oral sex. I am quite sure this is as much due to the emotions as it is the physical pleasure of having a slavegirl who gives the best head I have ever experienced.

"Master, how does it feel when I lick around the circumference of your cock near the base? When the ends of my hair brush against your skin? When my wet lips trail kisses from the base of your cock towards the head?"

I believe I have answered those questions.

23 August 2003 (long distance)

Katy and blowjobs by Master

I need to say up front that Katy gives by far the best blow-jobs I have ever experienced. By a very long way.

I have been trying to figure out why. On the face of it, her technique is much the same as other women's. In fact, her TMJ (although mild) should prevent her doing it as well as she does, as it prevents her from serious sucking for more than a few minutes. My cock is very thick, and so stretches her jaw muscles.

Her secret is that I know, beyond all possible doubt, that I have her full and undivided attention when she is servicing me orally. Pleasing me becomes, more than ever, the centre of Katy's universe – nothing else matters to her. Combine this with the obvious pleasure she gets from playing with it, stroking it, swallowing my copious amounts of pre-come (not to mention my spunk) and you can see why I declare her to be the best cocksucking slut on the planet.

23 August 2003 (long distance)

Love in the Mirror by Katy

Until last week, I didn't have a mirror in the bedroom. The one that came with my dresser was lost some time ago, and I never bothered to replace it. Master wanted one, and if you're guessing that it wasn't out of concern for checking to see if his tie was on straight, you'd be correct. I bought a simple full-length mirror and hung it on the wall across from the foot of the bed. It was a few nights ago that I realized that I can watch myself masturbate.

I was on the phone with Master and he ordered me to prepare the plug-in vibe and the hairbrush, and to lie on the bed with my legs spread. That's when I saw my reflection.

"If I move the comforter, Master, I will be able to see myself."

That pleased him greatly. He asked me to describe what I could see, and then ordered me to prop myself up with pillows to improve my view.

And then the play began.

It was an exhilarating night.

It was starting to see myself in the mirror. I'd never seen myself quite like this.

After Master ordered me into position, I could see up the length of my legs to the slit of my pussy. Above that, I could see the hills of my belly and breasts. Then, above a light chain collar closed with a lock, my face, topped with a tangle of sleep-mussed hair.

Master ordered me to watch, while I spanked each thigh and each breast. He noticed that my voice kept getting quieter – having the mirror was sinking me into subspace much faster and deeper than usual. I could see the blows falling on my body, my eyes widening in pain and then softening as it melted into pleasure. I seemed to feel everything twice, both as the masochist and the exhibitionist. But I wasn't watching a stranger. Not anymore. I was watching a woman that I had nearly lost and then discovered all over again. A woman I had fallen in love with over the past year.

Master found and loved her first. But then he taught me to love her too. She is beautiful in the mirror. A slut-goddess, a warrior queen. Had I ever really thought submission would rob me of my power? Impossible! This primal creature in the mirror was powerful beyond measure.

Master ordered me to come. First I doubled over, my eyes closed, as the pleasure washed over me. Then I remembered the mirror and lifted my face. Opened my eyes.

There was more play, with the vibrator, and as I was coming down, Master asked me to describe how it felt.

"Powerful," I said. "Sexy." I paused. "But that's not quite right. There's another word, right at the tip of my tongue, and I can't bring it to mind."

"Try," he ordered. I did. But it wasn't until we were talking of other things that it struck me.

"Free!" I said. I think I interrupted him, but he was too happy to say anything if I did. "I feel free! I'm me, I'm finally me. I can see me!"

It was what Master and I call a Breakthrough. We had many of them during the start of our journey, but as I've grown stronger and we've grown closer, we haven't had as many. But this weekend, in the middle of the night, I looked into my own soul and saw that the shackles are gone. The demons of guilt and fear and indecision no longer have a claim on me. As Master's slave, I am free.

I know you thought I was going straight to bed, Master. So did I. But after we hung up, I found a little extra energy inside to write this for you. How did you feel when I found the word "free" that night? How did you feel to know that your slut has fallen in love with herself?

23 August 2003 (long distance)

Love in the Mirror: Master's response by Master

Free? I have always said that I ask just two things of you: your obedience, and that you be yourself. You have long since given me your obedience. It is only recently that you have truly been yourself, and I think "free" is the perfect word to describe where you are now.

You have submitted totally to me, and within that you have found your freedom.

I have been waiting for this moment, yet I find myself almost overwhelmed with emotion.

3 September 2003 (long distance)

The greatest gift by Master

Katy is not my first submissive. She is without doubt the most submissive partner I have ever known. She may also be the most masochistic, although we are still exploring that.

What does it feel like to have a beautiful woman at your feet, whimpering and wiggling?

The purely visual impact is the quick answer. Watching and listening to an intelligent woman dissolve into a puddle of multi-orgasmic mush is incredible. I love seeing the orgasmic blush spread across her chest; hearing her whimpers and cries; watching the pleading look on her face as she begs for permission to come – telling me how she'll do anything for me (and means it); anything to get the release that orgasm will bring her.

But all that is as nothing when compared to the emotional impact. Katy is both beautiful and very intelligent, and leading on her this wonderful journey we have embarked upon is emotionally transporting. I once answered one of Katy's questions about dominance by saying: "Dominance and sadism aren't things I do – they're what I am."

Katy's submission (total surrender, even) allows me to be who I am. What greater gift could I receive?

4 September 2003 (long distance)

Crawling under you by Katy

When we are apart, Master and I talk at least twice a day. He gives me a wake-up call in the mornings and I put him to bed in the evenings. That's how the time zones work out, since he's 6 hours ahead of me.

Tonight's evening started, as it usually does, by me undressing as soon as I come in, kneeling by Master's side of the bed, and dialing his number. As soon as he said hello, I begged, "Will you collar me, Master? Please?"

I hadn't said those words in a while. I'd forgotten how powerful they are.

There are words to our collaring ritual that we always use. The variation is only slightly different when we are physically together. I kneel at his feet and press my breasts against his legs. He buries his hands in my hair and, if he pushes my head onto his cock, it's hard for me to tell because I'm eagerly lunging for it.

In 3D, he collars me while his cock is in my mouth. On the phone, I have to attach the collar. But we both can almost physically feel the connection between his cock and my mouth. Today he said, "Suck it, slut. Do what you do best."

That reminded me of his post about why he loves my blow-jobs and I melted. Both emotionally and physically. As he always does after the collar is attached, he ordered me to "Come now!" And I did.

Then I whimpered. "Use me, Master. Please use me."

"Not just yet," Master said, and I whimpered in agony. I had fallen into subspace so hard and fast, even more so than usual during the ritual, in memory of that post.

"Get the sheath and the twin bullet vibrator and crawl into The Cave."

The sheath is a leather knife sheath that makes an excellent spanking strap. The Cave is the walk-in closet. There's barely enough room for me to lie on my back with my feet resting on either side of the doorframe. There's really not enough room for Master to crawl in with me, but we manage it sometimes anyway. There are eyebolts to attach my ankle restraints to the points on the door frame and another one on the back wall to hold a chain going from it to my collar. I can't use the ankle bondage points by myself, but just crawling into The Cave and turning off the light makes me feel like a prisoner. Trapped. Helpless.

Being a prisoner is my oldest fantasy, predating my sexual awareness by many years. As a young child, I remember reading tales where someone was kidnapped and imprisoned and feeling warm between my legs. The first time Master chained me to the bed, he said my cunt was wetter than he'd ever known. Being in The Cave, though I'm not bound, still engages the prisoner fantasy. Just flipping off the light sends me another level down into subspace.

Master had me place one of the bullets just inside my cunt, then lie on my side with my legs closed to hold it in. Then he had me spank my left cheek. We do a daily spanking during each call, time and health permitting, but only occasionally is pleasure applied at the same time. Master knows this vibrator is intense. He also knows that I am a masochist and quite often come during a spanking, especially when he spanks my cunt. He, being a sadist, told me I was not allowed to come until he permitted, and said he might not allow me to come at all tonight.

This made me whimper.

The spanking ritual goes like this: Master announces how many strokes I am to receive and where I am to receive it – ass, tit, or inner thigh. On the left side, I count the strokes, and on each stroke Master says something to me. Something like, "You are a naughty slut and you must be punished". On the right side, Master counts and I say things. Like, "Thank you for the pain, Master."

Tonight was ten strokes on each cheek, followed by hard and fast strokes on the breasts. All the while the vibrator buzzed along in my cunt. I begged Master to give me permission to come. More than the desire to orgasm was the desire not to disobey Master and come without permission. Master said no, and had me switch from spanking myself to pleasuring my clit with the other bullet.

All while he was weaving the most delightful word-spell. Master has the sexiest voice you can imagine, and he can weave a fantasy out of mist.

At some point, he ordered me to come, again and again. And at some point he brought me back to reality and then back out of The Cave. I cleaned the vibrator and we talked and laughed about ordinary things. He was fading because it was after midnight his time. And sometime during all this, he asked what had brought on the mood I was in – especially submissive and clingy – and I said that when I heard him say that I was doing what I do best, I couldn't help but crawl under him.

I love you, Master.

5 September 2003 (long distance)

On making fantasies come true by Master

Katy has a mild vaginal dryness problem. It is somewhat less of a problem since she found her Master. Katy has never had children, which I am sure accounts in part for her exceptional tightness. This tightness, with the occasional dryness, coupled with my rather large cock, means we sometimes have to give nature a helping hand and use lube.

Stay with me. There is a point to the preamble.

The first time I chose to make Katy's oldest fantasy (the chained and tortured prisoner one) come true, was memorable, to say the least This scene was quite long, as I spent some time torturing her nipples, flogging her, scratching her. I also spoke to her, telling her how she was my prisoner, and that I was going to torture her, then use her for my own pleasure. Her groans and whimpers were the loudest I've ever heard from her.

At the end, when I entered her, it was like a hot knife going through butter. Her pussy was so wet, she was leaking onto the bed. I was ball-deep without effort – she screamed.

An amazing scene, and one that we will revisit.

25 September 2003 (long distance)

Disadvantages of Submission by Katy

I love being a submissive. I have been submissive all my life, and now that I have a strong Master, it brings me even more joy to be my true self.

However, there is one particular disadvantage to being submissive. My dog doesn't listen to me.

Why should she? It is obvious that I'm not the alpha bitch of the pack. It must vex Mutt greatly that an inferior bitch has control over doorknobs and leashes. We've been through a training course, and she knows all the commands, but she obeys them or not as it suits her.

Everything changes when Master is here. She recognized him immediately as an alpha male, and refused to meet his eyes for several days. Then, after an unfortunate incident involving rough sex and a broken table, Mutt became anxious whenever we created any kind of creaking rhythm.

The second visit, you could almost see the thought in her head, "Oh, shit, not HIM again!" But this time, her strategy was different. Whenever Master and I became close, Mutt tried to wiggle between us. At first we thought she was jealous of the attention that I was paying Master. But soon it was obvious.

Mutt wanted Master for herself. Mutt wanted to replace me as the alpha bitch.

Master is not a dog lover, but he tolerates Mutt for my sake. Mutt's designs to engage his affections are in vain. But she obeys any order he gives, all the while ignoring me.

Now that Master is gone, Mutt has returned to thinking herself the head of the pack and not listening to a word I say.

What's a submissive to do?

Monday 29 September 2003 (long distance)

Reasons why owning a slavegirl is a Good Thing #1 by Master

Katy is collecting formal business wear from thrift stores. Why? So they can be cut or ripped from her body. A scenario:

She comes home from the office. Someone is waiting behind the door. She is grabbed from behind and the door slams shut.

She knows it's me.

She thinks it's me.

It should be me.

Is it me?

A blindfold is pulled over her eyes and cuffs slapped on her wrists. The arms pinning her are strong. She cannot escape. She is pushed face down onto the floor. A knee in the small of her back pins her down.

A sharp knife opens the jacket from neck to hem. A rough hand tears her blouse from her back.

She's whimpering; perhaps crying. She struggles as her skirt is lifted and her pantyhose pulled down. The unseen assailant shifts position, grabbing her wrists and holding them tight against the small of her back as he moves between her legs and a well-lubed cock pushes at her tight anus. Insistent, demanding an entry that cannot be denied.

She is entered smoothly and slowly. Can she hear a grunt above her whimpering as his balls slap against her buttocks? Is she pushing back against him as he begins thrusting? Is the note of her little noises changing? She's being used like the piece of fuckmeat she knows herself to be. Did she just blurt out, "Fuck me!"?

He releases her hands now, knowing she's surrendered. She reaches back as best she can, grabbing him, pulling him into her. It is difficult to say who shouts loudest as she orgasms violently as she feels his cock explode deep inside her.

He lowers himself onto her, supporting much of his weight on his elbows. "Welcome home, my pretty slavegirl," her Master growls in her ear.

6 October 2003 (long distance)

First 3D meeting by Master

Katy and I had our first 3D meeting this February. My flight arrived at two in the afternoon. The airport is about a two-hour drive from Katy's place, so we got a hotel room. We didn't think we could keep our hands off each other for that long.

So we get to our hotel room and I immediately "attack" her. Nothing too serious as, after a seven-hour flight, I am in serious need of a shower and shave. To say that I left her weak-kneed and dripping from her slave cunt, would be something of an understatement. It was the first time she had been treated like the wanton slut and slave she is.

I then ordered her to return the luggage cart to the hotel lobby. She did, in something of a daze, while I got ready for the shower.

Before we met, Katy had expressed doubts about being able to masturbate in front of me. Her previous partner had laughed at her because she likes to masturbate. Interesting reaction from him, considering he hardly ever touched her.

Anyway, having thoroughly used her for the first time, I ordered her to masturbate while I took pictures. She did it without hesitation.

6 October 2003 (long distance)

First 3D meeting by Katy

The day I was to meet Master at the airport, it snowed. I allowed enough time to get all the snow off my car, and then I started carrying luggage to the car. I was pleased. I would be early, and have time to prepare the hotel room.

At some point, I left the door to the apartment ajar and Mutt took off. I panicked. She is not the smartest of dogs, and she doesn't have experience with crossing roads and such, as she's never allowed out without a lead or inside a fence. And I live very close to some busy roads. And she wasn't wearing her collar and tags.

So off I ran after Mutt, following her pawprints in the snow. Asking people who were shoveling out their cars if they'd seen her. The pawprints crossed over each other enough times that I gave up on that line of pursuit. By then the snow was mainly useful in ruling out areas to search. I kept calling her and eventually she ran right up to me like she was saying, "Look, Ma, no hands!" and I clipped the leash on her and hugged her tight and told her she was a good girl for coming when called.

During all the searching (about 30–45 minutes) I kept thinking "What if I don't find her? I can't leave until I do. Maybe I can call the hotel and leave a message for him. Oh, no, the reservations are in my name. Will they let him check in? They have my credit card, surely they will if I call and tell them it's OK. Or will they? How could I have ruined our first meeting by leaving the fucking door open?"

My "plenty of time to spare" turned into "no time to spare". Eventually I got Mutt to the kennel and set off for the airport. I made it to the hotel just in time to check in, and I saw that the airport shuttle was about to leave. So I didn't even go to the room. I simply grabbed my purse and one yellow rose from the bouquet I had bought for Master.

When I got to the airport, I removed my panties. The monitor showed his flight as "landed" but not "in customs". So I was shocked when I saw him. I recognized him at once. I didn't have the voice to call his name, and luckily in my confusion didn't scream out "Master!" I just dropped my bag and ran to him. We clung. I smelled him. He had sent me a T-shirt of his so I knew his scent. He whispered "Come now," in my ear, and I sank against him.

We touched and held each other continuously in between fetching luggage and calling for the airport shuttle to pick us up and waiting for it to arrive. Since I had a long coat, he was able to grope me discreetly and appreciate my lack of underwear. Me being cold-natured (and a slut), I was quite happy to be groped.

Some online couples are more careful when they meet for the first time and plan to just have casual no-sex meetings. That was never an option for Master and I. I left my hotel information with one friend, who called later to make sure I was OK.

We rolled the luggage cart completely into the room, and he surprised me by closing the door and pouncing on me. No deep kissing, as he wasn't very fresh after the flight, but lots of biting of throat and breasts and cunt. He attacked my cunt with his fingers and his mouth and then pushed his fingers into my mouth. I'm pretty sure my stockings were lost by this time, and my blouse was untucked. Certainly my hair was mussed and my face reddened by friction-burn from a face that needed a shave. And he ordered me to return the luggage cart to the lobby while he showered.

I don't know what the desk clerks thought, or if they noticed the difference between the me that went into the room and the me that returned. I didn't care either. Actually, it was my first taste of freedom. Of being *me*. It is a necessity that some of who I am can't be shared universally. I wouldn't trust my family or boss with that. But it is very good to be me in a place where there can be no negative consequences because no one knows or cares who I am.

Is that why there wasn't a moment of hesitation when Master ordered me to masturbate?

I used to only masturbate under the covers in the dark, preferably when the ex was sleeping or in another room. If he saw me, or guessed that's what I was doing, he would laugh at me. He was rarely interested in sex. When he did get in the mood, he seemed to feel that, since my appetite was so much greater than his, I should be grateful, and shouldn't expect niceties like foreplay or romance. In the last year, it was rare to have sex more often than once every four to six weeks. I told him once that I thought sex twice a day would be ideal, once in the morning and once at night. His response: "Are you trying to kill me?"

Master's response: "Unless one of us is sick, that is the minimum." And during both 3D visits, he has held true to that with me being the one to beg for naps towards the end of the visits (and him teasing me unmercifully about that).

I gave Master the gift of submission. But he gave me so much in return. His dominance, his love, his physical desire, but most of all, the freedom to be me. No wonder I had no self-consciousness when Master ordered me to masturbate. I was finally loved for being – and loving – myself.

16 November 2003 (long distance)

TMJ and fellatio by Katy

To give blow-jobs to a large cock will only make TMJ worse. I learned this the hard way and was forced to do without my recommended daily allowance of cock for several years.

This is a very bad thing for a slut who loves cock.

Thankfully, wearing a mouth piece at night for about a year has made me able to resume my slutty ways. But I still have to be careful not to overdo it. Chewing gum is out. So is hard candy. I still succumb to caramels, but never too many at a time. And it really isn't that much extra work to cut an apple into slices rather than chomping away on it.

When Master and I started negotiating together, one of the first things we agreed upon was that my mouth should only be for Master's use. Since he wants to receive blow-jobs as badly as I want to give them, he will not gag me. There's a kinky version of "you can't have your cake and eat it too" among Doms: you can have the gag or the blow-job. It generally refers to not being able to have everything at once, but in Master's case, if I wore a ball gag for too long, I might be impaired for weeks or months from giving head! That's not good!

Even with all these precautions, I can't deep throat. Never could, even with smaller dicks. Certainly not with Master's large and yummy tool. I can't even handle strong rhythmic thrusting for very long. And yet I give incredible blow-jobs.

My secret is that I am absolutely focused on giving pleasure. If you have jaw problems like me that keep you from being mouth-fucked too long, or you just want to vary your routine, try some of the following tips:

1. Take breaks to lick and nibble
2. Practice using your tongue in different ways, from a flat, wet lick to a pointed probe, to everything in between
3. Blow on wet skin
4. Suck on just the head
5. Hands, hands, hands . . . everywhere and anywhere
6. Nuzzle and lick the balls
7. If you have long hair, drag it over his cock and balls

8. If he has a foreskin, tease it, suck on it, probe underneath it (I could write another post just on how to make oral love to a foreskin)

9. Run your fingers through his pubic hair

10. If you can't suck him from cold to orgasm, then mix activities. He can fuck you until he's ready to come, then have you finish him off in your mouth. Or you suck him as long as you can, then he finishes with a tit fuck. Linear sex is dull. Mix it up!

11. As Dan suggested, use your hand on his cock as a way of extending your mouth for his pleasure and your safety

12. Most importantly, love his cock. If you love what you are doing, he'll love it too.

I wish your cock was in my mouth right now.
   Wouldn't that be nice, Master?

6 December 2003 (long distance)

The ax has fallen by Katy

Since late October, I've known that I would be denied orgasms for an undetermined period of time before Master's arrival.

He arrives in 11 days. He told me this morning that the ax has fallen. That he has had "December 6" in his PDA for several weeks as the day when I would be told.

I wish I could say that I accepted it graciously like a good slavegirl. But I didn't.

I'm not normally rebellious. I normally want so much more to be a "good girl" than I want any particular thing I might rebel over, including orgasms. The problem I had today is that I haven't been in subspace in quite a while. A combination of things (mostly it having been six months since Master and I have been together physically) has kept me from feeling as submissive as I like. Then last night, I went into an emotional Bad Place on the phone with Master over something very silly. Master hasn't been ordering me "Come now!" as often as he used to.

I expected something . . . different. I expected a phenomenal play session where he took me very deep before telling me not to come. Or perhaps him giving me a mind-shattering orgasm and telling me that was my last one. Or something. I didn't think he'd tell me first thing in the morning after a bad night.

So, I rebelled. Sort of. I cried. I told him I didn't necessarily want him to change his plans, because I want him to be in charge. It was sort of a rebellion because I didn't accept his plan whole-heartedly at first, but it wasn't really a rebellion because for me to have kept quiet and pretended to be okay when I wasn't would have been Many Times Worse. I'm supposed to tell Master when I have mental misgivings. Actually, it's a little stronger than that. I'm under orders to keep Master informed of my emotional state.

Master decided to take some time to think about what to do and I realized later as I was running errands that it isn't often that Master gives me an order that requires sacrifice. Normally submitting to him gives me far more pleasure than I give up. So I asked him to please not change his plans and said I was sorry for crying and not accepting it.

I love you, Master. I hope I haven't diminished the pleasure you will take in denying my orgasms.

6 December 2003 (long distance)

On surprising (and completely unexpected) reactions by Master

As Katy said here:

> "Since late October, I've known that I would be denied orgasms for an undetermined period of time before Master's arrival."

Simple enough, you might think, especially as we had spoken about it on a number of occasions over the last few months.

Katy has a strong desire to be a "good girl", and that is a strong part of the dynamic between us. She is eager to please, and I am careful not to abuse the power that gives me over her. She had several times said that she is also prepared to make sacrifices if I ask it of her and, although we have several times played with orgasm denial for a day or two, I have not otherwise asked her to do anything that she considers a sacrifice.

You may imagine my surprise when, on being told she was denied orgasms until we're next together, she went to pieces. Indeed, I was so surprised that it took me a few minutes to recover and I fear I didn't handle it as well as I might have during that period.

Katy said she was expecting "I expected a phenomenal play session where he took me very deep before telling me not to come", yet that is not how I did it in the past.

I suspect, as Katy seems to, that her reaction was caused by a number of minor things that had her in a slightly vulnerable place and I hadn't spotted that fact. So I must take most of the responsibility for it.

It is made *much* worse for me because Katy can't talk when she's crying. Consequently, we have to hang up and get onto ICQ, because she is able to type when she's upset. I hate that, it tears me up inside, because it make me feel like I am running out on her when she's in a Bad Place and that is abandoning my duty as her Dominant and partner. We deal with it by getting back on the phone ASAP. After Katy begins feeling better.

Once we are together, this sort of thing will be handled differently. Katy has to get off the phone because she can't talk, not because she wants me to go away. So, in 3D, we anticipate me snuggling with her while she cries, then we will talk. That will be much better. For both of us.

In the meantime, I wove Katy a verbal fantasy while she masturbated last night. She wasn't allowed an orgasm, of course.

30 December 2003 (physically together)

On giving all by Katy

Last night's play was intense and I went deep into subspace. The general rule of thumb is that, even if I appear recovered, I'm probably still not fully in touch with reality until I've slept. When Master is away, we talk on the phone every night, and on nights we have heavy play, I often go directly to bed after the call ends.

I was completely ready for bed after our play. Therefore, my befuddled mind thought of it as the bedtime spanking. I had given so much and trusted so completely that I felt quite vulnerable. But I wasn't close to being cognitive enough to say anything clearly.

There were two clues that Master might have seen (and this isn't assigning blame, this is something we looked at together to figure out how to avoid a repeat). First, when he asked if I wanted to watch a movie, I asked if I could brush my teeth first. I wanted to be ready to go to bed as soon as movie watching was done, but hadn't thought it through clearly enough to say so. Second, when we went into the bedroom, I asked Master if I could wear a T-shirt to bed. I've told him before that wearing clothes helps to blanket the nerve endings of my skin when I'm feeling overstimulated. I hadn't realized before that wearing clothes is also a subconscious way to protect myself when I feel vulnerable.

He asked if wearing a T-shirt would make my bottom feel better (I had mentioned several times how sore it was) and I nodded. He said, "That doesn't make sense," and I said, "I don't know, it just will." He gave me permission. I walked into the closet and was reaching for a T-shirt off the shelf when he picked up the hairbrush.

I froze, dumbfounded. "But I already had the bedtime spanking." I said it several times. He told me that the spanking before hadn't been bedtime, and that this was going to be very gentle. I couldn't get past saying the same thing. "I already had the bedtime spanking."

"Trust me," he said, and held out his hand.

This is the point where, had I been able to think, I should have said, "I trust you, but it's too much right now." I should have asked him to hold me until I knew what was wrong.

Instead, my very fogged-out brain got very confused. I *did* trust him. I knew the spanking wouldn't physically hurt me, much less harm me. I just couldn't give any more. Now he was asking me to give two things: asking me to trust him and asking me to take one more stroke. I had done that over and over, without him verbally asking, during the heavy play session. Now, when I was wrung out, he asked it aloud. Not asked, ordered.

I tried one more time "I thought I already had the bedtime spanking." He said again, "Trust me."

Thinking in subspace is very black-or-white. I was able to conceive of two responses to this: either acceptance or rebellion.

Either I take his hand, or I say that I don't trust him. The appropriate, nuanced response was beyond me. Safeword? It wasn't about remembering my safeword. I didn't even remember the concept of a safeword. I could see only two choices in front of me, and rebelling was impossible. So I took his hand and broke into tears, accepted the very light tap, and then had a meltdown.

I'd given everything and was completely empty.

I cried. Then we talked about it a long time – and believe me, talking about deep emotional issues is awfully fun when you're in subspace and can barely string words together.

30 December 2003 (physically together)

Sometimes shit happens – despite everybody's best efforts by Master

Like last night, after the events Katy just blogged about.

What Katy described finished at around 8 p.m. – too early for bed (or so I thought). We crashed out on the sofa again and chilled in front of some more documentaries from *Lord of the Rings: The Two Towers*. Just after 9, I told her it was time for bed.

We went into the bedroom, and I told her it was time for her bedtime spanking (one of our rituals is for her to be spanked when she awakes, and just before she went to sleep). She went glassy-eyed, and looked as though she was going to cry, and asked me why.

I explained that we always finished the day like this, yet she obviously didn't understand me. Remembering that she was still in subspace from our heavy play earlier, I reminded her to trust me. I did this because Katy has several times in the past become confused after play and, afterwards, when we conduct a post mortem, she has realized that she forgot to trust me. I assumed, based on the evidence past and present, that it was happening again now. I again told her to trust me, bent her over the bed, called her a naughty slavegirl, and tapped her once (very, very lightly) on her left buttock. Her butt, thighs and breasts had taken serious play earlier in the evening, and there was no way I ever intended to do anything more than a symbolic tap.

Everything was fine, right?

Wrong.

Katy started crying – not hysterically, but certainly with genuine emotion.

We talked things through for almost an hour, and the root of it was that she had gone so far into subspace after our heavy play and she really wanted to go to bed at 8 p.m. I hadn't picked up on it, as she had shown no signs of being in that place (it is usually very obvious). I had reached what I thought was the right conclusion, based on current and past data, and had merely confused her further when I didn't understand what was wrong.

I am not trying to duck my responsibilities here. Hell! I have a reputation of being a bit over-cautious in the kinky community. I do think this is one of those "shit happens" occasions. Why? Because I was doing my very best to supply good aftercare to Katy, but misdiagnosed the problem. Katy did her best to communicate with me but, being off in la-la land, couldn't find the words.

So, shit happens. We picked up the pieces, talked it through, and are OK – stronger, because of it.

Further thoughts: this is also a classic example of why safewords have their uses (especially early on in a relationship), but it is dangerous to rely on them. Katy became so upset when I wanted to give her the bedtime spanking that she wanted to use her safeword. She couldn't remember it. Worse, she couldn't put into words that she felt that badly.

I could have done a better job, of course. In my (slight) defense, I offer the fact that Katy and I have had just 40 days together in 3D during this year, and so I am still learning to read her.

11 January 2004 (long distance)

An answer by Katy

Back on December 31, a reader of Captive Heart asked:

> "Excuse me if I sound naive, but your relationship dynamic is so far out of my personal experience that I have trouble fully groking it. Katy, why did you have to ask permission to go to bed? does your submissive role really extend that far?"

I realized after I read that question that I left some rather important information out of the story. My bedtime is always 9 p.m. if I'm going to the gym in the morning and 10 p.m. otherwise. Exceptions may be made for special circumstances, such as a special event with others that we don't have control over the scheduling, or genuine illness or insomnia. Exceptions don't include staying up for a TV show or getting tied up doing something on the computer and forgetting bedtime. Bedtime comes, I go to bed. No arguments.

Now, without this information, I can see how the story might have looked extreme. What if he hadn't given me permission to go to bed? Is sleep deprivation for hours or days a form of play we use? Maybe there are people who play with sleep deprivation, but I would consider that very extreme play, in line with breath play (which we also don't do).

For Master and me, our physical and emotional health comes first. Before play, before pleasure. We may sometimes disagree on the means of protecting our health, but never on its priority. So Master would never keep me up past my bedtime without a very good reason.

In answer to your question, I never have to ask for permission to go to bed at the assigned time. It's only if I want to change the schedule that I would need to ask.

Another point is how much we enjoy the dynamic of me asking him for permission to do things, even when it's obvious to both of us that the answer will be "yes". "May I go to bed now?" is much more gracious than, "I'm going to crash – you coming?"

13 March 2004 (long distance)

When Master comes in my mouth by Katy

"How does it feel when I come in your mouth?" he asked.

First, there's the lunge. Since I have TMJ, I can't deep throat. I use my hand to act as an extension of my mouth so that his whole cock is being stimulated, and Master is careful not to fuck my mouth too hard if my hand isn't there to act as a safety block. But as soon as he starts coming, I can't help it. I drop my hand and lunge onto his cock, trying to take it as deep as I can. It's instinctive. Master told me tonight that he wants to come over my tongue sometime, but I think for that to happen, he'd have to be enough in control just before his orgasm to order me not to lunge. Even then, I'm not sure I'd be able to stop myself.

There's something deeply satisfying, in a way that's both sub-missive and potent, about feeling a cock pulse and twitch in my mouth. Feeling the hot spunk in my throat. Swallowing and consuming what I've drawn from his body with my lips and tongue and hands.

Sometimes I think of fellatio as a sacrament, on my knees before a holy altar. Sometimes it feels like he's feeding me, giving up some of his own life-force to nurture me. Much less common – even though we love humiliation games – it feels naughty. But usually, whether I've been a holy priestess or a dirty whore in our play until then, the sacred and the profane disappear when his cock touches my mouth. I become nothing more than an object, with no shame attached. In that moment, I exist only to please his cock. My mouth, my body, my entire being is focused on nothing more than sucking the spunk out of him.

And when I finally do? When Master comes in my mouth? How can I describe it? How can I put into words how it feels when my soul, intent upon a single goal, suddenly achieves its purpose?

The closest word I can find is "complete". I feel complete. I feel peace.

12 May 2004 (physically together)

Wake-up call by Katy

I am a morning person, but I hate waking up. Once I'm awake, I'm OK, but I hate the actual process of waking. This is where having a Master is a Good Thing.

When we were apart, he gave me a wake-up call every morning. I would whimper and beg for a few more minutes, and he would call me back a few minutes later. This might happen several times, but once 6.30 arrives, he'd order my sub ass out of bed.

Now, we actually have to set an alarm. Master gets up right away, makes a nice cup of tea, checks his email, perhaps does a bit of surfing.

Then he comes to wake me.

I still whimper and beg for a few more minutes, but now he can add a few swats with his implement of choice to help me along. Then there was this morning's solution which was very effective:

"May I have a few more minutes, Master?" (this was maybe the third or fourth iteration)

"No. I'm going to fuck you, instead," he replied. I was lying on my stomach. He grabbed my hips and pulled them up until I was on knees and shoulders and thrust into me. He fucked me hard, came quickly, and ordered me out of bed. I hadn't orgasmed. He didn't care. I loved being his object. And it did wake me up.

25 May 2004 (physically together)

How it happened by Katy

In March 2003 I wrote about some of the trouble I've had with anal play in a post about playing with a butt plug.

In November 2003 Master wrote about when he first actively lusted after my ass.

In January 2004, I wrote about how disappointed I was that my ass wasn't ready to be fucked during Master's Christmas visit.

Someone wrote (on a blog that is now sadly defunct) that, instead of training, I only needed to relax. I've been reading the book *Anal Pleasure and Health* by Jack Morin and, though he gives exercises to promote anal pleasure, they are intended to help relax those muscles. Ironically, by focusing so hard on those exercises, I was just increasing the tension. Every time I failed, it increased the stress level and tightened up those muscles.

Master and I decided to discontinue the training. Instead, he told me he would take my ass when he felt it was right. He would give me lots of orgasms and put me deep into subspace and play with my anus until it was relaxed. And then . . . he would just slip it in.

And that's exactly how it happened.

I was supposed to be going for a nap, but I was feeling needy, and I begged him to hurt me. I don't remember what he used. His hands, I think, and one of the riding crops. He had me roll over on my side and he snuggled up behind me. I was using the double bullet – one in my cunt and one on my clit. I could feel his hard cock resting between my ass-cheeks.

"Relax," he murmured as he adjusted his cock. "I'm not going to enter you yet. I just want to press up against you." The head of his cock pressed against my anus and it felt good. We rocked together, and I could feel that the head of his cock was sliding inside my outer sphincter. I moaned and he told me I was a good little bitch. It could have been minutes or hours. (He told me later it was about 15 minutes.) At some point, the pleasure in my ass grew intense, and I suddenly had to turn off the bullet on my clit. I think it was an orgasm, but it was a very strange one. It must have been using different muscles than normal.

"Katy," he murmured. "My balls are touching your ass."

I hadn't realized it. Somehow I had Master's entire nine inches in my very tight virgin ass, and I barely felt it. The muscles were so relaxed. Apparently most of the nerve endings are in the inner and outer sphincters. I couldn't feel the part of him that was beyond that – at least not directly. It was more of the pressure that I could feel against my cunt, and its buzzing occupant. I did feel him come inside me, although it may have been the pulsing at the base of his cock that I felt.

He says he might make it normal practice to use my ass. That he might save fucking my cunt for a special treat if I've been a very good girl, or if I've begged prettily enough.

That was exactly what I was afraid of before he took my ass. Now that he has, I want it more than anything.

I've felt more submissive since then – something I hadn't guessed was possible. I've been getting butterflies whenever Master calls me his "good little bitch". I can't wait for him to take me again. Harder. I want to be fucked in the ass when I'm tied up. I want him to flip up my skirt and bend me over the sofa when I've just arrived home from work. I want him to use my ass whenever he pleases, and without regard to my pleasure. I want him to fuck my ass while another man fucks my cunt. I want him to fuck my mouth, cunt, and ass in the same session.

Thank you, Master. Thank you for being patient with me. Thank you for knowing when I was ready, even when I didn't.

7 July 2004 (physically together)

On owning a slavegirl by Master

Having total authority over another person brings something with it: responsibility, not to mention accountability. Like any "good" dominant, I frequently analyse my own actions and reactions. Is what I am doing "good" for Katy and myself? That sort of thing.

During play, I only get to relax some of the time. Many of the toys I play with (the singletail whip and heavy leather flogger come particularly to mind) are capable of causing serious physical harm if misused. Katy, I suspect, wonders how I enjoy myself, when I have all this responsibility on my shoulders. I have tried explaining that "dominant" doesn't describe what I do, it describes what I am.

Heck, even our dog, and the monster dog belonging to our very cute neighbour, submit to me and treat me as the BigDog, or Alpha.

I enjoy/want/crave the power and responsibility.

Katy, meanwhile, is quite convinced that she has the better end of the deal – multiple orgasms; my total and undivided attention most of the time; an excellent cook (did I mention that?) etc.

Don't anybody disillusion her, please.

Cock Under Lock

D

4 January 2004

So it begins

I guess I'll get the intro entry out of the way. This blog is about my sex life with my significant other (my true love); let's call her E. After months of delving deeper and deeper into a progressively kinky sex life, it has culminated into my partial chastization. I say partial because I still get freed whenever she fancies. Sometimes it is to the benefit of pleasing her with my cock, but often I must pleasure her with other means whilst still locked down. Occasionally, if I am really good, I am allowed temporary parole and given some sort of release (sexually). She is starting out with short periods of chastising, moving on to longer ones. (She said she wanted to lock me up for all of Lent. Being Jewish, I didn't know what that meant. When she told me it was 40 days, I was in shock in what I had gotten myself into.) Now for the details. We already had a pretty kinky s/m-laden sex life. We both like to Dom and to Sub. I have set up some pretty interesting hitching devices in my bedroom. Sometimes she likes to violate me and make me her "Butt Slut". Sometimes she likes to relinquish that control and let me take over. Suffice it to say there's a lot of tying down goin' on.

Even though I we had/have tremendous amounts of sex, I would still give into my addiction to porno when she was not home. Once she commented on my constant self stimulation and it was perhaps hindering our sex life, saying, "I wish I could have you under lock and key." I mentioned that there were many devices on the Web.

That got her very excited and she insisted at looking at some as soon as we got home. We had been looking at chastity devices online, yet due to funds could not afford one at the moment (Xmas time). I then stumbled onto a page about homemade devices. After checking out some designs, I knew I could easily build my own PVC curve-type device. The next day after a trip to the hardware store I was in the business of building a kick-ass chastity device, which I presented to E later on that night.

That's the start. I will later blog on how that weekend developed. (Each day deserves its own entry.)

OK, that's it for now. Stay tuned . . .

4 January 2004

Day 1

I awoke on Friday morning with the most unsavory feeling. My body was attempting to give itself the daily morning erection, yet my restrained penis was unable to move anywhere. It was pressed into the end of the tube, fully swelled up. And the ring around my cock and balls was tight as blood tried to flow in and out. Actually the ring was the most excruiating part. As I surveyed my situation I got more excited thinking of my imprisonment, further delaying the subsiding of my semi-erection. Eventually as I walked to the bathroom things down there calmed down a little.

Urinating in the device is a somewhat humbling experience as well. At first I had to sit to pee. But later was able to straddle the toilet and let it flow like a faucet (which due to the shape is exactly how it looked). Dabbing up the little hole afterwards with a piece of toilet paper. I went through my day quite normally after that, except with the constant reminder encasing my penis, causing chronic cases of semi-erections and associated discomfort and pleasure.

That night E said I had been a good boy taking my medicine and that I would receive a small reward. She tied me to the bed with both my legs pulled back and suspended in mid-air. My arms tied spread out. I was fully exposed and unable to move. She pulled out "the swell guy", a Xmas present. Turning on the vibrations, she slowly worked it in. Once firmly inside she began pumping. At first it was only a little. She then lit a cigarette so she could leisurely enjoy the moment. The feeling of being so stuffed and filled up caused my cock to swell. It began twitching and causing the tube to move. I could feel pre-come start to ooze from my cock-head (which had built up from the constant excited feeling all day). Just as I was starting to buck and thrust my hips she started inflating more. I was riding the edge between pleasure and pain as my insides tried to accommodate the ever-increasing toy. I was on the verge of using our safe word, when she deflated the plug. Causing me to exhale a sigh of relief. She then started inflating and deflating more rapidly. I was really straining, feeling the pleasure but unable to do anything to my neglected member. I was in frustration hell. But incredibly turned on. She deflated the plug and pulled it out, replacing it with four fingers from one hand. She then proceeded to work in four fingers from her other hand. "Right now my hands are a spear shape" she whispered as she began to fuck me with them. E pushed and pulled causing my whole body to rock back and forth with her. I was getting stretched to my maximum. Just when I thought I couldn't take any more, she started twisting her eight fingers inside me. I was gripping her so tight that I could feel every twist and, even though it was pushing my limits, I was so turned on and hard as I possibly could be inside the tube. And just like that she said I was done. E untied me and led me into the shower, only to clean me up and lock me down again . . .

5 January 2004

Bitter Taste and an Early Release

Saturday morning I awoke with the same uncomfortable erection problem. My little guy's a fighter, and he persisted in wanting to get hard for a painful 15 minutes. All I could think about was how badly he needed to be touched by anyone or anything. Finally I gave up and eventually he simmered down.

The day went on as usual, except for the point during a walk to the store to get Diet Coke. I was making a joke referring to a porno I owned, and that E found somewhat repulsive, called *Ass Cream Pie*. At one point describing the kind of come-eating some of the girls do in that movie (read the description if you want to know). E was so disgusted by this, she said, "That's it! I'm tying you up and making you drink a shotglass of your own come. So you can know what it's like." I was turned on by this but also knew that I would not want to drink it after I came. But I was mostly turned on, and looking forward to getting some sort of release.

True to her word, when we got home I was promptly tied down again. She then decided that as part of my punishment I would have to watch the porno in question whilst I was immobilized. This went on for about 45 minutes. I was excited but unable to do anything to further my enjoyment. While this was going on, E just sat on the computer doing online shopping and emailing. Eventually she proceeded to unlock the chastity device. I was already semi-hard but, once freed, became almost instantly erect. She started teasing me with light strokes, making me increasingly more rigid. I was as swelled up as I've ever seen myself. If that wasn't enough, she inserted the Tristan butt plug into my ass. She left the room for a moment and returned with a glass. I couldn't hide my simultaneous embarrassment and arousal. Then came the lube.

I couldn't believe how incredible it felt to be stroked like that after being denied attention for a day and a half, plus I kept catching glimpses of the porno. My hips started bucking and my thrusts were meeting her hands, all slick with lube. Sensing my closeness, she used one hand to grab the glass. She put the head of my cock inside the glass. Almost jerking me off with her hand into the glass. I shuddered and loudly moaned as I came. I watched as the glass filled with semi-clear fluid. At that point I really didn't want what was to happen next. (Why is it that right after a man ejaculates he doesn't want anything remotely to do with sex, especially anything kinky that might have been getting him off in the first place?) Regardless, I knew better than to refuse her.

E had a bit of a smirk on her face as she brought the glass to my mouth. "Drink up," she said. I tried to squirm away but she moved the glass towards my head and started to tilt it. I begrudgingly opened and swallowed it down as quickly as I could.

Gooey battery acid. That's the only way I can describe it. I swear that must be a taste that one cultivates. Because I was repulsed. I was later informed by E that depending on what you eat it tastes better or worse. I wasn't eating a lot of fresh fruit lately.

Anyway, I had taken my medicine like a good boy and was

washed and cleaned while still tied down. The plug stayed inside me as she moved about the room to do day-to-day things. Eventually coming back to me with the chastity device. As she lubricated my cock and the device to make it easier to slip into, I quickly became hard again. I don't know if it was just to get my cock into the tube or if she was feeling generous, but she expertly jerked me off again. This time I sprayed come all over my stomach. I was cleaned again and finally put inside the tube and locked down once again. It was to remain this way till Sunday night still, or so I had thought . . .

5 January 2004

Prisoner escapes again

So. I pretty much thought that was it for a while. At least until Sunday night. After the shower we did about 3 hours of *Pride and Prejudice* on DVD. E was still turned on from the treatment she gave me, and was craving some attention herself. Like I said in an earlier post, we are both switches, meaning we each enjoy both ends of the power exchange. I was feeling pretty naughty at that point, so when she asked me to "do stuff" to her, I had some pretty elaborate plans in mind.

I first tied her in the same position she had me in only days before. Arms stretched out and legs suspended mid-air and pulled back. Probably somewhat akin to what it looks like at the gynecologist. She was fully spread out, and unable to hide her shaved pussy or asshole. I took out my mind gear machine. Something I've had for a while but had rarely used. This would give her the ultimate in sensory deprivation and and relaxation. Slipping on the goggles and headphones, I told her she was about to have her limits pushed too. I could tell she was extremely horny and it wouldn't take long to give into her first orgasm. But I had further plans than that. I pressed play on the program and started her off.

After caressing her body for several minutes, I worked the pocket rocket on her clit. Watching as she tried to move her body up and down to get a better angle on it. Then I decided it was time to start getting down to business. I grabbed the silver stud and replaced the smaller vibrator. I removed the small plug in her ass and replaced them with one and then two of my fingers. I could feel that she was loosening up and she was really enjoying the fingers inside her. I started twisting my fingers just as she had done to me. I commanded her to tell me when she was coming, which she did almost immediately. I began working my two fingers in and out of her deeply, while she came about as hard as I have seen her come. I was surprised she was enjoying it so much, this deep and stretched. The vibrator was making slurpy, skinflapping noises on her pussy, which almost furthered her humiliation and hence excitement. She came for about two minutes solid as I whispered dirty things in her ear. At the end of this orgasm something unexpected happened. She screamed, "I need you now. I need your cock inside me. Inside my ass." I was taken aback (we rarely try anal because she says I'm too big for her) and asked if she was sure. "Yes! Get my keys. I give you permission. GET MY KEYS!!"

I clumsily looked around the room, almost killing the moment before I spotted them. Thank God. Promptly I freed my cock, which again got almost instantly hard.

There she was, fully spread out in front of me. I lubed up my cock, thinking to myself, there is no way I am not getting this in there. I pressed the head against her opening, put the vibrator back on her clit (but at the higher speed) and started pushing and pulling back slowly. My little guy wasn't giving in at all and stayed like steel. My head eased inside her. I couldn't believe how tight and good it felt. I could tell by her eyes rolling back in her head that she was digging it, and could take even more. I decided to take advantage and really "fuck" her with my full length. We went on like this for about ten minutes or so, longer than I thought she could take me in her ass. I was really thrusting in and out, although only with 3/4 of my cock. I could tell she was enjoying it but also ready for me to come. I was so turned on, looking down and seeing my shaft so deeply in her tightest of openings. I gave a few more strokes and finally exploded deep inside her asshole. Her pussy twitched as my come erupted inside her. Pushing her over the edge again.

We stayed locked like this for a minute or so. I eventually withdrew and watched as my come dripped from her asshole. I said, "There's a real ass-cream pie right there." She was not

amused by this comment and took a mock swing at me. We laughed
a bit and then headed off to the shower.

Instead of locking me back in, She said "I want to cuddle with
him tonight" referring to my penis again, not me.

What could I do but oblige . . .

5th January 2004

Sunday Night

What was to be my original day of release became one of full
imprisonment. E is moving into a new apt, so I had much of the day
dealing with chores related to that. I was hoping that if I acted
really good, I would get some kind of special attention. Alas, in the
end, she was the only one that got "the treatment".

We got back to my place, had a shower and were about to watch
Sense and Sensibility. (Can you tell we are on a Jane Austen kick?)

Before watching the movie, E confessed to me a little fantasy she
had the other day. I had to coax it out of her with persistence,
because she was more than a little embarrassed about it. She
wanted to be tied up and forced to watch a porno while I "did
things" to her. This is quite shocking because she finds most of my
pornos repulsive. But I think that was part of the whole turn-on.

I was really looking forward to this. A chance to push all her
humiliation buttons, and perhaps work her into another frenzy
where she wanted my cock again.

I blindfolded and gagged her, chained her spread eagle to the
bed, and put on one of my more graphic, over-the-top pornos,
Seven the Hardway.

I took the blindfold off as the credits started to roll. Starting out
slow with the pocket rocket on her clit again, I grabbed her by the
hair and made her look up at the TV, telling her if she looked away
she would get a lot worse than she expected. I had her watch about
15 minutes this way, all the while telling her what a "naughty girl"
she was for liking such graphic porn. At the point where they
started the double anal penetration, I flipped her over so she was
face down/ass up right in front of the TV and retied her this way. I
now put the Hitachi magic wand on a pillow right underneath her
pussy. I told her to rub against the vibrator and try to get herself

off. She was straining because it kept moving, but that only made it more fun to watch. Noticing that she was looking away from the TV, I again grabbed her hair and told her she better not look away. This was emphasized by half a dozen hard smacks on her ass. Her cheeks were rosy red as I started to go to work on her asshole. First using the silver stud and then moving onto my fingers. Once again I could feel her loosen up as she rubbed her pussy on the head of the magic wand. I knew she was close to coming and told her to announce when she was. She tried to speak, but the ball gag mumbled her speech. However, I knew she was coming. I had two fingers inside her ass and started to stretch them as wide as I could in there. My hopes were moving towards another round of full-blown anal sex. She came so hard, for a solid few minutes. At the end she was exhausted, but I told her she would have to take the treatment for the whole movie's length. I did allow her a cigarette and Diet Coke break, while she was tied up of course. We then moved the next and final scene of the DVD. I retied her in the exposed gyno position, reinserting the small plug in her, and placing the Hitachi on her clit. Again I held her by her hair and ordered her not to look away from the TV, but now I was going have to be harder on her for not obeying as much as I liked. Removing the plug, I again worked two fingers in, but this time she wanted it deep, and practically impaled herself on my fingers and started grinding. I was taken back by the wanton display of complete whorishness. I knew she was ready for more.

I reached for the Tristan plug (which was pretty big for her before) and I started to ease it in, telling her she was going to be a good girl and take it all for me. There was some effort involved on her part. But she got most of it all the way in. I told her I was sorry but she deserved this, and gave the plug the final push. Her eyes widened with a sort of shock, yet almost instantly glazed over with a pleasure/pain kind of high. I knew that I was really on the edge of her boundaries. But I wasn't done. I took two fingers from my other hand, and worked them into her super-wet pussy. It was tight because the plug was almost working against my hand. She was getting it from all ends, plugged, fingers inserted and the magic wand. The Wand started making those slurpy skin flapping noises again as I ground it on her pussy, all the while fucking her really hard with my fingers. I knew this was the one. She came, and came, and came and came. It must have been a solid five minutes of orgasms. I was giving her my nastiest treatment and she loved it. She was now done. She begged me to stop, and I obliged, even though I think there was at least another 15 minutes left of the movie. But I could tell it was cuddling time, and I like that too.

So we had more Jane Austen and sleepy time with no relief for little D.

Maybe tonight . . .!

7 January 2004

A Very Lucky Boy

OK. My mood did a 180. Here's why and how.

When I got home last night I was still very frustrated and very pouty. E was doing more online shopping for her new place. I was beginning to wonder if my burning need would be acknowledged. I could tell it wasn't that important to her.

Finally, she got off the computer, sat down next to me and informed me of her decision. I would be freed, but she wasn't feeling that Dom-like, and instead she wanted to be tied up. I eagerly agreed. I didn't care how I got it, just so long as I did. Besides, I had a lot of pent-up aggression and frustration, of which she was the most obvious target.

On pulling off the chastity device, she agreed to allow me time to modify it so it could be cleaned easier (that was how the end of my night was spent).

I wasted no time. Immediately I got out the wrist/ankle restraints, rubber blindfold, and ball gag. It must have been an all-time speed record for attaching these babies. I laid her out so she was tied spread eagle, but with a pillow underneath her ass. Lying there all splayed and gagged, I knew she was really in for it. Reaching down between her legs, I used both hands to spread her pussy lips and, while she was fully exposed, I lightly tongued her opening.

I then started with lightly pinching her nipples and tapping her clit with my forefinger. I leaned over, whispered in her ear that I was going to make her pay for denying me the past two days, and began kissing her through the ball gag. I could sense her excitement as she started moving her hips to hump the air. Out came the Hitachi. I set it to the lower speed and proceeded to rub it up and down, from her clit to her increasingly glistening lips.

My cock was aching, it was so hard. I got over her, and straddled her chest. My cock inches away from her mouth, I removed the ball gag. "Open wide," I said, which she readily obliged. I sensed submission was taking over her. Instantly, she took 3/4 of me down her throat. "Keep it wide open." I pushed more and could hear gagging sounds. I then leisurely began fucking her mouth like I would fuck a pussy, all the while keeping the Hitachi buzzing on her clit. For ten minutes I kept this up, hearing gurgles and choking noises coming from her throat. When I felt I was close to coming, I pulled out and moved down to her so my cock was inches from her shaved opening. "You're going to feel this cock so deep inside you." A few squirts of lube and I was fully embedded in her silky smooth pussy. Building up momentum, I started to work my fingers inside her asshole. She was taking it all with gusto only a true slut could. I decided to push the envelope a bit. Straddling one of her legs and keeping my cock inside her and the magic wand on her clit, I reinserted my ring finger and pinky in her ass, and worked my index and middle finger into her wet cunt. "You're being stretched out little whore. How do you like it?" Moaning noises escaped from her gag. I built up vigor and intensity, until I could tell she was coming. "I want you to tell me when you come." I think she was saying that she was, but it was impossible to decipher.

After she had a few prolonged orgasms, I withdrew and repositioned her. Her legs were then moved so they were suspended in mid-air and pulled back. Leaving her pussy and ass in full view. At one point while repositioning she tried to fight me, so I smacked her real hard on the ass. This riled her even more, and I actually had to really strain to keep her down and retie her. I was scared of what she might do if she got out. Eventually I got her where I wanted her. I proceeded to fuck her in this position. But not just fuck her, pound her with all I had. I wanted to make her pussy hurt. A few times I went in so deep, so quickly that she jerked with pain and shock. Grabbing her thighs I pulled her in closer, as I continued my rabbit pace. I felt like I was going to come a few times so I had to slow it down.

My cock was so hard I felt I could have pulled a truck. I was also feeling really dirty. I started to rub the head of my cock against her recently stretched asshole. She moaned a bit, and I knew what I was going to do next. I relubed my member, and started to ease it inside her puckered hole. Surprisingly, she didn't seem to dislike this at all. I could feel her sphincter relax and let my head slip in. Pushing further, I had at least half of my shaft up there before I eased up. Taking a few minutes I let her relax around my cock as I slowly worked it back and forth. She was getting more turned on, so I again put the Hitachi on her clit (high speed this time) to really max it out. "I'm coming," she mumbled through the gag. My pace increased. "I'm going to fuck your ass like I fuck a pussy," I breathed in her ear. By this time most of my cock was inside her. I pushed her legs back even further and eased in, my hips touching her hips. I was truly buried inside her. She continued orgasming heavily, as I began pistoning in and out of her. By the end I was fucking her like I fuck her pussy. A sly smile crossed my mouth as I remembered only weeks ago anal sex was as much of a possibility as me winning the lottery.

I think she came for like seven minutes or something, as I moved in and out of her asshole. She screamed, "I want you to come in my ass. I want to feel your come. Please!". As if on cue, I erupted inside her. The spasms wouldn't stop, and I felt like I came a gallon. I left my cock inside her as she continued to come. She just wouldn't stop. The spasm in her ass pushed my cock out, and it began to drip thick, milky come.

When she had enough, I took the vibrator off of her. "I'm almost embarrassed about how much I came. That was so good! I can't believe you pulled that off."

The joke of the evening became my response to her statement that it didn't hurt at all. "Well, when you do it right. It shouldn't hurt," I quipped.

She then proceeded to mock me 1/2 hour for that.

As promised, she gave me a night off to modify my chastity device and let my penis recover. We'll see what happens when I go home tonight.

10 March 2004

What's going on?

It's been a while since I've blogged. Partially because I was real busy last week and partially because there wasn't a lot to blog about. I'll try to update you on the important bits.

I was locked up from Tuesday morning till Thursday night. I remember E and I had sex that night at my house, but it wasn't anything out of the ordinary – just plain great sex. For those keeping score at home, it was once on the bed and once on the chair at my computer desk (which by the way has been getting more action lately and has started to fall apart, breaking at the most inopportune moments).

We hung out until Saturday night, when we had a little friction in our relating to one another. I think it was a combo of male complacency, *Grand Theft Auto Vice City*, and female hormones. We decided to take a couple days off of hanging out. I went home, unlocked (yes. There was some viewing of the porno collection).

The break turned out to be a good thing. By Monday, we were both aching to be back with one another. I headed back over E's last night, and that's when things got interesting again. While smoking a joint, I suggested the idea of breaking out the bondage gear, that I had thoughtfully brought over to her place several days earlier. I had barely finished my sentence, when E cut in, "Yes!! Will you tie me up?"

Exactly what I wanted to hear. I was feeling really horny, and knew that I wanted to fuck her for a long time, and I wanted to fuck her like the inner-slut that she is. We showered, I shaved her pussy, fucked a bit while in the shower, got out, dried off, and we smoked a joint while I prepped the bed for the festivities.

I had initially laid her out in a spread eagle position. Blindfolded, pink wrist cuffs and ankle cuffs. I don't know why, but I was already rock hard and felt my needs overriding hers at that precise moment. I positioned myself so my cock was right above her blindfolded face. "Open your mouth for me." E complied and I put the head of my rigid cock into her mouth. "I want you to keep it open and relax." I began to push 3/4 of the length of it down her throat. I heard a gurgle and pulled back, only to push harder again. I wanted to hear all the gagging noises. I casually began fucking her throat, taking care to back off when she looked like she couldn't handle it. But it was all under control. Recognizing her for her slutty willingness to serve, I leaned over and began tonguing her clit, while my cock was still in her throat. We 69-ed like this for a while. Every so often my cock would slip out of her mouth, and she would have to bob around (blindfold) to find it again and somehow get it back in her mouth, no-handed. This was simultaneously entertaining, a complete turn-on, and I hope a bit humiliating to her.

E was being a good little whore. It was reward time. I grabbed the magic wand and placed it on her clit (low speed) while I repositioned myself facing her with my cock right at mouth level. I proceeded to tease her clit and pussy lips with the wand, while she feasted on my shaft. Whispering what a "pretty little cocksucker" she was, and other naughty bits.

I'd been having this idea, and I thought now might be a good time to try it. I unhooked the clips that were holding the cuffs. I told E to move on to her stomach. I clipped one wrist to the opposite leg behind her back, and then did the same with the other pair, leaving her in a hogtied position. It was my fantasy to be able to fuck her throat like this. Yet logistics were difficult and it made it hard to breathe for her. Not to worry, leaving her in this position I put her first on her side and then later on her back. This turned out to be a most excellent position for fucking. She's basically holding her legs all the way back for me. It wasn't long before I was lubed up and slipping inside her. My cock felt like kryptonite. And I alternated from fucking her real slow to pounding her the way she likes it. Some moments I was appreciating her wet pussy swallowing the full length of me, other times I was fucking her so hard that she was near tears and gasping that she couldn't take it. Yet she wanted more. Go figure. I was fucking her like this for a long time. It felt so good I didn't want to come. But eventually, during one of my jack-hammer moments, I couldn't take it anymore. "I'm going to come all over you!" "Please. Please do it." I pulled my cock from her, already feeling myself spasm. Jets of white come shot all over her stomach and tits; she was opening her mouth, trying to get some in there. I practically passed out on top of her, I came so hard. I had to take a few moments to recompose myself and get off of her. Both of us later acknowledged how transcending that experience was. Our sex is almost always amazing. But sometimes it approaches the celestial. I swear I love this girl so much. But the sex is only one of the reasons.

I thought that might have been it for the night. But like an hour later we were going to watch *Best in Show*. We started kissing and caressing. Before long I said, "I think I'm ready for round two." E agreed. We started with her on top, in case her pussy was sore. Again my cock surprised even me with its rigidity. E rode me for like 15 minutes before I flipped her around to mish. I laid into her again with all I had. Thrusting so my hips slapped against hers. The sensation of fucking her so intensely and our eyes locked in each other's gaze was incredible. Whereas before was bondage slut time, this was "lovemaking", for lack of a better word. We kept this up for a while. Between strokes E whispered nasty things in my ears. Telling me what a good boy I was and how much she loved my cock in her. I was feeling close, and started making noises. E breathed, "I want your come. Give it to me. I want to taste you." Hearing this put me over the edge. I made some kind of weird animalistic noise and pulled out of her trying to get my cock into her mouth as quickly as I could. The tip felt so sensitive as E's lips engulfed it and started sucking my juices. All I could do was make inarticulate beast noises (probably to the dismay of her new neighbors) as she swallowed it all.

I was done after that. Not just done with sex, but pretty much stayed there like a drained immobile mass. I don't even remember the lights being turned off or falling asleep.

14 March 2004

Fin

I feel like I owe everybody an explanation of why I haven't been blogging as of late. The short story is that E and I broke up again. That happened last week.

After our last break-up I thought things were improving. There was a lot of amazing sex that accompanied this too. I kept telling myself I have to blog about that I have to blog about this. But a busy schedule and lack of inertia during my free moments kept me from documenting it.

I miss E horribly and I'm worried that I might never have a relationship that is so fufilling. All I can do is hope that I will find such happiness again, either with E or without her.

I'm sorry that there won't be much more steamy content up here anymore, barring some twist of fate or incredible luck.

Thanks everyone for visiting and supporting us.

22 March 2004

Whoa Nelly!!

Once again it is proved to me that it ain't over till it's over. I had pretty much resigned myself to the fact that things were done between me and E. In fact I was getting downright angered by her refusal to even see me so we could talk about stuff. Imagine my surprise when she showed up at the club where I was playing on Thursday night. We talked, had some cigarettes, had some drinks, I played, and yes, we went home together.

I won't go into the details of that night, but I will let you know there was some hot drunken sex, at which point I had her half falling off the bed, spreading her pussy as wide as she could with her hands, while I thrust all the way in and pulled completely out. Leaving her pussy twitching at the emptiness where my cock had previously been. The sex was hot, hot, hot, but what was even more pleasurable was her agreement to attend a special party with me on Saturday night.

Friday day at work I was soooo tired, but I was elated inside. E and I wrote love notes back and forth to each other and met for lunch. We both needed more and made plans to meet back at her house. Let me just say this, Friday evening was the beginning of a weekend that will from now on be celebrated as a personal holiday.

I was waiting at E's place when she got home. She said that she missed me so much and thought I deserved a special treatment. She informed that she was going to play with me and tease me all night until I couldn't take it any more. E changed out of her work clothes and donned some ultra-sexy attire for the evening's festivities. She put on a black sleeveless fishnet shirt, black sheer tight boxer briefs (mine but they looked so amazing on her. drool!!), and a pair of knee-high boots. I stripped down to my undies. I couldn't believe how hot and sexy she looked. I just wanted to rub my hands all over her and bury my face beneath her pussy and ass. Her ass looked to die for, by the way. Before she even touched me I could already feel my cock twitching. We made out and had some general petting before the real session began.

Occasionally she would lightly brush my cock with her hands or pinch my nipples. Just teasing. Never allowing me to really enjoy the sustained pleasure. At one point she was lightly rubbing her pinky finger into my pee-hole, driving me absolutely crazy. Out came the restraints. E asked me to put down the black rubber sheet we have. She stripped off my "panties" and began fastening cuffs on all my extremities. Then my ankles were tied off to opposite ends of the bed. I was pretty stretched out and spread wide open. She then proceeded to secure my wrists to their respective ankles. A chrome cock ring was worked onto little D, once I could control myself and let my erection subside a bit. E inspected her handwork, and decided I was secure enough. I felt as exposed as a woman might at a trip to the gynecologist's office. I had recently shaved all of my body hair. E remarked on this and said that my opening "looks like a girl's asshole". This sent a wave of delicious humiliation throughout my body.

She decided that it needed a little something in it for starters. She produced the Silver stud and easily worked it into my waiting ass. She then began to work the Hitachi magic wand over the shaft and head of my penis, getting it to an increasingly hard, turgid, state. "Don't you come!" she warned as I began moaning. "You have a long time to go before you get to come." I promised her I would control myself and try to please her. This went on for 20 minutes or so. During this time E would give me hits of pot or sips of Diet Coke. I didn't know how I was going to hold out. Precome was dripping from the head of my cock when E decided to take a break. She went into the bathroom to do her make-up, while I was left bound with my twitching member.

E emerged from the bathroom looking even more incredible than she did before. Her make-up was smoking! If my hands were free, I would have furiously stroked my cock to orgasm instantly. That's how good she looked. She decided to take it up a notch. Digging through the bag of toys, she pulled out a collar with leash, the inflatable butt plug, a huge bottle of lube, a leather slapper, a pyrex dildo, black rubber gloves, and a black rubber strap-on dildo. "You're getting the full treatment tonight," she said with a sly smile.

"I think it's time for a bigger toy. It's been a while since you've had ass-stretching class. You must be tight up there." E replaced the small silver stud plug with the larger inflatable/vibrating plug. She turned up the vibrations as she eased it in. "Good boy. That's it." The plug slipped all the way in, and my cock swelled even more. The collar with leash was then placed around my neck. E giggled with excitement when she realized how much fun it was to pull and choke me with. She then secured the leash to my restraints, leaving a mild choking effect. She slowly began inflating the butt plug. She would pump the bulb a few times and then stroke my shaft. Pump some more, stroke some more. Then she began inflating it to full capacity, only to let it instantly deflate again. The feeling was one of being fully stuffed to fully cavernous. She repeated this over and over again. I was groaning in ecstasy. This went on for who knows how long. It felt amazing and I could feel its effects filling my balls with come. After quite a long time, E decided to take another break to order some food. She of course left the butt plug inside me, filled to medium capacity.

"You're going to have to answer the door for the delivery guy," she informed me. After seeing the look of fear in my eyes, she said, "Well. I'm not answering the door like this. So you have to go down like that." Eventually she conceded to let me wear a bathrobe. Still, that didn't do much to hide the cuffs or the collar around my neck. She also let me remove the plug before we ate. While waiting for the delivery guy, she let me lick her pussy. I got her so hot after five minutes, that I was allowed to fuck her. With the stipulation, of course, that I do not come. I fought against coming and fucked her as hard as I could until her buzzer rang. So when I was paying the guy I wasn't sure if I should be more embarrassed about the restraints poking through the robe or the tent I was pitching in the center.

It was really fun to be seated at her kitchen table in my slave gear while she looked like a stunning goddess. We ate and afterwards smoked a joint.

I must say at this point I was already having the time of my life, and didn't think it could get much better. I didn't know of the incredible crescendo to come.

E led me back into her room. I was told to get on all fours. I watched over my shoulder as E put on her black leather cowboy hat. I was so captivated by how hot she looked in her hat and boots. Like a real cowgirl. I just didn't know yet that I was going to be her pony. She tied me up inverted to how I was before. Wrists to ankles but this time my ass was fully spread and exposed in the air. "Look at my little girl's asshole. I'm going to fuck you now like you fuck me." I couldn't see everything but I could hear the clanging of buckles and adjustment.

When I finally did see E, I was blown away. There she was, the sexiest cowgirl, but this time she had an eight-inch black rubber cock between her legs. She offered to take off her boots so she wouldn't accidentally spur me. I declined because danger is my middle name. E stood up on the bed and positioned herself so the head of her cock was rubbing my asshole. "Is my little slut ready for this?" she whispered as she eased the cock inside me. My ass was fully stretched from before and had no problem taking it in. She then thrust all the way to the hilt, breathing in my ear what a "good boy" I was. This was heaven. E increased the pace of her thrusts, bucking in and out of me. She would occasionally reach down to stroke my rigid cock. I couldn't believe how good it was. I felt a tingling in my penis and when I looked between my legs I could see droplets of pre-come oozing from the head.

I begged E to free me so I could touch myself. Once she released me, I instantly handed her the leash to my collar. She got the hint and started pulling hard. I was in ecstasy as I began stroking my aching cock. E began pounding my ass hard as she pulled me back with the leash. It was an incredible sensation. I felt like I was truly being used. "Do you like it when I fuck you like this? Fuck you hard, like you like to do to me. You're my little pony. Aren't you?" She was pistoning in and out of me in jack-hammer motions, slapping my ass, and grabbing my hips, and pulling hard on the leash. In all actuality she was fucking me like I do to her. Bravo!

My orgasm was getting to the point of no return, and I don't even know what kind of things were coming out of my mouth. All I could do was take it while I visualized how this might look from a third person perspective. Me getting fucked doggie style as this hot cowgirl has me by the reins, whispering dirty things to me as I take every inch of her rubber cock.

"That's it, come for me. Come for me, you dirty boy. Jerk that cock off!" That was my cue. Almost immediately this incredible groan escaped my lips and streams of hot white come shot out of my cock. I felt like I orgasmed for a complete minute as E continued to fuck my ass. Slowly she eased her pace, and eventually pulled out of me. "That's a good boy. Did you come hard?" I made some kind of incoherent yes noise and she seemed to be pleased with herself. As I looked down at the rubber sheets, there were copious amounts of white fluid. It looked so hot to see all of that white come pooled on the black rubber sheets.

"Holy shit! We've been having sex for seven hours!" I heard her say. Sure enough I looked at the clock and did the math. Sure enough. Seven hours, give or take some time for dinner and weed. I was drained physically, sexually and mentally. Or, a better way to say it . . . I was spent but content.

E and I slept really well that night! Little did I realize that things were just getting started . . .

23 March 2004

Peepshow Party

So, now you know about Friday night. I alluded earlier to a special party that I asked E to. Here's that story.

If you don't already know, I have a rubber fetish which has been contagious for E. We've gone to fetish balls and we both like it. NYC doesn't have as many good parties as one would think, so when one comes along your ass better be there. Along with being bummed about our break-up, I was also despondent about missing what could have been the sexual event of the winter with the one I loved. Fortune smiled upon us, when it healed our wounds right before this event.

When I told E about this party, we started scheming about what to wear. I chose to go in my black rubber pants and shortsleeve front zip black shirt. E opted to première her black rubber cat suit. I was salivating as I visualized how hot she would look. Also what was exciting about the suit was its crotch-thru zipper that allowed many possibilities for naughtiness.

Saturday night came. I had anticipatory butterflies in my stomach. This was not just a well promoted fetish party, but also a *rsvp-only* play party. I knew that both E's and my desire to perform and be the center of attention was going to make this a night to remember.

E looked to die for in her black rubber cat suit. It accentuated every curve. As I cleaned and polished it on her body, I thought to myself, "Holy fuck, am I lucky. I'm with the sexiest girl in the world." She was like a black shiny rubber doll. She had a riding crop in her hand and she glistened like an Indy pace car.

I slid on my rubber, fixed my hair and we headed out into the night.

We arrived shortly after midnight at the private loft, said our secret password to the bouncer and the doors swung open. It seemed that our timing was perfect. The place was just beginning to fill up and people were already getting frisky. There was a pillow room, a quasi-dance room and the rest was like a dungeon. There was a St Andrew's Cross and various implements laid out, as well as TVs with hardcore S/M videos playing.

E and I settled in as we watched a girl being roped to a chair. Her Master did some intricate knot work, leaving her neck arched back, mouth wide open, and unable to move a single muscle. We had some drinks and smoked a joint while taking this in. I noticed an attractive blonde girl in lacy black lingerie with her boyfriend checking out E. I whispered this in her ear. When E met the other girl's gaze, she immediately turned away in shyness. It was really cute. E was too scared to walk over and talk to her, so we watched while another girl came up to the blonde, started talking, and then began kissing her. Once again E's face turned crimson. It was adorable to see her being so coquetteish. I asked E if she would like to walk around. We checked out some of the other rooms and eventually settled into a couch and cuddled.

It wasn't long before the blonde girl showed up again; this time when her eye met E's, she walked over. She introduced herself as L and her boyfriend introduced himself to me as D. Immediately the girls began talking about girly things and bonding, while I chatted up the boyfriend. After about 15 minutes or so, I asked if they felt like seeing what was going on in the other room. We walked by girls and boys being spanked, tied, sucked, licked, you name it. The party was really gaining momentum now. We found an area by a wall in front of the St Andrew's Cross. E and L continued talking, but now I noticed their hands were occasionally touching each other's body, and they were moving closer to each other. I saw L put her hands up to hold E's face as she began kissing her. It was on!

L continued to kiss E, as she explored her body with her hands. E reciprocated, rubbing all over L's exposed flesh. E looked so hot in her catsuit. Things were getting more intense. She rubbed the riding crop behind L's back and then pulled her closer in. L responded by slowly unzipping E's catsuit. The contrast of E's beautiful white breasts coming out of the black catsuit was beautiful beyond compare. L freed both of E's girls and started slowly, lightly teasing her nipples. What was even sexier than this were the smiles on the girl's faces as they explored each other.

L moved the zipper further down E's torso until her freshly trimmed pussy was exposed. I watched as L dug her hand inside the catsuit and began rubbing E in her most private parts. Moans of pure delight escaped her lips as L kept petting and rubbing. I got behind E and began moving my hands over her shiny derrière and back. I reached between E's legs and pulled the zipper the rest of the way so that L could have better access. I did however catch part of her pussy-lips with the zipper, which abruptly broke the mood and pissed E off.

Whoops! After being severely chastised and spanked as punishment, E and L resumed. L had E sit on the dresser. She began kissing her again, slowly moving her lips down her body. In no time L's face was between E's legs, and I could tell from the look on E's face that she knew what she was doing. E smiled and cooed as L used her mouth and fingers on her. E's breathing became heavier as she clutched L's head between her thighs. E handed D her riding crop and he began using it on L's bent over behind. Yet this wasn't enough for L and she moved her panties down to her ankles so she could feel the crop on her bare ass. L continued to lick and suck E, as she bent over even more, inviting her ass to be spanked. This scene was getting core of the sun hot. D handed me the riding crop so I could spank his girlfriend's ass, as I watched her eat my girl's pussy. L kept at it for quite a few minutes. Before long E was heaving and thrusting to meet L's tongue. "Ahhh. I'm going to come!" she screamed. And with that I saw L pick up the intensity as E began to shudder. It must have lasted 40 seconds or so, and then I just saw a beaming smile on E's face. L rose up and passionately kissed E again. I can't even tell you how incredible this was to watch. I felt like I was high on ecstasy or something, but this was a sex high.

It was now E's turn to reciprocate. The girls traded places, with L sitting on the dresser and E in front of her. E began by softly kissing her while fondling and exposing her perky little breasts from her bra. Slowly E's tongue worked its way from L's mouth to her nipples, down her stomach. L's panties had long since been abandoned on the floor, E's tongue licked down her freshly shaved mons and buried itself in the soft warm folds of her intimate flesh. E was gradually building up momentum. I could tell by the look on L's face that she was in heaven. I knelt down and got behind E. I was stroking her hair and rubbing her all over. I whispered in her ear, "I think she likes that." E stopped licking for a second to tell me how hard L's clit had gotten in her mouth. "She likes when I suck on it." L was making all kinds of pleasure noises, but suddenly her breathing and gasps got more urgent. Then she began to shake and tremble while more groans erupted from her. D said to me, "I think your girl just made mine come." E moved slowly back up to L's face. They both had the happiest smiles on their faces. They continued to embrace and kiss. I excused myself to go the bathroom, after asking L and D to watch over E.

On the way to and from the bathroom I saw more kinky action. Men getting whipped by girls, girls with other girl's fingers inside them, guys sucking guys, naughty nuns, transvestites, you name it. I was surprised not to see any barnyard animals or Maori tribesmen in the mix. I came back sitting against the dresser. We started talking and then kissing. To the left of me a woman knelt between a man's legs, sucking his engorged member. To the right L and D were petting on each other. Next to them a naked guy in a cape had another guy kneeling before him sucking his cock. I began to kiss E harder and while rubbing her up and down. She began lightly stroking my cock through my pants. It felt sublime through the rubber.

I started moaning and she could see the desire in my eyes. "Do you want your cock out?" she purred. I nodded and made some incoherent "yes" sound. E reached into my pants and removed little D, although by this time he wasn't so little. I was rock hard from all the action I had witnessed and was still witnessing. E pumped my shaft with one hand while she tickled the head with another. I felt like I was made of iron at that point. E moved her mouth down to take the head of my cock between her lips. While still lightly pumping, she flicked her tongue and wet mouth all over me. Eventually we worked ourselves into a rhythm, where I was fucking her mouth and hand. This felt amazing, but was even better was being able to take in what was going on around me. It was like watching a show, but also being part of the show.

I noticed now that L and D had followed suit. D was sitting on the dresser next to E while L was working his cock. It was too much! Really the feeling was one of freedom and being alive. But it was also animalistic urgency. I began pumping harder into E's mouth. Fucking it like I would fuck her pussy. Pushing in hard only to pull all the way, and repeat, and repeat. Crowds were gathering around us to take in the action. I counted at least four single guys jerking off around us. While this was not a turn-on, it did enable me to control myself from coming just then, and keep the action going. So thank you, weird jerking-off guys. I continued to fuck E's mouth, while L kept sucking and pumping D's shaft. After 5 minutes more of this, I decided I would not come at that moment and asked E if she wanted to smoke a joint.

We took a little smoke break and talked with L and D. It was really fun to get to know someone after sharing that kind of intimacy. They were really cool and we had a nice rapport going. E wanted to go pee so I accompanied her to the bathroom. While in there I was telling her how good my cock felt in her mouth, she countered! "Yeah. That was nice, but I want it somewhere else right now." I told her that something could be arranged and led her back into the main room.

We walked back over to L and D. E was talking to L, while I was behind her rubbing up against her latex-clad body. L was facing E, rubbing her hands over E's slick suit. D said, "I think round two is about to begin."

E and L started passionately kissing again. I reached for the zipper that started right above her ass-cheeks and zipped it down between her legs, once again exposing her dripping wet pussy. My cock was still hard and slick from E's saliva and my sweat. As E and L held each other, kissing, I pulled E's hips closer to mine and eased my cock inside her. She was so hot by this time that it just glided right in. I started at a leisurely pace, just enjoying the feeling on sliding in and out of her wet cunt, and looking at her slick, latex-clad ass. Just a tiny bit of pale white skin was visible through the zippers of the suit. The contrast was unbelievably sexy. I continued to fuck E as L held her and kissed her. I could hear L whispering in E's ear. "He's got his cock inside you. Is he fucking you good? How does that feel?" The sound of this sent E into serious passion mode. Her moans were getting increasingly louder. I started thrusting harder and faster, working into the pace that E loves. L looked me in the eyes, and with a devilish grin she commanded, "Fuck her harder! C'mon. Fuck her!" Then she grabbed E's hair and pulled her close. "You like getting fucked hard like that? You like that cock? Show me how much you like it." E was making noises I never heard from her. I was giving her everything I had. All I could hear were moans and the sound of rubber slapping against rubber. My cock was absolutely pistoning in and out of her. I thought I might break her, I was giving it to her so hard. The intensity was at a fever pitch. But every so often L would shoot me a sinister little look, and I would want to fuck E even harder. This went on for a solid 15 minutes or so.

Still I couldn't come. Maybe it was the guys jerking off around me or maybe it wasn't about the coming. Whatever it was, I felt pretty satisfied and spent by the time we started winding down. It was getting close to 4 a.m. and E mentioned she was tired. We told L and D that we were getting sleepy. They asked if we wanted to grab a bite, and both of us realized how hungry we were and agreed.

We all got our coats, jumped in a cab and headed to the coffee shop in Union Square. I was a bit worried about heading to a trendy persons' joint in our fetish gear. But E was in top form and was like "I'm just gonna have to show those people what's up." And so it was. We got some dinner, talked, and exchanged contact info. What was really funny is that this was L and D's first play party, yet both E and I thought they were total pros. I guess some things are just innate.

I think we all had a really good time. And who knows? We might just see them again some time.

28 April 2004

Hedonism Weekend and Under Lock Again

There is a lot of ground I have to cover, but think it might be better to summarize most of it and go into detail on a few matters.

This past weekend E and I had another mini-hedonism fest. It started on Friday night. We partied with some different recreational drugs than we usually do. We were up till 4 a.m., you figure it out. E wanted some sexy pics of her taken for the blog. E dressed in black panties, black bra, knee-high black boots, black leather cowboy hat, and a black collar with a silver leash dangling from it. She looked magma hot! We snapped a few pics inside, and then E put on her black leather overcoat and we headed out into the drizzly night. We shot in rain soaked streets, subway entrances, and anonymous doorsteps. E would shimmy out of her coat to near nakedness and I would play shutterbug. I like how they came out, but E is a bit more picky than me, so these might be for private use only. When we returned home, we were both treated to orgasms by the other.

Saturday night, I played a show in the Lower East Side. E brought along her friend, R, and mentioned to me earlier in the evening that her friend might be up for some intimate playing afterwards. When we got back to her place the plan was to start out by playing Sexy Uno (rules to be posted in the future). We played a few hands of Sexy Uno, but E was getting impatient that the game was moving too slow. She made the suggestion that we cut to the chase and tie R up. R changed into something looser and more flowing, we then blindfolded her and tied her spread eagle to the bed. For some reason I don't really want to go into all the details of what we did, but I will include the highlights. It was fun domming someone else with E. She and I would be working on R's clit and pussy, talking about her in a clinical tone, almost like she wasn't there listening. We would comment on what a responsive subject she was, and note any noises or tell-tale pleasure sounds she would make. At one point E was fingering her and using the Hitachi on her, E's ass was sticking out so I took the liberty of licking it while rubbing her clit with my thumb. This led to me lubing my cock up and thrusting it into her already wet pussy. I fucked her hard for a while, while E ate R out and vibrated her clit. R wanted the blindfold off so she could see. As she watched she told me to fuck E harder, to which I readily complied. Later E slipped a butt plug inside R, commenting on how easy she took it and what a "butt slut" she was. I continued to fuck E while almost straddling R's tied leg.

I don't think R ever came. It was her first time being tied up, and I imagine she was a bit nervous. After a few hours of play we wound down with some joints and bong hits. After R left, E and I continued to play by ourselves. Again it was like 5 in the morning before we both nodded off to a post-orgasmic slumber.

On Sunday E needed her place to be thouroughly cleaned. She called the maid service. Which is actually me in a French maid's uniform and heels. E thought it was lovely that the dress rode up and hardly even covered my cock. Any time I bent over my ass was a target for E and her riding crop. I dusted, vacuumed, mopped, did dishes, emptied the garbage, pretty much did it all. All for my beautiful mistress and employer. E thought I looked so pretty she put lipstick on me and took pictures. She now wants to post them on her blog. E did an inspection, and when she was fully satisfied with the maid's job, she opted for a special kind of payment.

I was tied with my legs spread wide open towards the end of the bed. E hiked up my dress and exposed my throbbing member. "Look at what a little slut you are. You know a nice girl doesn't wear such a short skirt, and leave all her goods hanging out." E went into the bathroom and came out with a Q-tip and a bottle of lube. "I'm going to fuck your pee hole with this," she announced with a coy smile. I was both excited and scared, knowing that it would hurt, but in a good way. E lubed up the hole of my urethra as well as the rest of my cock, and slowly eased the head of the Q-tip inside the small opening. It felt so strange to be penetrated there. It didn't even hurt that much. My cock grew more stiff as she started fucking me with the Q-tip and jerking my cock with her other hand. She would push in deeper and deeper until more than half the Q-tip was inside my cock. The sensations ranged from invasive to exquisite.

The big turn-on was being violated that way. As she fucked me harder and deeper, my cock swelled. I loved watching her churning away. I knew orgasm was imminent. I told her I was about to come. She picked up the pace, and right as my cock started twitching and shooting she pulled the Q-tip out. I came, copious amounts of fluid mixed with lube. "Don't be a dirty girl and get any on your pretty dress." E returned with a towel and wiped me up before setting me free. All and all, I loved it. New terrain for me and E. We both know that it is a sensitive area, and must be treated with much care. So I advise anyone interested in that type of play to research it beforehand.

Now to the lockup. A few weeks back I had told E about another Peepshow party coming up this weekend. E was on the fence about going, but eventually relented with the stipulation that I wear my chastity device from Sunday up until we are at the party. Now this alone is pretty tough, but I had also got into deep hot water with E over an unrelated issue. Not only was I going to be under lock, but she was now fully determined to not give in at all. This was on top of the plethora of spankings with a paddle and riding crop I was to endure.

So it was, after the urethra fucking, I was cleaned, and locked back up. E then had me bend over the bed. My naked ass was pointed up in the air, when she began smacking it with the paddle. She was giving it to me harder than she ever had before. I must have taken over 50 hits with it. I was relieved when she stopped, but only momentarily. She picked up the black leather riding crop and made me forget all about the paddle. I could hear the crop swishing through the air before it would land on red, stinging ass. E gave me another 50 with the crop. This instrument was far more brutal, and all I could do was scream into the mattress as she swung away. When it was over, my butt was so red and raw I couldn't sit and it still was sore a day later. I will only say that I got what was coming to me.

15 June 2004

And Then There was Just Static

E and I broke up. Sorry. I'm not even sure if there will be any future posts on this blog.

Thanks for having been with us out if you are a regular reader. If you are a newcomer feel free to browse the archives. What else can I say? Check back a little later, no telling what the future holds.

30 June 2004

180

Hmmm, Logging into the new blogger interface, I noticed that it shows the sum total of posts your blog has. I was surprised to see that there are only 26. It feels like there should be a much higher number. I know that there would be if it wasn't for my chronic periods of apathy and E's and my *repetitive break-up syndrome*. Yes. That's right. We have a disease, and the crux of it is that we hard time staying together, but we have a much harder time staying apart. This one felt like it could be permanent (which would have sucked), but I think we are on the way to patching things up and possibly starting from a new outlook of honesty, acceptance and respect. At least I hope, and I know E does as well.

Monday night we had a bit of a blow-out on the phone, ending with E never wanting to see or hear from me again, this being the result of a careless, hurtful comment I absently let spill from my lips. I apologized profusely by phone, mail, and other means.

I didn't hear from E till the end of the next work day. After a lengthy instant messenger conversation she agreed to see me, to at least talk about stuff face to face.

I think we were both pretty guarded when she came over to my place. Kiss hello on the cheek, eyes downcast. As we talked and expressed ourselves, the physical distance began to disappear. Hand-holding led to caressing, and as we reached the conclusion that we both feel a hole in our hearts and lives without the other one, we embraced. I can't tell how everything else just melts away when I feel E in my arms. It is so natural and nourishing. It feels as necessary as oxygen. Yet I wasn't able to admit slowly suffocating without it. I love her so much. I told her this last night, but I will tell you all. I would and have wanted to marry her ever since I started dating her. I just know that my life is much richer for being with her.

Anyway, as we both professed our love and cuddled it led to the much anticipated and never overrated *make-up sex*. I was considering going into details here, but am going to hold off for a couple of reasons. Most of all I consider this kind of lovemaking and therefore more personal. I can't emote what it feels like when you reconnect profoundly with someone that is so special to you. Also when I blog I more or less like to write about the really dirty, naughty, hope-your-mom-never-finds-out kind of sex. What happened last night is more like the moments in life and nature when you recognize as being truly beautiful.

So, when things get sweaty, lubey, rubbery and saturated with our own fluids again, I won't hesitate to share 'em with y'all.

22 July 2004

Endgame

It looks like things are pretty over between E and I. I really tried so hard to make this relationship work. I think towards the end I just lost steam, and resigned myself to the fact that it was a losing battle. While I am not too chipper at this point, it's too disheartening to go through the emotional turmoil anymore. My brain and my heart are finally on the same page. My cock is another story. *C'est la vie.*

I don't know if there will be any more activity on this blog. But who knows? A lot can happen from out of nowhere.

So once again I say, "Thank you" for all your comments and support. It was a pleasure to be able to share this with you.

12 August 2004

New Blog

I started a new blog. It's not a sex blog, for that would require someone else to have sex with. It's more of personal diary than anything else. Maybe it will evolve into something sexy later. I don't know yet. Anyone that is interested can email me and I will send the link.

Newlywed Satisfaction

The First Entry

5/11/03

The first entry. Woohoo.

Forgive my lack of enthusiasm, but I haven't been getting any the last few days and that hasn't exactly put me in a good mood. Both of us are stressed with the exams coming up in about two weeks, and realising that we know shit and are probably going to fail this exam.

I've decided that I need a place to vent my frustrations, to share my thoughts and views with whoever cares to read them. Yes, my husband is there for me to vent to, but sometimes I need an audience of more than one. And lucky you. You get to be it.

That's it for a first entry. Maybe more later. We'll see.

An Intro to Me

6/11/03

I suppose I should post a short introduction of myself. I am a 21-year-old married female, hailing from the sunny tropical island called Singapore. I am currently slaving my butt off reading in an unnamed university in Singapore. My husband is also a student, reading his final year of physics.

I have been married close to one year now, and the newlywed bliss is starting to wear off a bit, which is sort of why I wanted to start this weblog. I'm really bad at keeping a written diary, and since I spend a lot of my time on the internet surfing and writing emails, I thought I might be more conscientious in keeping an online diary updated. Plus, as mentioned in yesterday's post, I get to have an audience. The point of this weblog is to keep track of my thoughts on the progress of my marriage, sex life, and other stuff that I might just feel that I want to talk about.

OK that's it. More tomorrow. I promise.

I am a Nympho

7/11/03

I think I'm a nymphomaniac. I crave sex almost constantly. The more I get, the more I want. I guess it's almost like a drug high, only that unlike heroin, I don't need more sex just to get the same high, I just get higher and higher with more sex.

My husband does not understand my insatiable sexual appetites. This puzzles me somewhat as I have laboured under the delusion that if a woman constantly craves her man, it must mean that her man is definitely doing something right. Correct me if I'm wrong though. I haven't had exactly that much experience when it comes to dealing with men and sex, having slept with only one man in my entire life.

The difference in our sexual appetites bothers me.

Firstly, because I'm so much hornier than he is, I feel the need for pleasure even when he's not really in the mood. But he takes offence when I try to masturbate. He misses the point completely that it's not that he doesn't satisfy me. I'd trade my handjob for his cock anyday. So now, I've got to do it in secret, which puts the guilt factor into the picture. But if I don't, I tend to get cranky, and I take it out on him, which leads to even less sex.

Secondly, I get insecure about my own sexual abilities. This could be sort of a flipside of my Hubby's point of view. Sometimes I feel like maybe I don't make sex fantastic enough for him to want it as much as I do. God knows I try to do everything he wants me to. And he tells me I'm fabulous in bed. But still, the nagging doubt is there.

My appetite for sex has sometimes led to arguments. He has

accused me occasionally of wanting him around as my walking, talking, breathing dildo. But that's when I've become really cranky after not getting sex for a couple of days. Other times, he teases me about it, and how much I boost his ego, wanting him so much. And then he'll indulge me. And ooooh, does he indulge me!

I am a nymphomaniac. And it's all his fault.

Sacking the Sack

14/11/03

I have had it with condoms.

I hate those rubbery things. He hates it more. It's gotten to the point where he's avoiding full-on sex just because he hates the sensation of the condom on him, which means that I've got to thoroughly exercise my repertoire involving my hands and mouth. Sometimes we go without using one, but only if I'm sure that it's not my fertile period.

Unfortunately, I'm fertile right now, which means that he's avoiding me like the plague. And I'm in dire need of a good fuck with all the exam stress that's been piling up. With the exams starting tomorrow, I need to get my muscles unclenched. And he won't oblige me. AT ALL!

So. Since we're not getting much going on without some form of birth control, I've gone to see my doctor about putting me on the Pill. I've always thought that going on the Pill would mean that I'd go see the doctor, we'd talk a bit about my options, and then she'd write out a prescription for me to take to the pharmacy. But no, I had to go for a PAP smear, and a pelvic exam. And I only get the prescription when the results for the smear come back in two weeks.

That means two more weeks of playing cat and mouse with my boy.

Two weeks is bad enough. The doctor then tells me that I've still got to use a condom for the first month I'm on the Pill so that the hormones will stabilise and stop my body from ovulating. My mind froze.

That means six more weeks of playing cat and mouse with my boy.

Oh, God.
Help.

Butt Matters

22/11/03

I love having my butt fondled. The feeling of having my cheeks squeezed and massaged is sometimes enough to make me go over the edge. Which is why I have a nightly ritual in which my hubby rubs moisturising cream on my butt. I don't really need the moisturising cream on my butt, but he does it for me anyway, sweet thing that he is.

I've got to tell you, my butt isn't really all that fantastic to look at. It isn't perfectly pert, tight or round. It jiggles around if I jump up and down and I've often got to buy jeans that fit around my butt so I've got a lot of space round the waist, so I can't wear hipsters.

But I love my butt. And nothing, NOTHING, makes me feel as good as when my husband caresses it, telling me that he loves it. Nothing makes me feel more sexy than when he wedges himself in between my cheeks and tells me how much he wants to fuck it right there and then. Nothing makes me feel more sexy than when he grabs my ass in public. Oh, and how naughty I can get when he threatens to spank me. With a hairbrush.

50 Things

4/12/03

I'm back! Thanks to those who've been checking back every so often to see whether I've got anything new up! I'm sorry it took so long. I've had to recover a little from shell shock. I couldn't think of anything but chemical equations and mathematical formulae for a while, and I'm not too sure you want to hear about those!

Anyway, I've been noticing a lot of '## things about me' on the weblogs that I've linked to. Since I haven't actually let on much about myself, I figure why shouldn't I post some about me. So here goes nothing . . .

1. I am 21 years old.
2. I am studying to become a chemical engineer.
3. I hate it.
4. I'm probably going to end up teaching after graduation.
5. Although if Hubby pulls in a big enough salary, I'd rather stay home and take care of the kids.
6. We want at least two kids.
7. But not right now because both of us are still in school.
8. We fuck a lot though, to make sure we're in shape for the main event:)
9. I've been pregnant (accident) before but I lost it at seven weeks.
10. I was relieved when I lost it.
11. I felt guilty for feeling relieved.
12. No one except my hubby knew about it. Now, you do.
13. I love fucking.
14. I am a nympo.
15. I like it best doggy style.
16. I have multiple orgasms.
17. The record is 26 in half an hour.
18. I'm not sure that's accurate because my brain went numb for a while and I stopped counting.
19. I am very vocal during sex.
20. I stay with my parents.
21. I have learnt to suppress my "noise" because of number 20.
22. I love watching my husband just before he comes.
23. I'm proud of my ability to give good head.
24. And that I swallow.
25. With relish.
26. I like to pretend that I'm a porn star while I'm doing that.
27. I can be satisfied making my husband come, without getting any sexual favours in return.
28. But not too often. I'm a nympho, after all.
29. I've only had one serious relationship before I met my hubby.
30. I met him two weeks after that relationship broke up.
31. On ICQ.
32. My first serious relationship was really innocent.

33. We didn't even get around to holding hands.
34. I told my hubby he had to meet my parents before he could take me out.
35. He won my heart when he actually did it.
36. He is the first person I've ever slept with.
37. We were together for almost two years when we got married.
38. We got married in Dec 2002.
39. I was a virgin.
40. The first time was on the floor.
41. It hurt.
42. I didn't bleed. So much for my mother telling me that all virgins bleed the first time.
43. I had my first orgasm the third time we had sex.
44. I think that's when I became a nympho.
45. I am never more content than when my hubby strokes my hair when we're both falling asleep in each other's arms.
46. Watching my hubby sleep when I wake up in the morning is one of my favourite things to do.
47. I play computer games a lot, especially *Diablo II*.
48. Currently, I'm trying to finish *Final Fantasy X-2* on the Playstation 2.
49. I'm waiting for hubby to finish with his *ProEvolution Soccer 3* on the PS2 so I can get on with my game.
50. I've got to go help my mom, so this is it for Part 1! OK. I've gotta run. I'll post more stuff about me regularly, Tata!

First Anniversary

15/12/03

Sorry again for the long break in between entries. I've been away in Kuala Lumpur, Malaysia, on an annual "visit-the-relatives" trip. I've got a set of grandparents and a couple of aunts and uncles living there, although most of my relatives are here in Singapore. Most of those in Malaysia I see only once a year, and the last time I saw some of them was at my wedding.

Coincidentally, I celebrated my wedding anniversary there.

Waiting for midnight to come, and greeting the arrival of a new day, (and a new year of marriage) with a loud raunchy round of fucking. Felt like the first few weeks of marriage, when we hardly ever left the bed; we were fucking like rabbits all the time. I'd very much have liked to spend the entire day in bed doing nothing but fuck, on that very special day, but duty called and I had to get out of bed to go visit some more relatives.

And then we got back to the hotel, and we fucked some more.

I don't remember if we ate anything that day. I was just stuck on the idea of getting back to the hotel room and getting back into bed. It's so rare that my hubby is the one who's ripping my clothes off, pushing me into the bed. Straining to get inside of me. Can anyone honestly blame me for wanting to take advantage of that?

Well, my first anniversary didn't involve dinner, flowers, chocolates. But it involved lots of my favourite activity, and I think that was romantic enough for me;)

The Pill

22/11/03

I've just completed my first week on the Pill. It's not as bad as I thought it would be. I've been warned of bloating, massive weight gain, low libido, higher blood pressures, and basically turning into a perpetual PMS monster: I'm not really seeing any of it. There's no weight gain. Yeah, I think I'm retaining a little water, but the only visible effect right now is that it's making my boobs appear bigger and bouncier, which hubby is having a lot of fun with right now. My appetite has actually decreased, I have half portions now for all meals and I still feel pretty full. I'd say that's going to do wonders in the long run for my diet. Decreased libido? Nah. Same as usual. Only now, hubby is actually complying a little more since the pressure to use the condom is off;)

It's such a relief to have actually started on the Pill. When "the accident" happened, we were using condoms as birth control, and I hadn't noticed any leaks or such. Apparently, such "accidents" happen quite a bit, when I saw the doctor about it. I couldn't really trust using a condom after it happened, that's why I turned to the Pill. The Pill is supposed to be much more effective, and it helps make sex that much more enjoyable without the rubbery feeling of a condom.

I think I've just found a new best friend.

Afternoon Nap

2/1/04

When you get back from your errand later, I will be in the doorway waiting. Naked. I will drag you in by the shirt collar, devouring your mouth as I kick the door shut behind me. I don't care how many shirt buttons I pop, as long as I get your shirt off as soon as possible with one hand while the other gropes at your fly, rubbing the growing bulge in your pants.

I will shove you to the floor, tearing any clothes that remain on your body with my teeth, so hungry am I to get to you. Throwing your briefs in the corner. I relish the sight of your erect shaft. Taking the tip of the head in my mouth. I will proceed to lick, nibble and suck you. I will cover every single inch of your cock with luscious kisses, and surround it with the hot wet velvet of my mouth. Pausing only to take some breaths, I will make you beg me for more. I will make you grovel for completion.

When I have you panting for ecstasy, beyond dignity, then will I sit on you, sliding your hard cock between the throbbing lips of my wet pussy. Slow, hard strokes will I give you, squeezing with my inner muscles. You will beg me for faster, harder. You will grab my hips, forcing me higher, faster. Your hips will slam into the cheeks of my buttocks, forcing panting breaths and moans from me, which will only drive you on. I will turn around so that you can see your cock sliding in and out, in and out. And with one last moan, you will succumb to blessed release, your hips thrusting. And there we will collapse, entwined in each other, for an afternoon nap.

Blather

15/1/04

Time does fly by, doesn't it? I realised that the last time I posted was about a week ago, and it certainly hasn't felt at all like one whole week. More like a couple of days. Maybe it's because I've been doing at least a couple of hours of overtime every day, there's so much testing to be done! It's an accelerated project, so I think everyone's pretty much stressed about it, and everyone's on my back to get the results as fast as possible. It's like "I want the results yesterday!" Though sometimes, it's really impossible because the samples for me to run my testing on don't come in from inventory until next week! I feel kind of sorry for my supervisor. She's the coordinator for the whole project, and anything that screws up gets put on her shoulders. I'm trying to help her as much as I can, but seeing that I'm only on apprenticeship there's only so much I can do!

I'd be cranky and tired, doing all this work, except that hubby's been having a great run lately. I think it's the *Kama Sutra* that I got from my friend. We've discovered "The Elephant". I'll see if I can find a link to a picture of this position and put it up here. Actually, it's not all that different from doggy style, but it's added a little more spice. And lately he's been reaching for me in the middle of the night, half asleep. Not that I'm complaining, I love this attention! I'm feeling so wonderfully attractive and happy, and all this sex is helping me get through the day at work. I wake up fresh and all glowy; and I can't wait to get home at night. Ooh . . .

I think tonight I'll try another one of those positions that I've never tried yet. Or two. Or three.

Make-Up Sex

18/1/04

I love make-up sex. Really, I do. Sometimes I'll start a fight just so we can get around to having make-up sex. Obviously, sometimes that backfires on me. But today was just one of those happy days when things turned out the way I like them to. *grin*

I don't remember what the fight was about any more. Today was a really hot day, the kind where you just perspire without really doing anything. And on days like that, it's not very hard to get on my nerves. Something that hubby was doing very well. I know he did something to really tick me off. I think it was him refusing to get off me. Usually, I like him lying on top of my back while I type on the laptop lying on the bed. But today, it was just so hot and sticky and uncomfortable, so I told him to get off. And he didn't. And then he started tickling me. Which ticked me off even more because I was trying to concentrate on the game I was playing.

Basically, things just escalated from there. Suddenly we were at a point when we were yelling at each other. I must have said something to really piss him off as well (I have a tendency to just shoot my mouth off), because the next thing I knew, he'd grabbed my hair, and was twisting it around so much it hurt. He slapped me around a little bit, not enough to bruise me or anything, but just enough to show me I'd really pissed him off. And then he put me in a headlock.

I REALLY wasn't too happy at that point. So we got into a little wrestling match, with me trying to get loose and him trying to keep me locked up. So he's pulling me really close to him, and then, I feel his hard cock just poking into my butt. He flips me over and tells me, "You know, you're so damn cute when you're angry."

In short order, our clothes are off and all over the floor, and I'm riding his cock hard, fast and furious, while he's yelling obscenities at me. Grabbing and squeezing my butt-cheeks, raising his hips to slam into me. Sucking so hard on my nipple, just the way I like it. And just when he's about to come, he pulls me down into a bear hug so I can't move, and have to rely on my vaginal muscles to keep up the pace. Thank God for Kegel exercises.

Afterwards, it's quiet time, with us facing each other. Him stroking my hair. Me stroking his facial stubble. Fight's over now. Everything's back to normal. And we've put things back into perspective. We're crazy about each other, so everything else isn't really that important.

I don't know how couples who say that they don't fight keep the relationship alive and happy. I think it'd be so boring. Life together without make-up sex? I'll pass, thanks.

Post-Valentine Musings

16/2/04

Well, Valentine's Day has come and gone. Not that it matters much since my hubby doesn't believe in celebrating it. He thinks that he can show me his love every day, why pick one particular day to do it just because everyone else is? I can't argue with that since he does come up with his own Valentine's equivalents occasionally, when I'm least expecting it. And he pampers me every day so I guess I can't really complain. I remember thinking that some of my girlfriends only get picked up from work to get taken out to dinner on "special" days, while he'd show up out of the blue, travelling out of his way just to escort me home. I know how lucky I am, coz I've heard lots and lots of stories about how guys tend to forget to do these small things once they've got the wedding band on their finger! ;).

For me, it's Valentine's day whenever he.

1) sends me an SMS telling me he loves me.
2) gives me a backrub without me asking when he knows I'm tired.
3) sits through watching *American Idol* with me even though he thinks it's a stupid show.
4) cuddles me awake in the mornings.

I figure he's right. Why wait for Valentine's day when you can make it happen every day?

Sunday Morning

24/2/04

I woke up Sunday morning with a very stiff cock waving in my face.

"Suck me!" comes the order, while he slaps me around the face with the object of the desired attentions. Sleepily, I open my mouth obligingly, getting a very rude accelerated awakening when he grabs my hair and shoves his cock right down the back of my throat, eliciting a gasp and tears to my eyes.

"Ooh, yeah, suck that, bitch. Get on your knees."

I didn't really have much of a choice, him pulling my hair that way. So I do, And when he lets go of my hair, I slap him. Before I get down to business again.

I swirl my tongue round the tip of his cock. It drives him nuts when I do that. He moans and tries to shove my head down over his shaft but I slap his hands away. I like to take my time. I work my way slowly down, enveloping him in my warm, moist mouth, sucking him first gently, then harder, and harder, the groans coming from him driving me on to bring him even more pleasure.

"I want to come in you."

He pulls my head away, and throws me on my stomach, and enters me from behind. Quick fast thrusts and he's soon done, finishing with much shaking and "Fuck!"s.

He collapses on top of me, and we drift off to sleep again, on a lazy Sunday morning.

Bath Time

23/3/04

It's been the longest time since hubby and I have made love in the shower. It's one of the things I miss most. When I stayed with my mom, we had a bathroom attached to our bedroom which we didn't have to share with anyone. Now that we're living with his mom, we don't have our own bathroom any more. His family is really conservative, and I think it'd send my mother-in-law into shock if we went to shower together. We don't get much time alone in that house, so there's not much opportunity to do that when no one's around.

I really miss bathing with him. I miss running my hands over his back, giving him a slippery soapy massage before sliding my hands down between his thighs and playing with his balls. I miss sucking on his cock while he stands under the shower to wash all the soap off. I miss him turning me around to cup my breasts in his hands, bending me over and slowly entering me from behind. I miss coming with the water pelting at our backs.

Excuse me while I go find a bathroom now. I've got to go "relieve" myself from all the memories.

Payback

30/3/04

I haven't had sex for three days, and I'm so horny right now. I just want to go home and rip his clothes off, throw him in the shower and have him do it to me doggy style in the bath tub, warm water swirling around my knees and hands, running down my thighs. I want to feel his pelvis slamming into my butt, his hands on my breasts, his head buried in my neck. I want him to make me moan and scream, overwhelm my mind with animalistic passion. And I don't want him to come. At least, not yet. It's payback time.

Yesterday, he made me give him a hand- and blow-job. I wasn't allowed to touch myself at all, both hands had to be concentrating on him the whole time. Evil bastard. After he came, he slept for all of twenty minutes before waking up and making me do it all over again. Same thing. The first time, I'd already gotten so horny, and not being able to touch myself drove me nuts. So the second time round, I was begging and begging him to fuck me, to let me ride him. And he wouldn't let me. And I still couldn't touch myself. After that he fell asleep again, with his arms wrapped around me, so I couldn't even sneak in a quick one. Took me ages to fall asleep.

Oh, he's going to PAY.

Outburst

3/4/04

I'm so frustrated right now! He just won't go down on me! I'm in the middle of some petulant selfish anger right now, all because he won't eat pussy when I suck his cock all the time. Someone please tell me what I can do!

To Eat or Not To Eat

8/4/04

Threatening to not suck his cock until he eats pussy is not working. For one thing. I can barely keep myself away from his cock, so even if I don't suck it, I fuck it anyway. We've fucked at least five times in the last three days. And so he says with so much fucking, he doesn't really need me to give him a blow-job anyway, he's completely happy with just sex. Hmph.

It's really driving me nuts now. While I'm not complaining about the frequency of sex, nor the quality of it, it's just stuck on me that he won't eat my pussy! I guess it's more of a "why won't he do it for me?" rather than a "I need it real bad" kind of deal right now.

He's gone down on me once before, during the first few weeks of marriage. While I didn't really find it all that fantastic, it did feel kind of nice, and I'd really really like him to try it again. I know it's not because I taste or smell bad down there. I taste myself all the time on him when he wants to come in my mouth. He's got this psychological barrier that tells him that "down there is gross". Which really irritates me when he brings it up because I could say the same thing about his dick and I've gotten over it.

I guess all this is really normal, but I do wish there was some way I could solve this. Any idea how to change his mind? Or to make me stop thinking about making him do it?

Sleeping Pill Me

19/4/04

I'm a happy woman right now. Hubby hasn't been able to sleep well the last few days. So he's been fucking me until he's exhausted enough to fall right off into a nice deep sleep. I'm not that worried though because after that I know he gets his eight hours of uninterrupted sleep. And it's nice that I'm a solution to his insomnia, rather than his depending on some pills to put him to sleep.

So with the last few days being as good as it is, I stopped thinking about having him eat my pussy, or exploring possibilities with someone else. As Frank said in the comments to my last post, an orgasm is an orgasm, no matter how you come by it. And with the number I've been having lately, I don't think I really need to look for more sources :)

Tease

23/4/04

I think there's something about me lately that's been driving him to distraction. Maybe it's my hair growing longer and as a result my waves are becoming more defined and alluring to him. Or maybe it's my skin glowing lately after I started on a new skincare regime. Or maybe it's just that my male colleagues at work are paying some attention to me.

The last week or so there's been lots of buzz going around about so-and-so thinking I'm attractive and such. I've had a few engineers who asked me out for dinner and a drink after work, but they backed off after I told them I'm married. There's also a new guy at work security personnel. I think he's gorgeous, and I suspect I'm developing a crush on him.

Obviously, I've been milking all this that's been going on in the office to get my hubby crazy-jealous. Aren't I just evil?

Good Girl

27/4/04

Yesterday, I stepped in through the doorway at home and was immediately enveloped in a big bear hug, before being swept off my feet and carried into the bedroom. Hubby dumped me on the bed, pinned down my wrists, and started to cover my face with kisses, punctuating every kiss with sweet mumblings. I am ashamed to admit, the first thing that went through my mind was "What's he done now?" but that thought rapidly flew out of my head when he pressed his hard cock, which I felt through his shorts, into the crotch of my jeans.

Feeling him so hard for me just made my pussy start dripping. It's just such a turn-on knowing that my hubby wants me like that. I wanted to get my hands in his shorts, to stroke him. I wanted to have him in my mouth so I could suck on him. Most of all I wanted him in my pussy, pounding away at me until all coherent thought left me. So I started to untie the drawstring to his shorts.

And he slapped me.

"You're a naughty girl. You didn't have permission to touch him. Bad girl."

He tied my hands above my head with a towel, and took off his shorts. His cock was so hard, so inviting, my pussy started to ache. I wanted him in me so bad. He started running his cock down my cheeks, around my face, slapping me every now and then with it.

He started moving down to my breasts, and sandwiched his cock, now slick with pre-come, between them. Sliding himself slowly back and forth while he squeezed my breasts together, caressing my nipples with his thumbs.

He straightened up and started kissing me hard again.

"Do you want it?"

nod nod

"Do you really want it?"

nod nod nod

"What do you want?"

"I want your dick inside me. I want you moving in and out. faster and faster, making me come. I want you to fill me, get deep inside me. I want to feel the waves when you come inside of me, the feel of your come oozing out of me."

Laughing, he pulled my jeans off and threw them on the floor. And with one swift motion, he entered me. Oh. I was in ecstasy. Then he started moving slowly. In. Out. In. Out. So slow. So excrutiatingly pleasurable. He builds up speed until he's pumping hard, his crotch slamming hard into mine. I felt the build-up in my body and knew I was going to come.

And then he stopped.

"Time for dinner, naughty girl."

I was left speechless. And angry. How dare he deny me!?!

Before I could say a word, he leaned over and kissed me.

"I did need to punish you, you know. That's for being a naughty girl. If you're a good girl, maybe I'll let you come later."

So we ate dinner. And watched TV. And all that time, I was just thinking about how I could be a good girl for him so I could get dessert. And he knew it, the smirks he threw at me the whole time we were watching TV.

"Come here, babe."

I went over to him and sat on his lap. He pushed me off on to the floor.

"Suck me."

I pulled his shorts off, took his already hard cock in my mouth, and sucked him slowly. Sliding my mouth up and down, the way he likes it, my tongue tickling the little notch right under the head. He grabbed my hair and started moving my head faster and faster, letting out little moans which only made me want to please him even more, to make him moan even more. I was getting so wet again just hearing him moan. He pulled my head up, reached down and pulled me onto his lap. He took my underwear off, and sat me down on top of his hard dick, thrusting upwards as I slid down, bringing a gasp to my lips.

"You like that, bitch? Huh? You like that?"

He thrust faster and faster, matching my own rhythm as I rode him facing each other. His hands on my butt tightened while his eyes fought to stay open. I knew he was going to come, and the thought brought me to the edge. I felt the pulses of pleasure ripping through me, my pussy contracting around his cock. He drove hard into me, clenching his butt and I felt him spurt his hot come into me, my pulsing pussy eagerly devouring every drop he could give me.

I collapsed in his arms, as he stroked my hair.

"Good girl."

Service (Fantasy)

10/5/04

This is something that popped into my head during one of those days at work when nothing seems to be moving. It got me so horny visualizing it in my head. I'm definitely going to try my luck persuading hubby to play with me on this one!

He stepped tentatively in the shop, glancing furtively over his shoulder. He'd never been in one of these shops before, with the lewd neon signs advertising their goods. Turning, he nearly fell over the shop assistant. who'd come up to see if she could assist him in any way.

"Oh! I'm so terribly sorry!" he said, blushing furiously.

She laughed. "It's OK. Can I help you with anything?"

He turned even redder. "Um . . . well . . ."

"Oh, come on, there's no need to be shy. I won't bite . . . unless you want me to, that is." She winked at him saucily.

"Um . . . Well . . . My girlfriend and I . . . well . . . we . . ."

The shopgirl leaned forward on the counter, her arms positioned to push her cleavage into prominent view, her mini skirt riding up her ass.

"Yes?"

"I need condoms," he sputtered, embarrassed beyond belief,

eyes transfixed on the girl's perfect globes, his hands itching to grab them, caress them, suck them.

"Well, now, was that so hard to say? Come on then, we'll get you set up," she said, eyeing the growing bulge in his pants. She walked around the counter, grabbed his hand and took him to a corner of the shop, where condoms lined the walls, in their colourful wrappers.

"Right, then, what size do you need?"

He shrugged helplessly.

"Well, then. I'll just have to measure you." she said, putting her hand on the bulge in his pants. She silenced his protests by kissing him.

"Shhh . . . this is all just part of the service here. We want to make sure our customers are fully satisfied with the products they purchase."

She kneaded his cock through the cloth of his jeans, feeling it get harder and harder, straining to escape the confines of the zip.

"I can't tell what size you are from this. I'm going to have to let you out."

Slowly, she unzipped him, allowing his erect cock to spring free. A drop of pre-come glistened on the head.

"My, my, that's a big boy we've got there. Let's size it properly, shall we?"

She got down on her knees and flicked the tip of his cock with her tongue. She took the head in her mouth, sucking gently. He, overwhelmed with shock and the experience of it, leant back on the counter to steady his shaking legs. He couldn't prevent a moan from escaping as she started to move down the length of him, taking his entire shaft in her mouth.

She felt him grow harder and bigger in the heat of his passion.

"Well, if a little mouth can make you bigger, I'm going to have to determine your size a little more accurately."

She hitched her skirt up around her waist, and he could see that she hadn't any underwear on. Her pussy was glistening with juices, just begging to be fucked.

"Come on, big boy. You know you want to," she said, wiggling her ass at him.

He reached for her, pulling her ass into his crotch. She moaned, feeling his hard throbbing cock sliding over her pussy lips. With one swift thrust, he pushed himself into her velvet depths, a moan of ecstasy escaping both of them at the same time.

"Oh, my God, that's the biggest one I've ever felt yet. You're going to tear me into two."

He pumped faster and faster into her, reveling in the experience of his first fuck. He couldn't believe it felt this wonderful, the tight, velvet softness of a warm moist pussy enveloping his cock. The animalistic noises she made while thrusting her hips back at him were so erotic he could barely stand it. Within minutes, he felt his balls churn, and with one last hard thrust, he shot himself deep into her.

"Mmmm . . . I think I know exactly what you need."

She straightened up, smoothing her skirt back down. A trickle of white come started dribbling down her leg, which she scooped up with her finger and put in her mouth. Turning, she reached up to retrieve a box from a high shelf, allowing him a last view of her creamy ass. Watching her, he could sense the beginnings of another hard-on.

"I think you'll find these to be your size. You're a lucky boy. We don't usually sell much of these; they won't fit that many people. That'll be $15 for the box. Thank you sir, have a nice day. Come back soon, we're always willing to please with the service!" she said, giving him a wink, before turning her attention to another bewildered-looking young man walking into the shop.

Memories

4/6/04

Yesterday, my hubby's aunt got married in a religious ceremony. It was beautiful, bringing back lots of memories for me, of my own wedding a year and a half ago.

I remember waiting anxiously for my hubby to arrive, half afraid that he'd gotten cold feet and wouldn't show up. Every minute passed with agonising slowness. I remember the feelings of relief and joy when he showed up early. The euphoria when we were pronounced man and wife.

But, most of all, I remember the hurried unzipping of clothes to get to our naked bodies, being flung on the floor. Passionate kisses, frantic groping. The initial pain and then the uplifting pleasure of him thrusting into me.

I'm pretty much sure he remembered the same thing, because we relived that memory last night when we got home. Only I got much more pleasure out of it than that first night. So I guess memories of my wedding night are just going to get better and better.

My Pet

7/6/04

I love my hubby's cock. I am utterly possessive of it. I've told him before that if he ever gives over use of his cock to any other woman, I'll bite it off.

I am totally fascinated with it. I have spent hours between my hubby's legs while he slept, just looking at it. Looking at him flopped over his leg, his balls hanging loosely under him. It gives me an insane urge to pet it, stroke it, suck it.

I love watching him get hard and develop a slight tilt to the left as I hold him in my hands. I love feeling him grow harder and longer in my mouth while I run my tongue up and down the length of it swirling around the tip. I love the salty nectar that pours down my throat as my hubby rams his cock further into my mouth.

But definitely, most of all, I love feeling the head of his cock teasing the entrance of my pussy, the feeling of him entering me with one swift thrust. The feeling of him coming inside me, the walls of my pussy stroking him as he pumps and ripples within me.

He's a good little pet, my hubby's dick. MY pet. My preciousssssssssss . . .;)

Jumping the Gun

7/6/04

I always knew that if I'd met the right guy, I'd want to get married young. Hubby had the same idea. Only, both of us hadn't really planned on getting married this young. We already knew that we wanted to be together, but had planned to get married after graduation. Then one day, our parents sat us down and had a long talk about us. Our families are pretty much conservative, and premarital sex is a huge no-no. But they also understood that Hubby and I had needs and urges that probably couldn't be contained for very long, and they wanted to avoid any hanky-panky, as they put it. So they offered to pay for the wedding, and to continue to support us while we finished up our degrees.

Of course Hubby and I jumped at the chance. Getting used to married life without any financial commitments sounded like a really good idea. It meant that by the time we had to go out and look for jobs and handle car and house payments we'd have hopefully gotten over the initial awkwardness of married life and the tension that it can bring. Also, it meant we didn't have to foot the bill for the wedding;) And yes, it meant we could have sex.

Getting married so young has been exhilarating. Wedding rings on our fingers, we proved that we wholly belonged only to each other, and to any children that might result from our union. I am the envy of my single friends because I have found my soulmate, while they're still struggling with the rollercoaster of emotions in search of theirs. He is the one person I hide nothing from, who knows every single thing about me. He is my fuck-buddy and my lover, and I love being his slut.

It's brought new perspective to our lives. The drive to do well in exams and get good qualifications is there. We know we've got to get suitable jobs that will provide for us and our family, and we know we've got to do reasonably well so that we could pick a position that suited us.

On the other hand, getting married has ripped me away from my friends. We aren't on the same wavelength anymore. Our priorities are wildly off tangent. They're thinking about taking six months off after graduation to travel before settling down in a job. They worry about where to go and how long to spend there. I'm worrying about getting a job and paying for a house. I'm out of that carefree life where I don't have to worry about anyone except myself. Much as I view my wedding band as a visible declaration of my love and commitment to my husband, many of my friends see it as a ball and chain. Some have commented that I think like an old woman. I see it as having taken the next step in life, leaving them behind. But on that next step, I'm one of the youngest there. Most women in

Singapore get married in their thirties. I'm the "baby" of the group. They don't really believe that I take my married life, my husband and my commitments seriously. So sometimes, it's a really lonely life for me. I'm stuck neither here nor there.

Hubby, on the other hand, has it easier. His friends are pretty much like-minded, and are serious about their current girlfriends with marriage in view. So they kind of understand him and his worries. So in that sense, he's not as alone as I am.

I'm not really all that sad about no longer relating as well to my friends. I've got everything I need with my hubby. But sometimes it's nice to get an alternative view, or to have someone who can help me figure things out, especially when I can't turn to my hubby (when he's mad at me). So thank you, for reading and commenting!

All in all, I wouldn't have changed a thing. There've been some rough and painful times, but in the end it's entirely worth it, just to have my hubby stroking my hair in the morning to wake me up.

Teddy, if you're reading this, I love you.

Undate

17/6/04

I'm baaack! :)

I've finally finished with my apprenticeship! Now I'm back in school, mugging my brains out for my final year. Being back in school means I have more free time for mid-afternoon fucks in between classes . . .

I also turned 22 this past week. Hubby gave me the most glorious time the entire week leading up to my birthday. He was ripping my clothes off at almost every opporunity, and fucking me in all my favourite positions and places. He said he'd better get as much of the sweet young thing I was before I turned into an old crone. He really got spanked for that one.

So, basically just a short update on my life at the moment. More sugar and spice in my blog soon, now that all the technical shit is being purged from my system.

Wet Dream

23/6/04

I woke up in the middle of the night yesterday feeling inexplicably horny. My pussy was throbbing, feeling so empty. I knew I wouldn't be able to get back to sleep until my pussy's hunger had been satisfied.

I rolled my snoring hubby over onto his back. His cock was already half hard. I took him in my mouth, sucking him slowly. I felt him grow harder and longer, hitting the back of my throat. I could taste the salt of his pre-come. He shifted slightly on his back, letting out a soft moan, and I knew he was ready for me.

I straddled him, using his wet cock to play with the lips of my pussy. I was already wet, and the feel of his head sliding across my clit was gorgeous. Settling the tip of his head at the entrance of my pussy, I slid down his cock. He moaned even more, thrusting his hips higher to drive his shaft fully into me. I rode him slowly, savouring the feel of him pumping in and out of me, feeling the waves of pleasure course through my body. I moved faster and faster, feeling his hands tighten on my waist, guiding my movements. His hips slammed into me as he thrust himself upwards. burying himself deep in my cunt. With a small cry he came, as I did.

I collapsed on top of him, amused to note that he was still sleeping. He probably woke up thinking that he'd had one hell of a wet dream.

Lonely

26/7/04

I am in pieces right now. I'm feeling neglected. Hubby's stuck to his Playstation 2 most of the time now. The last few weeks it didn't seem so bad because I was studying and I thought he just probably didn't want to disturb me. Now that the exams are over and I'm free as a bird until school starts again, he's still stuck to his PS2 and I'm twiddling my thumbs watching him whack demons for the 13875th time (exaggeration, I'm sure, but it feels like it).

And then there's the sex. I get attention when he wants sex. Me, being the nympho, wants more sex than he does. So I'm getting rejected a lot. I'm hearing the "I'm too tired" phrase all too much recently. I want to strangle him. He stays up till four am playing his stupid games, not paying me any attention and then he wants to complain he's too tired? How can a machine replace me?

So, taking advice from a few friends that men needed to have things spelled out for them. I spelled it out for him. Several times. And I did it nicely too. It achieved zero. It got me really upset. And then I got the "Get over it or I'm going to get really pissed at you" look.

This was several days ago. After getting the look, I've basically had to pretend that everything is fine. If I even start to bring it up, the look comes back in full force. I have to smile, and suppress all the anger that's just building up in me every single day that goes by. It feels like he doesn't care how it's breaking me up inside.

This all just makes me very very sad.

The Rain Has Come!

4/8/04

Well, the dry spell is over. Last night I got fucked at bedtime. I guess maybe he's forgotten how good fucking can be because he reached out and grabbed for me again first thing this morning. But, since it's been a few days since we last had sex, it was all over pretty quick. I didn't come, but the knowing that he really did like sex with me made up for it.

Also, I think I've come up with some compromises for us when he's playing his PS2. I've just discovered his vibrating joypad. So now I can plug it into the second-player, sit back and just go along for the ride;)

One a Day . . .

11/8/04

About a week ago, I put my foot down and told hubby that he had to get used to the idea of having a nymphomanic wife. And that if he wasn't up for once-a-day at least, then he'd better learn to live with the fact that I will end up masturbating to get myself off. And not always in front of him where he can enjoy looking at me, either.

Amazingly enough, this has prompted him to jump to fill the daily quota. And more. If I had a carry-over system, I believe he's filled the quota to the end of next week. But of course, I'm not letting him cheat me of enjoying my pleasures every day.

I know I probably took a risk in putting my foot down. On one hand he could have gone totally cold on me, figuring that I was telling him that he didn't satisfy me at all. On the other hand, he could take it the way I really meant it. That he was so de-fucking-licious that I couldn't get enough of him and it was driving me crazy. He, of course, took it to be the latter. I guess it must have pumped up his ego so much, he's just roaring to go now.

I'm really having so much fun!

Reunion

24/8/04

Life is truly hectic at the moment. I'm just starting my final year in the university, and having to work on my final year project is taking up a whole lot of my time. The upside is that I'm away from Hubby a lot during the day, so when it comes to kiss, cuddle and fuck at bedtime he's all eager to go. I get to bed tired, fall asleep even more tired but really happy and sated. OK, that's it for personal update on my sex life for now. Juicy post on the way soon, I promise!

Last weekend, I went to my 10th year primary school reunion. In Singapore, kids graduate from primary school at age 12, and then they go on to secondary school. It's been 10 years since I graduated from my primary school.

So far, I'm the only person to have gotten married in my class. Which leads to the inevitable "So early! So how did you know he was the one?" I don't mind being quizzed about what it feels like to be married, how much I enjoy sex etc. But it does get awkward when people ask me how I knew my hubby was the one for me? These usually from friends who are wondering whether their current partners where the ones they were meant to be with.

I hesitate to tell them that I really just knew, that it was a gut feeling that this was going to be the man I wanted to spend the rest of my life with. The man I wanted to father my children. The man I wanted to knock any potential rapists over the head with a baseball bat and carry me off to safety. Six months into the relationship, I knew. He, apparently, knew the first time he talked to me. I'm not comfortable telling them this. I also know people who have been undecided about their partner for years, eventually settling down with them, and having stable happy marriages. They didn't have the feeling of certainly that I had.

Often, I'd spout off the generic answer of "It depends on the individual." Just as often, I get dirty looks right back. "You didn't help me much, dammit!"

So how do I do this?

Submissive Reflections

Sarah

http://submissivereflections.blogspot.com

Monday 24 November 2003

I guess this is where I start to let you all out there know about us. Hi. I am Sarah. He is Mac. Mac knows about this blog. I asked permission to be allowed to post here. He granted it, as long as we retain our privacy and as long as I am honest and I enjoy my time here. He understands my incessant need to dissect our relationship, even though He has no wish to do so with me. He may read this from time to time and I know that He will only be angry over what I write if it is a lie.

So, us. We have known each other for four years but have only been involved for just over one year. How we went from friends to lovers was really a simple thing that never really changed who we were, just allowed us to acknowledge it for the first time.

The first time we had sex was a week after He had kissed me and accepted that I was His. It happened to be my birthday. Neither of us were waiting for it, it just happened to be the first chance we had to be alone together as work was keeping Him busy and out of town. When He came to my place He simply said hello and bit my neck and pulled my skirt up and my panties down and pushed me to the floor and fucked me. There was no foreplay and no words of tenderness. It was just a matter of raw hungry sex. Within minutes He withdrew from me and turned me to my stomach, pulling me to my knees and hands while growling at me to "present" and whilst I was still trying to get my bearings I felt His cock press against my ass. I felt so incredibly turned on. He slid His cock slowly inside my ass, stopping when I clenched and gasped, then pushing into my ass again. I couldn't believe He was ass-fucking me without a word being spoken about it between us. When His cock was fully inside me He lay over me and bit my shoulders and neck. He used one hand in my hair to pull my head back and reached for my mouth with His tongue. I closed my lips over it and sucked on His tongue and He came in my ass, growling and grunting and filling me with semen. He collapsed against me and I collapsed against the floor and He kept Himself inside me while He licked and bit and sucked at my neck. He whispered, "Happy birthday Princess," in my ear and I felt like I was the luckiest girl alive.

When we talked about it later He told me that He hadn't asked if I liked anal sex because His kind of woman preferred not to be given options. He also knew that I would do anything to please Him, and that had been what pleased Him. Had it repulsed me, He said He would have had to rethink what He wanted as anything that did not make me "pant with lust" would not please Him either. I remember feeling tinier than I had ever felt when I was lying wrapped up in His arms. I had never felt so safe and protected and loved. I remember thinking that it was the best sex I had ever had and I didn't realise until the next day that I actually hadn't come.

Tuesday 25 November 2003

There is someone else that I should introduce to everyone as she is a very important part of our relationship and I am sure she will pop up often. Her name is Emma. (Emma and Sarah, I always think they sound so pretty together.)

I met Emma during sex, although it was not sex with her. She was just watching. Emma is soft and gentle and loves being a woman. She is the type of woman I adore. We became lovers fast and friends soon after. She doesn't live with us and she has a life and relationships outside of us but she never brings any of her outside life to our bed. Most of the time we are like two giggling little girls being naughty together. It is a relationship I cherish.

Mac thought it was important for me to have Emma in my life because He felt He couldn't offer the gentleness and the girlish giggles that I can share with Emma and He wants me to have it all.

He admits though, that I am not the only one who gains from our relationship with Emma.

For example: there was a day Emma and I had planned to spend together. We had shopped and lunched and gone back to my place for some afternoon decadence. We modelled new clothes and played with new makeup and giggled quite a bit. We played with each other's hair and we kissed. We lay side by side on the bed and we kissed. We talked and we kissed. Somehow the topic got around to Mac's cock and then to how He preferred to fuck and finally Emma told me that she had never had a man fuck her tits. Emma has beautiful breasts and it surprised me that no man had ever tried to get his penis between them. Emma was blushing (but that could have been because my fingers were between her legs) and I was grinning and I told her we would have to ask Mac to do it for her. She told me she wouldn't know how.

I jumped off the bed and grabbed some baby oil off the dresser and poured the oil on her breasts. I sat over her belly and massaged the oil in, adding more when I felt like it until she was a very slippery girl. I grabbed a lipstick and did my best to paint her nipples deep dark whorish red and showed her how to hold her breasts to be fucked and told her that Mac would prefer to come in her mouth once He had started to come.

She then grabbed the baby oil and did the same to me painting my nipples red with the lipstick too. We then spent time rubbing our oily bodies against each other, loving and kissing, licking, tasting, exploring, discovering gasps of enjoyment and moans of pleasure. Her body is a treasure of sensual delights.

By the time Mac arrived home He found two very dishevelled girls filled with lust and love waiting for Him with oil- and lipstick-smeared breasts. We knelt on the bed and bowed our heads and cupped our messy breasts in offering. We both tried very hard not to giggle when He commented on the state we were in and I waited until He was quiet. Then I asked Him if it would please Him to fuck Emma's tits.

He hesitated for a moment. I think He wasn't sure if He wanted to use us Himself or watch Emma and I pleasure each other.

In the end, He did both.

Monday 1 December 2003

I have been thinking about what Mac gets out of our relationship. Mac has always said that He is dominant, but not "A Dominant". We don't have rules, He doesn't give orders, and if I do call Him sir or master it is done in absolute cheekiness and likely to send me into a fit of giggles.

In saying that He doesn't give orders, I should add that sometimes, rarely, He does insist I do as I am told. These occasions usually occur as I am on the verge of becoming hysterical about something. At those times He will take complete control until I am calm and able to think clearly. He does this because I have an enormous ability to do myself great damage and He will not allow me to hurt myself.

He is, of course, very dominating. People notice it about Him immediately. He is the guy that is centre of attention at the party, the one that people look to for approval, and the one that people want to notice them. He is self-confident, (read that as arrogant), intelligent, witty, and an outdoors sportsman to boot and I have seen the mood of a room change just because He has walked in. (Can you tell I adore him?)

So what is it He gets out of my submission to Him if He has no need to control me? I have asked Him this and His answer is that it is something that I need, that I am not happy without, and He enjoys my happiness. He likes to fill my needs, as much as I love to fill His pleasures.

He has had sex with unsubmissive women, He has enjoyed sex with unsubmissive women, and He has enjoyed relationships with unsubmissive women. He doesn't feel that a woman has to be submissive to meet His needs. So why does He enjoy me so much? To put it into the words of Mac, "I don't need a cold beer at the end of a hot day, but damn, it makes the day a hell of a lot better when I have one."

I would have to say that one of the most intense sexual experiences that He and I had together had nothing at all to do with control, or domination or submission. All it had to do with was us.

We were lying together on the bed in the middle of the afternoon, talking and laughing and watching the clock as we were expecting people over in an hour or so. He reached for me and pulled me over

Him and I gladly took Him inside me. I always love the idea of making Him come, and doing it just before having friends in the apartment would be just delicious. I would be able to smell Him on me all afternoon.

We made love, kissing, caressing, just enjoying the feel of each other and when He could tell I was about to come He asked me to wait as He was nearly there too. Two more strokes and I was whimpering and He said, "Fuck it, come for me and I will be ready next time." I came, and suddenly He did too and I giggled and He shook His head at my delight and pulled me to Him. He stayed inside me and moved enough to keep Himself hard and before long I was ready to come again and He held me close while I did. Then He came and again He stayed inside me and we both came again.

I was breathless and totally caught up in Him, as He was in me. We turned so that I was beneath Him and I wound my legs around Him and tangled my fingers in His hair and we kissed and kissed and I loved Him so damn much I thought I would burst. I came again and He came, then I came and He did too. I was amazed, His body would tense and shudder in the midst of grunts and growls and His cock would stay hard and inside me and He was coming as much as I was and we were both lost in each other's pleasure. I don't know how many times I came and I don't know how many times He came but we were still very caught up in each other when we heard voices outside.

Our friends had arrived and we both dove for clothes, Him cursing and me racing to the bathroom to clean up. We stayed very close to each other that afternoon, almost always touching, the connection between us still very strong.

After everyone had gone He told me that he had never experienced anything like that before, He said it was almost like He had become a part of me and could feel everything I felt and me coming was enough to make Him come too. I have never ever known a man to be able to come as much as He did that day.

It hasn't happened for us again since. Sometimes I curse the friends for turning up when they did. Other times I think it was a good job they did show up, or we might not have come up for days.

Then again, would that have been such a bad thing?

Tuesday 2 December 2003

I would like to use this post to answer a question that I also answered privately to the one that asked it, what makes being shared good for me.

The first thing that comes to mind is that Mac is in control, the whole time. No one touches me and no one comes near me unless He decides it will happen. I surrender all I am and all I have to Him. I place my trust in His hands and know that He will not fail me. If the situation feels wrong to Him, or if there is something or someone that is making me uncomfortable, I know that Mac will take me and walk away. There have been times that we have done just that.

I also know that Mac takes a lot of pride and pleasure in the fact that His girl is so desired and wanted by other men and women. He finds it gorgeous that I trust Him so completely that I give myself up to the lust during these "adventures" and lose track of everything around me except the man or woman I am pleasing. It fills Him with a need to take me and make me His again. He is never as gentle or loves me as carefully as He does after the sex and the sharing has been the roughest. He understands that after being used for other's pleasure I need to be His princess again.

But also, there is the pleasure I get from it myself. And I do get a lot of pleasure from it. It makes me feel so beautiful to be so desired, to be the object of so many people's pleasure and I have to admit to a certain validation I feel, waking the next day, knowing that there are people waking up and thinking "what a delicious little slut that Sarah was, wish I could have her as mine."

That brings me to a little bit of wickedness I would like to share. Mac and I had travelled to the city and spent the night in a hotel. We were there to attend a reunion of His old team mates.

I woke in a playful mood and tried very hard to entice Him into sex. In the end He sat across my tummy and pinned me to the bed and told me that I had to behave. He grabbed a rope (funnily enough, we usually have some close by) and tied my hands together, then tied them above my head to the bed. He covered my eyes with a blindfold (something else we keep close by) and made sure it would not slip off and that I could see nothing. By this time I was already wet with lust but what He said next made me gasp and heightened my desire.

"We are going to have an adventure."

Usually I am given time to prepare myself for our adventures. Mac will call me from work and tell me what time to be ready and what to wear, and I am left shivering in anticipation all day. To be tied to the bed and have it announced was new and it thrilled me.

"Two men," He said. "You will see neither, and they will not speak to you or give you any clue as to who they are. They will be allowed to fuck you any way they choose, but they will not be allowed to hurt you. You will never know who they are, but both will be at the party this afternoon." He waited until I said "yes", and then climbed off me and I could hear Him getting dressed. He told me He would see me in a little while, and He left.

I don't know how long I waited but my cunt was throbbing and if I had use of my hands I would have been masturbating. I lay there, relaxed, knowing they would use me and wanting it to happen.

When the door opened, I smiled. I could hear someone undressing and a man lay over me and thrust his cock into me and I knew from his breathing that he was already about to come. I pushed my hips up to meet His thrusts and I licked my lips and I begged him to come for me and he did, showering my pussy with his semen.

He dressed quickly and he left and when the door closed behind him I felt a little empty and hoped that I wouldn't be left alone for too long.

The door opened again. Two large and rough hands handled me very deftly. He turned me onto my stomach and push-pulled me onto my knees, my upper body resting on my elbows. He guided his cock into my cunt and thrust into me a few times, then he withdrew. I felt him press against my ass and I wriggled back against him while begging him to fuck my ass. He did, roughly and painfully and I moaned and begged him for more. He slid his fingers beneath me and rubbed the first man's semen over my clitoris and I came, whimpering into the bed. He grabbed my hair and pulled me back onto my elbows and ran the fingers from my pussy down my cheek. I turned my head and sucked on them greedily and he growled and he came, filling my ass with hot spurts of semen. I thanked him quietly and he left.

When Mac came back to the room, He surprised me by telling me that the first man had asked if he could fuck my mouth and Mac had agreed to allow it. I was thrilled at being asked for again, and thrilled that my permission was not sought. I belonged to Him.

When the man came in he climbed over my chest and sat with His cock at my face. I licked him and suckled at him and he came all over my face as well as in my mouth. I thanked him and he left again and I waited not sure what was going to happen next.

This time when the door opened I knew it was two people. Mac told me to relax and untied my hands from the bed, though my hands were left bound together. From the size of the hands that shifted me across the bed I knew the second man was with Him. I was positioned with my hips on the very edge of the bed and the man lifted my legs up his body and slid his cock inside me. He pounded at me, roughly and urgently and I arched my back and came, begging him not to stop.

I felt the bed move near my head and I was not surprised to hear Mac's voice say, "I want to put my cock in your mouth now." I turned my head to take His cock and for a while I completely forgot everything else while He growled and filled my throat with His semen. I tried to swallow but I could feel it trickling from my lips.

When His orgasm was complete, He shifted down beside me and whispered in my ear, "Make him come, baby. Make him come hard." And I remembered that there was a man still fucking me. I twisted my legs around him the best I could and tried to pull him over me. He allowed himself to fall onto me and Mac quickly untied my hands. I pulled this stranger to me and I kissed him, surprised that he did not hesitate to kiss me back due to the other men's come that was on my face. Between each kiss I begged him to come for me, fill me with his come, I want it, I need it, please give it to me, and I kissed him again, long and slow and deep and He groaned and he bucked and I felt his orgasm shudder through him. He swore and I later thought that it was funny that the only word I heard from either of them was, "FUCK."

When we were alone, Mac kissed me and held me and told me how pleased He was. He made love to me and called me His princess and His angel and I felt very cherished and I fell asleep wrapped up in His arms.

When He woke me later He told me I could wash my face but I was not to wash away any semen from my thighs or pussy, He wanted me to feel the come still on me.

When we arrived, I was nervous and excited and half convinced that He was lying about them being there and I think He sensed this because He leaned over and told me that He had spotted them the moment we had walked in. I spent the evening feeling all eyes watching me and throbbing with absolute lust. Everyone settled down to watch a video of a game they had played and Mac found a chair and I made myself comfortable at His feet.

As the video was about to start He leaned forward and whispered in my ear. "They are watching you, baby, and they know what a slut you are."

Just thinking about it still makes me shiver with lust.

Tuesday 9 December 2003

Yesterday I was so angry. If there is one thing I cannot stand it is being talked down to. I am an intelligent female with thoughts and opinions of my own and I am completely capable of expressing them without degrading anyone. I went out with some friends because being at home alone was depressing me. We were sitting around talking about dating when one of the divorced men in the group, Robert, said that he couldn't understand why all the women he dated were looking for "father figures". I asked what he meant by that and he said, "Women that need help in making the simplest decisions, you know, the ones that want you to approve of everything they do. I have a daughter and do not need to raise another child. I prefer strong women."

I asked if he thought that women who need a loving supportive relationship were weak and he said yes. Everyone else had pretty much fallen quiet. Mac and I do not make a big deal out of His position in my life. I don't refer to Him as Master, or announce I am His submissive, but at the very least most of my female friends are aware of the dynamic that passes between us and realise that I will defer to Mac before making a decision so all were watching this exchange in interest.

I am always very careful when choosing the words I use in a discussion. Mac often says it's like being savaged by a slaughtered lamb. I told Robert that in my opinion, women that need a loving relationship are no weaker or stronger than anyone else, they just function best that way.

Robert said, "OK, Sarah." "If you say so, Sarah." "I must be wrong, Sarah." "You are right, Sarah." And that's when I started to lose my temper. I told Robert that I would like to have an intelligent conversation about this, but that was obviously impossible and I started talking to someone else. Ten minutes later when I got up to go to the bar, Robert followed. He said he was sorry, that it was just that I had attacked him with my opinion and that he just didn't want to argue with me so he had agreed. I told him that there was no attack, I offered my opinion and hoped it would spark a conversation but his treating me like a child had precluded that. He said that he would leave me alone as I was obviously angry. I ordered my drink and when I turned back to him, he was gone.

When I went back over to our friends, I overheard Robert telling them that I had told him to take a hike and that I had treated him like a child. And that's when I really got angry. I pointed out that it was he who had started saying, "OK, Sarah, yes, Sarah, you are right, Sarah" and that he had been the one to suggest leaving me alone; I just hadn't disagreed with him.

Robert announced that he was tired and left quickly and I was furious. He didn't even have the balls to admit the truth. He made me feel inadequate, not because he feels submissive women are weak, but because he treated me like I didn't count. To me having my opinion dismissed like that and then being deceitful to our friends is much more of a weakness than admitting you need to lean on someone to make the world right for you.

I think it's fair enough that Robert does not want to date women that he feels depend on him too much. It's great that he understands that he can't handle that. I just think it is a shame that he sees this trait as a weakness and I was hoping to point out that to another man it could be a delicious plus to the relationship. I guess you can't make someone see the woods for the trees if they don't want to look.

So what did I do in my anger? I went home and rang Emma and she listened to me rant and whine then she suggested we go out for some fun. Mac doesn't mind if Emma and I are a little wicked together, so long as we share the details with Him and as long as we don't put ourselves into any danger. Emma knew this horrible little dive of a bar where we could go and misbehave as much as we wanted.

Emma and I look kind of amazing together. She is fair and blonde, I am olive-skinned and brunette. We are practically the same size in height and in weight, although I am slightly curvier than she is. We both wore short black skirts with stockings and high heels and I had on a tight sleeveless top with a black lace over-shirt, Emma had on a tight red shirt that showed off her cleavage and gosh she looked yummy.

We had a great time flirting with a heap of different men and playing at being coy little sluts. Eventually Emma singled one guy out and I mainly watched while she teased and cajoled and convinced him the offer she was making was for real. We eventually got the guy into the alley behind the bar and while he was still protesting the lack of privacy Emma freed his cock from his pants and he got really quiet. She bent over to look at his penis up close while she was stroking it and she said, "Mmmm, pretty cock," while glancing wickedly at me. I had to bite my lip so that I didn't break down in a fit of giggles. She told me to come look and I knelt and started to stroke him too. Emma got to her knees on the other side of his cock and we started to kiss him and then my tongue touched hers and I tried to kiss her around his cock. All I wanted was her tongue in my mouth. We watched each other kiss and lick and stroke his cock and balls and he was more just a toy we were playing with than a man we were pleasuring, but that didn't stop him from coming pretty quickly. He came on Emma's face and shirt and we both giggled when he did.

Emma and I stood up and I licked at the semen on her cheek and slid my tongue into her mouth and once I started kissing her I didn't want to stop. I murmured to Emma that we should go home and the guy cleared his throat and we both looked at him, a little startled. I had forgotten he was there. He asked if he could come with us and Emma said no. He said he would pay and Emma and I burst out laughing. We told him thank you but no and we walked out to the road and grabbed a cab.

Emma spent the night here last night and she has just borrowed some of my clothes for work.

It's not the first time Emma and I have used a guy as a toy to enhance our own excitement, but it was the first time we did it without Mac there. I have a feeling that when Mac gets home from

His trip, Emma and I will be told to show Him exactly how we did it.

I can hardly wait.

Sunday 21 December 2003

I am hungry.

I watch Him move around the room unaware of all that I am thinking and feeling. He smiles at me with the air of One without a care in the world. He stands casually in His blue jeans and crumpled shirt waiting for me to reply and I smile sweetly and hope that my eyes do not give me away. He doesn't know that the tables have turned, that the prey has become the predator. I want to feed.

He used me yesterday for His pleasure and I still feel the marks of His hands and the bruises from His teeth and it is not enough to slake the gnawing in my stomach, the ache in my groin. Lie still, my darling Male, I promise this won't hurt. I want nothing more than the groan from Your lips and the semen from Your balls. Fuck foreplay, who needs it? Not me, I don't care if You touch me, I don't care if I come. I could take care of that without You. I know where my clitoris is. I don't need You to show me. It is You that I want, Your lust that fills me. I want to fuck. Give me Your cock and I will empty Your balls of all You have and still I will want more.

I want the builder from across the road that caresses each piece of wood as he drives a nail home. I want his young apprentice, the one that blushes each time I say hello. And I want the other guy, the one that doesn't speak but looks at me like he is hungry too. I want to rut with them like a dog in heat. I want to take their cocks inside me and force each of them to spill. I want to drag their semen from them again and again until I have it all. I want to make them growl and shudder and spurt. I want to fuck them over and over again until they are spent. And then I will still want more.

I want to be taken to Your rugby club and offered up to the players on Your team, those giant men awash with adrenaline and testosterone. Strap me to the table and sacrifice me to their lust. Let them dirty me with their muddy hands and mark me with their sweaty scent. Let them use me. Let them drive their cocks into me until I scream for them to stop while begging for just one more. One more cock to spill inside me, one more set of teeth to mark my tits, one more set of balls to empty. Please, just one more? Let just one more call me slut and let me revel in the way the word rolls from his lips as his cock pulses and I feel his seed empty into me. I need them all so deep inside me, deeper than ever before. I need their semen to spill from me as new men take me. I need to be drenched in come. I need their pleasure. I need.

The hand at my neck startles me back to reality and I blush as I realise He can see the words on my screen. "So my girl is hungry," Mac's voice hisses in my ear as His fingers trail down to cup my breast. My head lowers and I am too embarrassed to speak. His teeth nip gently at my neck and His thumb plays across my erect nipple. "Is she?" He asks gently but firmly stealing any control I had and causing my body to throb with lust. I nod and He grins at my lack of voice. "Finish your post, and then come to the bedroom. I think it is time I fed my slut." I shudder as He walks away. The tables have been righted. I am the prey once more.

The meal shall be delicious.

Friday 2 January 2004

I had a former boyfriend that always wanted me to tie him up and rape him. This was always a hard thing for me to do as I always felt so out of control. How do I rape someone? Should I humiliate him? Call him names? Hurt him? The best I could do was tie him up and have sex with him, which hardly makes it rape. I always felt like I was faking it but I did my best to please him. I just thank the powers that be that he never asked me to hurt him. I can imagine it now.

SMACK
  Him: ouch!
  Me: Did I hurt you? Was it too hard? Should I do it softer? Do you want me to stop? I am sorry. I didn't mean to hurt you.

I am sure it would have destroyed any mood we had created. I just cannot hurt anyone. On the other hand, I like a certain amount of pain. I am far from a pain slut that can be tied up and whipped and belted and caned and flogged and so on and so forth. Nor do I need a lot of pain to get the endorphin/adrenaline rush flowing, but slap my face or use a fine whip on my breasts and I will beg for more.

When I first started masturbating, my fantasies were of punishment. It was wrong, it was dirty and, if I touched myself, it had to hurt for me to enjoy it. My orgasm was always achieved to appease an imaginary Him that would kiss me and tell me what a good girl I was to do as I was told and all my sins would be forgiven in His pleasure.

Mac is different to me, as one would expect. He never had fantasies of domination, or fantasies of hurting anyone and He once told me that the best way to make a woman want to please you is by making her come hard many times until she wants nothing more than to wind her fingers through your hair and wrap her legs around you and make you come. At the same time He has always taken the lead in His sexual relationships and never thought about taking a submissive role either. Mac just assumes that He is in charge of pretty much everything He does and, strangely enough, people go along with Him.

So why is it that Mac gets a sexual rush at the sight of His girl on her knees, tear-streaked and begging Him to hurt her more? I think what He gets a rush from is the fact that I am so obviously aroused. My whole body becomes one giant erogenous zone and a single touch will leave me gasping for breath. Yesterday, I was halfway to this point before We even started.

Emma put the cuffs on my wrist and did them up, but left them unhooked from each other, then we went to the bedroom where Mac was waiting for us. He kissed me fully on the lips and then put His hand on top of my head and I sank to my knees at His feet. He told me to take off the top then He hooked the cuffs together in front of me. Emma stood behind me and knew that she was there for support should I need it.

Mac said, "Offer me your breasts," and the words thrilled me. I did my best to cup my breasts with the cuffs on and I presented them to Him.

"They are Yours."

"Yes," He said. "You belong to Me."

I smiled softly. "Use me as You will."

He smiled too and told me to raise my arms above my head and keep them there. I did as I was told and He used the fine leather whip we own on my tits. The pain went deep inside me and found its way to my throbbing clit. I cried and I bit my lip and shook my head for Him to stop and when He did I pleaded with Him not to stop and so He gave me some more. Emma held my hands up when it became a struggle for me too and I leant my head back against her lower tummy and arched my breasts towards the whip and my mind swam, my whole body on fire with the pain from my tits.

When He felt I had reached a point that was enough He tossed the whip aside and grabbed me by the hair and pulled my mouth to His cock. He forced Himself inside my mouth and fucked me roughly, making me gag and choke. He came before I could relax to His rhythm and more of His semen spilt from my lips and dripped from my chin to my breasts than I could manage to swallow. My breasts stung from His come, deepening the ache within me. Mac leaned down and covered my mouth with His and He kissed me deeply again. He helped me to my feet and suggested that Emma use her mouth to clean me.

Her tongue against my abused skin made me sob both from the pain it caused and because I could hardly stand her touch. I needed to come and I didn't want any more stimulation until I could. I begged Mac to allow it but He said He wanted to fuck Emma. He unhooked the cuffs and told me to make Him come first, and then He would let me have the orgasm I craved.

I watched while He kissed Emma and she took His cock in her hands and started to stroke it. He pulled off her top and took down her panties and pushed her back towards the bed. I could see that He was already hard. He ran His unshaven jaw over Emma's tits and I whimpered as I imagined Him doing the same to mine.

"Get on the bed, Sarah," He demanded and I obeyed, hardly even thinking. He told Emma to "present" and she rolled to her stomach and raised herself to her hands and knees. He pushed Himself into her and I knelt behind Him and reached between His legs to stroke His cock and her clitoris as He fucked her. He leant forward over her back and I licked His balls. Emma grunted each time my fingers touched her clitoris and Mac was grunting with each lick of His balls and I was whimpering, so desperate to come. Emma came, shuddering and groaning and I moved my hand so that my finger pressed into Mac's ass and I timed it to His thrusts into Emma and He growled and shuddered too, His semen oozing from her with His final strokes. He moved from her and I sat on the end of the bed, still whimpering, unable to find the words I wanted to ask again if I could come. Mac slid off the bed and pulled me to my feet, spinning me around so He could hook the cuffs together behind my back and then He pushed me to my knees again with the bed at my back.

"Do you want to come, slut?"

More whimpering.

"Do you?"

All I could think to do was nod.

"There is only one way to make a slut like you come instantly," He said.

He pulled my head up to look at Him and He slapped me.

"Slut."

"Whore."

"Cunt."

I took the three hard slaps to the face and I braced myself for more but He stopped.

"More," I gasped.

"Enough," He growled and then He reached between my legs and slid His hand inside my panties. His other hand reached for my neck and pushed me back against the bed, His fingers closing over my throat. I tried to gasp for air but couldn't draw breath and He rubbed my clitoris and the world started to go black around the edges and He whispered in my ear for me to come.

I don't know the words to express properly what happened next. I came but it was so far beyond coming that I don't know how to describe it. It was almost like my body exploded into tiny pieces and each of those tiny pieces were coming independently and yet I could feel each tiny part orgasm. Somewhere in there Mac let go of my neck and drawing in a breath was like coming all over again. He kissed me and again I exploded in ecstasy. Mac was telling me He loved me and I could hear Him and I knew what He was saying but the words made no sense and my body just kept piling pleasure on pleasure on pleasure. I started crying to release some of the enormous emotion I was feeling and Mac kissed away my tears. He unlocked my hands and practically picked me up off the floor and laid me on the bed. He lay beside me and pulled me to His chest and stroked me while my body kept shuddering over and over.

It took a long time for every touch to stop sending me into another orgasm and Mac wouldn't let me go. Emma laid behind me and they both talked to me gently and it made me cry to feel so much love. I don't know how long it was before I started to drift off into sleep but after a while I jolted awake and asked Mac if it was ok for me to sleep and He smiled at me and kissed my eyes shut and told me to rest.

When I next woke Emma asked me if I wanted some orange juice and I couldn't think if I did or not so Mac told me to drink it and I did. Emma asked if I wanted a bath and again Mac told me I did so I had a bath. When I got out Emma helped dry me and Mac carried me back to the bed and Emma climbed into bed with me and we tangled ourselves together and Mac sat in the chair at the end of the room and grabbed a book. I watched Him for a while from Emma's arms and He felt me staring and looked up at me.

"It's OK, baby, go to sleep. I will watch over you." It felt right to have Him there and I drifted back to sleep. I didn't wake until late last night and I read the comment Mac had left on here and I cried with happiness.

My breasts still bear the marks He put on them yesterday. There are tiny fine lines of broken skin as well as redness and some bruising. They are sore and yet I hadn't wanted Him to stop. I could have taken more pain from Him, I wanted Him to hurt me more, I wanted Him to slap me again and again but He wouldn't. There is a point He will allow me to reach but He will not go further than that. He pulls back and sometimes it frustrates me that He does but He always says that He has to be true to Himself first so that He can protect me from myself. I have learnt that when Mac says "enough" He means it and no amount of begging or pleading will change His mind.

Today, with the way that I feel, the aches I have, the soreness of my breasts and my face and throat, I am glad that I have a man that doesn't want to hurt me. I think that if I had one that took pleasure from hurting me I would not know when to stop and I would end up really damaged. The marks He left on me are superficial and will probably heal faster than I would like them to. I cringe to think how much I would let Him hurt me if He liked it.

Mac helped me piece yesterday together for here. I remembered most of it, but not what order everything happened in. Emma was probably more involved but in all truth my concentration centred on Mac and myself (sorry, Emma), as He was the one in control, the one I needed to please. I was still very grateful to have her there.

We don't have sex like that often; Mac just knew that with the mood I was in it would be easy to push me into heightened state of arousal and it was. He took full of advantage of it and gosh, it was so good.

I am glad we have a day to rest. All wwe have to do is lie around on the couch and read books and watch television.

Oh, and of course I will have to take care of His cock, if the need should arise.

Smiles.

Saturday 17 April 2004

I went out because I miss the interaction. I went out because I was looking for some fun. I wanted to find someone who could make my nipples ache, my pussy muscles clench, my mind wander. I went out because Mac wasn't home again and Friday nights are hell when you are on your own.

I sat with friends. The ones I knew would be there. We talked and we laughed and we had a good time. There was no flirting with them. It is hard to impress people that know you so well. Besides, the inevitable "Where's Mac?" dampened any fun that started there.

I cruised the bar, looking for a set of eyes that didn't turn away. I was definitely hunting, but for what? Sex? Nah, I can get that any time. Dominance? In a way, because I crave that like a thirst. What I really wanted was desire, I wanted to be wanted. I wanted to feel his lust. I wanted him to take me to a point where my hunger was such that I wanted to kneel before him and beg him to take me home. I wanted someone that would tell me no. I wasn't looking for someone to go home with. I wanted to ache for something I can't have.

Mac always used to be the one to tell me no. He could make my nipples harden with a casual glance and force my muscles to clench with just a word or two. He played me like a well-tuned instrument. No, more like an orchestra, bringing forth the responses from each section that He required. He used me as His toy, taking me to the very edge and letting me dangle my feet over, but never allowing me to fall. He told me once it was the dance that made the night worthwhile. He wasn't interested in the ride home.

So dance we did, often and decadently, enjoying each other's responses. He always sent me home alone. I wanted that again.

I went home disappointed. There was no one there that could hold my gaze, let alone someone there that knew how to dance. I trudged up the stairs and headed towards my room when I noticed Mac slouched against the doorway of His study. I jumped, both from the surprise of Him being there and from the tiny thread of guilt that ran through my mind. I felt so naked under His gaze. My nipples hardened.

"So," He said quietly. "Did you find what you were looking for?" He shifted to slouch more comfortably.

How the bloody hell could He know? Am I that transparent?

"No," I whispered, staring at the floor. He chuckled.

"Didn't think you would." A pause. "Well, I have work to do; don't stay up too late. You are still not sleeping right. I want you in bed soon."

My muscles clenched.

"Will You come to bed too?" I asked hopefully.

"When I am ready to I will, girl."

My muscles clenched again. He turned away to go back to the desk. I watched Him move, wanting Him, needing Him, knowing what He would say.

"Mac?" I asked tentatively and my breath caught in the moment He turned back to face me. He can still do that to me.

"Sarah?" He answered while His blue eyes sparkled.

"You still make me ache for You."

He took a moment to drink me in, His eyes darting over my breasts, to my groin, the length of my skirt, my stockinged legs and high heels before returning to the desire etched upon my face.

"I know," He said and turned away again to sit at His desk.

Bastard.

I love You so much.

Thursday 6 May 2004

I woke to an insistent tugging on my hair. I frowned and groaned and buried my face into the pillow. I heard Mac chuckle and I felt unreasonable anger at His joy in annoying me. He tugged again, hurting me slightly. I struggled and growled, wanting Him to go away and let me sleep. He tugged once more and I came out of the pillow to tell Him to sod off, but He was quicker than me and easily turned me to my back. He moved across my chest and sat on me, pinning me to the bed. His effort had been negligible.

I wriggled beneath Him, trying ineffectually to escape. He chuckled again, raising my ire.

"Bastard," I hissed and He slapped my cheek. It warmed my skin without really hurting but the surprise of it caused my pussy to clench and I gasped.

"You may call me Sir," He stated. I looked at Him with a mixture of amusement and defiance. He locked His jaw and I saw He meant it. "Well?" He asked.

"Bastard, Sir," I replied coldly and He threw His head back and laughed.

His cock lay hotly between my breasts, both of us very aware of it against my skin. I raised my head slightly so I could see it before resting back against the pillow.

"Is this what you want, girl?" He stroked His cock arrogantly, milking the pre-come to the tip.

I was annoyed. I knew I shouldn't be but, damn it, I had been sleeping. I was tired and irritable and it was the middle of the night. He wanted to have sex and I was just supposed to give it up because He wanted it. I didn't feel like complying. I really just wanted to pout.

"No." I said it loud and clear. I said it with an air of authority. I said it with meaning. He slapped me, three times, one after the other, with much more strength to them than the first. The heat spread out through my groin. Tears welled in my eyes but I refused to let them spill. I raised my hand to scratch at Him in return but He captured both my hands easily holding them in one of His hands as He slapped me again. I whimpered.

"I told you to call me Sir. Watch yourself, girl." He took my hands and placed each into a cuff that were connected to each other around a bar in the headboard. I didn't struggle. He had subdued me enough for the moment. When He was satisfied with the fit He sat back on my chest.

"Now," He said, stroking His cock once more, "is this what you want?"

My eyes narrowed; my mind was boiling with anger, blanking out the throbbing between my legs.

"No," I hissed and I looked at the ceiling, refusing to meet His gaze. He threw His head back again and laughed. He placed the head of His cock against my cheek then moved it across my face, marking me with His pre-come. I closed my eyes and tried to block the warm stickiness out. He chuckled again. He slid down my body like a cat stretching out in the sunshine and brought His mouth up close to my ear.

"I am afraid, my darling girl, 'no' is a luxury you don't have a right to." He slapped me once more, harder than any that had come before. "And you will call me Sir. I will not tell you again. Do you understand?"

I shuddered with anger. His absolute arrogance that He could take from me whatever He wanted made me want to scream. The confidence in His eyes made me want to scratch them from His face. His grin mocked me, teasing my anger to a new height.

"Yes, Sir," I answered through clenched teeth.

"Good girl," He chuckled.

I stared at the ceiling and breathed.

He played with my body. His fingers squeezed my nipples without pinching. His cock pressed against my thigh and not my groin. I squirmed against these almost, but not quite, intense sensations. It was driving me crazy. His teeth grazed my breast and I tried to push my skin harder against His mouth. He moved away.

I could smell Him and I could smell me and I hated my body for betraying me the way it did. I ached for Him to take me, I ached for Him to use me, I ached for His body to be inside of mine. He kissed my face, licking His pre-come from me and taking it to my lips. I opened my mouth to accept it from Him.

"Tell me you want it, little one. Tell me you want my cock." His voice melted inside my mind, my tormentor had become my seducer again. His lips nuzzled against my neck.

"No . . . Sir," I whispered. My voice faltered.

"I told you, girl, 'no' is a luxury you don't have."

He forced His legs between mine. I gasped and struggled against Him. He slapped me and easily spread my legs wider with His own. I struggled harder, adrenaline making me stronger than I should have been. He laughed at my efforts and knelt between my legs, forcing them up to my chest. He leant forward and His cock tore into me.

He released my legs, knowing that I wouldn't lower them, and He lay over my body, fucking me with ease. I twisted and turned beneath Him, my hands pulling at the cuffs. He fucked me hard, each stroke deeper than the one before. The pain of Him filling me caused me to cry out each time He pressed inside me.

"Tell me you want it, slut," He growled into my ear.

"No, Sir," my breath caught.

"Tell me you need to be fucked, little whore."

"No . . . Sir," I gasped. His hands captured my hair and exposed my neck to Him. He licked my skin, tasting me. His mouth sucked at me, bruising me. I arched back, raising my hips to His.

"It's not yours any more, girl. It's mine. You gave it up a long time ago. You are mine. Give me what belongs to me, slut. Give me what is mine." His voice ordered, demanded, filled my mind and wiped out everything else.

I writhed as He overtook my body. My hands clenched into fists inside their bindings, my fingernails bit into my palms. I grunted with the strain of the pleasure that controlled the movement of my muscles. I wrapped my legs around His back, drawing Him further inside as my orgasm filled the world around us.

"Good girl," He whispered into my whimpering mouth. "My good girl."

"Don't stop," I moaned. "Please don't dare stop, Sir."

He smiled and reached above me to unclip my hands. My fingers tangled in His hair, dragging His lips to mine. I devoured Him in my hunger, my need for Him.

"Please Sir, come for me? Please come. I want it. Please?" I begged. He grinned at me.

"Do you really think I am going to make it that easy for you, girl?" He turned and pulled me over with Him. I sat over His cock. He held my hips, controlling my thrusting. He teased me, not allowing me to fuck Him the way I needed to. Not letting me fuck Him with abandon. His control was frustrating me and He knew it.

He slid His hand up my body, touching my chin and tilting my head back. I held this position. He slapped my tits, firm slaps that reverberated into the muscles inside me.

"You are such a little slut," He said. "You are such a little whore. You will do anything for me, won't you? Anything to please your Man."

"Yes, Sir" I gasped as He slapped my tits again. My whole body felt like it was throbbing. I raked my nails across His stomach. "Harder? Please? Sir."

He sat up and I quickly fed my breast into His mouth. I convulsed as He took the nipple between His teeth and ran His tongue back and forth across it. I called Him "God", I swore at Him and I pressed His face harder against me as my body was rocked with orgasm again.

He released my nipple and I released His head and He lay back against the bed. I fell over the top of Him, capturing myself with my arms before I landed on Him. His hands went back to my hips, controlling my movements once more. My hair fell about us like a curtain.

"I love You, Sir," I whispered and He let my tongue slip between His lips. I pulled away from Him just enough for Him to see spit dribble from my mouth to His. He groaned and His body stiffened beneath me. I leant down and sucked at His neck, bruising Him the way He had done to me. His hands dug into my sides, pulling me down harder against Him.

"You know," He said when we finally came up for air. "You really have very little control over that slut inside you. Especially when you are being dominated and controlled."

"I really was mad at You," I countered.

"I know, but I really wanted to fuck you and I wasn't about to let your temper tantrum get in the way."

"And what if I really meant no?"

He laughed. "Like that is ever going to happen."

I grinned. "It might."

"Yeah, well, when it does, someone had better send the devil a warm coat because it will be mighty cold down there."

I snuggled down into the bed lying on my back beside Him. He turned and cuddled up against me, His head near my breast. I twisted His hair between my fingers and He started to drift towards sleep.

"Mac?" I whispered, "I love You. Sir."

He smiled against my breast. "Shut up, Sarah. Go to sleep."

I smiled and closed my eyes.

"Good girl," I thought as I felt my mind slide.

And I was.

Red Whore

Fucked by the Teacher. Alone.

I'm lying in bed wearing the same thin tank and flannel bottoms, thinking of you grabbing my hand and forcing me to hold your cock last night. I begin to pinch my nipples through the shirt and squirm a little, thinking of how you pulled it down and sucked them last night.

My pussy starts to wetten up and I snake my fingers down my pants – lightly rubbing my clit – thinking of how slutty I can be . . . how I make your cock stiffen so easily. I rub myself harder and yank my pants down around my ankles so I can spread wide and see the red-haired pussy you so love to look at. I pull my shirt up above my tits and stare down at them. My nipples are hard and sticking out – needing someone – at this point, anyone – to suck them hard.

Then, I open a book that has a nasty scene in it – a male high school teacher with a ruler has a female student stay after class. He locks the door. He tells her that her shirt is too tight. She has large breasts, and he keeps staring at her tits as he asks her if she knows what wearing that tight shirt does to men.

He takes the ruler and points it toward her nipples and they harden. He licks his lips. He rubs the ruler on her nipples and begins to breathe harder. She puts her hand over her breasts, and he pulls them away and starts to massage them while pressing his cock against her leg through his pants.

He shoves her back on his desk and pulls her skirt up, licking her thighs near her panties. He sees she's wet. He starts fumbling with his suit pants and removes his dick. It bounces like a spring on her thigh.

She struggles a little, but he tells her, "Do you know how much I've wanted you, sitting there each day? You cocktease, you slut . . ." and he fucks her . . . takes the ruler occasionally and spanks her thighs, then puts the cock back in and fucks her hard. He pulls out when he's done and squirts a load of come all over the ruler.

I rub myself to the point I am dripping all over the bed, squirming around, and thinking of you doing that to me.

When I came, I am looking down at my tits and saying, "You want these titties, don't you??"

When I Think About You (three) I Touch Myself

The problem with swinger websites is that you can't really figure out who will rock your world in the context of a group situation.

Here's the deal. It's easy-easy to find one guy who'll work well with W and me, because it's all about *me*. If I like the guy, I fuck him. If he's really good, I fuck him more than once. (In the several years we've been doing this, we've probably met three guys that make that cut, B being head-and-shoulders above the rest.)

But if I want three cocks or more, it's tougher. That's when you have to do it at an "on-premise swing club"*. These places are much more conducive to a gang-bang or circle jerk. And we generally make our best friends there. How ironic.

Problem is, I will admit something – I have a hard time coming in public. While I love attention like it's cocaine, the rush I get from being watched by strangers as I'm being fucked is entirely different from wanting to come. It's more of a performance. Most of the time, I come later talking with W about what a slut I was.

---

* Before you gasp with horror and claim that all these clubs have old, fat people in them, let me set you straight. Reality is, there are clubs all over the US that cater to all types of people. I'd say the average age of the patrons is 30–50 years old. Yes, there are physically unattractive people that go, and very attractive people, also. But I've never been to one where we didn't have a ball. Or two.

So, let's say I really want to spend some time with three cocks — not performing, but in my bedroom with several hours to spare. In that case (believe me), everyone has to like each other. You can't have someone who's "cocksure" (I love that word) trying to "thrust" his way into my perfect orgasm. Otherwise, I'll shut down. W can confirm: when someone's over the top, I stop.

Bottom line is, I'd really like B to fuck me, X to be in my mouth, and W to stand and stroke. Someday, let's do that. We just need to identify X.

I Think I'm Gonna Kiss a Girl

I upped the fantasy-ante today and emailed the girl who made W come. He looks at her pictures and they drive him wild.

She and her partner (bi-male) have contacted us many times asking for a date, but we've never acquiesced because I've always been skittish about playing with other women.

Once, we were at a party and hit it off with this gorgeous Spanish couple. Talk led to flirting, with me making the other guy very hot. I started sucking his cock and looked over to see the woman sucking W, who was really getting off watching me. Then, I straddled the guy and started riding him, and I looked over, and the woman did the same (the little copycat). I was mesmerized watching her ass as she moved on him.

I made the Spanish guy come very quickly, and afterwards, I expected W would, as usual, come to me and finish off. But he'd apparently come exactly at the same time as the other guy. For some reason, I had this tiny little nervous breakdown for a second. The couple didn't know it . . . we graciously disentangled and I headed for the bathroom. W could tell something was wrong and followed me in.

I don't think I said anything; I just looked up at him and burst into tears. He held me while I sobbed, and we cleaned up and went back to our hotel. Of course, the next morning while we made love, the only thing I wanted to talk about was her pussy.

So that's pretty much it in terms of our experience with other women. He's had a blow-job here or there, but it can be disconcerting for the blow-job giver, because he's always intently watching my activities and doesn't, um, reciprocate.

But I think this couple might be fun. I'm just worried about one thing. What if she wants me to lick her pussy? First, I don't know how. Second, I don't even like it that much.

Actually, it begs the question: is she like me? If so, it will be all about her.

My head hurts.

Can My Boys Open Their Minds? Doubt It!

B called me today. His voice was softer, more sexy than usual.

He was calling to let me know that our earlier conversation left him distracted. I made him to promise to go home and write me (exactly) what he wanted me to do for him on the weekend – even the stuff he's maybe afraid to say – and then stroke himself and make it come. And of course, write and tell me about it.

B's hot, he's got it all. W's the same – brilliant in a Kennedy sort of way. I have a penchant for men who are smart, sexy, and true gentlemen.

Together, B & W make an enticing pair. In public, I am convinced that others look at us and assume they're the partners, because it's rare to have such male beauty (booty) in the same place.

So, I'm trying to convince them both that *it's OK* for me to rub their cocks at the same time and perhaps *let their cocks touch* for a quick pic . . . seriously . . . my TONGUE will be in it, for God's sake!

But they each just laugh at this and say (in the same, alpha-male way): "Umm, NOT happenin'!"

I contend that if I sign a non-publish disclaimer and demand it as what I want (what I need!) that they might give it up. I'm hopeful. The contrast of black and pink cock is just too sweet.

Orgy Weekend, Part 1

I'm going to give you this weekend's recap as it unfolded. I encourage you to swallow the whole thing and not skip over the mushy parts because you're looking for a) my first fulfilling sex with a woman; b) descriptions of the fucks I had; c) the considerable exhibitionism I displayed; or, d) pictures of above. I'll be giving you a), b) and c) on Orgy Weekend series, I promise. d) To be provided in the medium of words.

One note: This blog started as a private journal years ago. I write what I remember, but W and I are always amazed at the details that move to the front of my memory versus his succinct, detailed recounts. See, it's like he's watching a movie. For me, I'm **in** the movie.

Also, for me, there is nearly always an element of shock after we do this. I sometimes forget a major element of the story, because for me, it's not a "story." It's a lifesaving experience that teaches me a lesson every single time. I'm always, always "looking for the lesson."

Early Friday Evening

W & I invited B to join us at the hotel for private time before we all headed out to the party. W went down to the lobby to "read a book", while I met B and took him upstairs for a little while. W's imagination is one of the sexiest things about him. The sweet torture of imagining me for a few minutes alone with B, and being able to trust my loyalty to our relationship, makes him stiff as a board.

B arrives in all black, looking as dashing as usual. He walked in the hotel, and as I saw him, I started to greet him with my big smile and a "hello," but he put his finger to his lips. "Quiet."

He walked slowly towards me in the lobby, W sitting down near me. He stopped, looked me in the eyes, took my face in his hands and slowly put his mouth on mine, snaking his tongue deep inside. It was full, wet and it sent electricity to my pussy. He gave W a hug, and then B and I immediately left for the room.

I looked back at W, imploring him to not wait too long (I had a feeling B and I couldn't make this first encounter in a few weeks last very long).

I was wearing black thigh-high stockings, black leather boots, a very tiny skirt, and a low-cut black halter top cinched below my cleavage with a cream satin bow. Atop, a staid black topcoat finished off the ensemble. (Hey, I can't prance around the lobby without some covering myself or the employees will get all silly and wonder what's up.)

As we walk to the room, we're chatting about how nervous I am, how I need to go to the bathroom when we get there, how B needs to go, too. (Told you, it's a very good friendship, too.)

Once there and restroom visits are accomplished, we find ourselves standing in the bedroom of the suite, looking at each other intensely. We've never been alone. We've never been able to kiss like we're alone. It starts urgently and never subsides.

My coat was already off, and he's feeling my nipples through the thin halter. I'm against the wall. My skirt is up. The panties are roughly pulled over. My tits are pulled out of the halter on each side. His mouth is on my nipples.

He's on his knees. His face is buried in my pussy. My hands are on his shaved head. I'm moaning. Next thing I know, he's laid me on my back on the bed. His cock is sticking out of his pants and it's beautiful . . . it's mine . . . it's hard and huge and he's looking at me.

I tell him I need it inside me that very moment and he plunges it in and I'm in heaven – his mouth is back on mine, his breathing is where I want it – labored, fast – and then he starts his whispering, his questions. "You like that, baby? You want that?" he repeats quickly, over and over. (The answers were yes and yes, signified by my moaning.)

Then, and only then, did I hear the faint click of the main door shutting. It seemed like an incredibly long time before W came up. His presence was fuzzy; I was so absorbed with B's rhythm and pressure on my cunt. I told B I wanted his come on my titties (yes, sweeties, I know. I always ask for that early on. It's what I love. The come).

I hear the camera in the other room, the beep that sounds when it's powering up. But I can't wait, and I'm in full-on Redwhore at this point, talking my sweet/sexy/nasty/slutty talk as B's excitement becomes less controlled.

By the time W makes it to the bedroom, B is ordering me to move my halter and skirt so it's not mussed for later, and he's outside my pussy, stroking loads of extremely white come on my chest and tits. (Later, we find come on my face, in my hair, and pretty much everywhere.) W is fine, and we relax as we move from the bedroom to the main area to prepare for the party and catch up on life. I remember looking across the room at W and being startled (yet again) by the absolute catch in my throat whenever I contemplate his love for me; how deeply he wants to make me happy and fulfilled.

No pictures were taken. There wasn't time. W contends he only waited 15 minutes, and while at first B and I were incredulous, B kicked into male mode and checked his watch. Damn if W wasn't correct.

Time doesn't fly when you're having fun sometimes. On early Friday evening, it crept deliciously into another dimension and became irrelevant.

Orgy Weekend: Part 2

I'm doing something that I hate to do right now. See, I loathe performing any activity (or for that matter, thinking any thought) that doesn't feel good. I like being happy. I love being Me and making the world smile. I love it dearly.

And conversely, I detest that I have to write about what a fuck-up I can be, but I owe this to myself, mankind, and most important, W. The "lesson learned" in this recap was as basic, yet serious, as paying bills on time so you don't have services disconnected. I mean, you gotta live. Sometimes I ignore the basic premise and forget what I'm here for.

Later Friday Evening: How I Fucked Up

We traveled to the party in separate cars and I was as heady with my sexy self as ever. The Friday Parties are always more intimate; less crowded.

W and I chatter some about the sweet encounter with B. We arrive and enter in our considerable glory. It's always a treat for us (and for the crowd) to see friends and begin to misbehave so quickly. The beat of the music always sends me into overdrive, and the adulation of strange men makes me strut like a peacock. I work the room quickly when we arrive at these events.

I kiss my dear girlfriends and survey the crowd to see who, that night, gives me an immediate rush.

Side note: Interestingly, my immediate fuck-thoughts on men are rarely what rock my world five hours later.

Bizarre confabs are a norm in swinger clubs. You never know who might be married but with another partner, who might be a slave performing for his/her Master on the other side of the room, or who might simply be a fucking weirdo. Just like in real life, working the crowd is a must, and utilizing discernment is key to success. When you're in a loving relationship, you play off each other and allow yourselves to trust the partner's instincts, too.

W and I never play alone. We also never seem to synch up with the wrong person because we get off to each other, so it has to work for both of us.

But, there's this bad, bad thing about me. I love gin. Actually, I love white liquor, period. But when I'm on the gin, I am simply **slutty**. I am as uninhibited as ever. I am fearless. And I can sometimes be thoughtless and mean.

You may have guessed – tonight, I'm drinking gin. I'm on a roll. I'm dancing, smiling; early on changing into an outfit that is downright nasty. I'm prancing around in my boots and stockings with a barely-there negligee that works entirely as it should with my curves. My popularity (especially under the influence of Bombay Sapphire) astounds me.

I fuck repeatedly with abandon in the back rooms and then re-enter the dance room with increased drunken abandon. I'll let W bore you with the hot details of the encounters, because the evening ended so horribly that I can only recount my own lesson from it. Since the ending is eventually happy, someday we'll revisit, I'd assume.

So, late in the evening (early in the a.m.), W and I decide to leave. B, by the way, was all over the party and was beautiful, as usual. He noted my giddiness occasionally with both admiration and a slight "Are you OK, darling?", but as I said, I was on a roll. Anyway, W left to retrieve his shoes from another room and I told him to meet me at the bar so I could say goodbye to my friends.

While at the bar, one of the men and his lady whom I'd played with earlier were there. I'd made him come in an astounding way, according to the both of them. He was having some hang-ups on coming, and was ever-so-delighted to have gotten a nice porn fuck out of the evening with me. Given my fetish with affirmation, this made me all the more charming.

Somehow, at the bar, our short discussion led to her taking his cock out and beginning to suck it. I, feeling very powerful, looked him dead in the eyes and started to talk about how good his cock felt, and how much he needs it to came. The next thing I knew, my head was back, my gin was spilling to the left of me, and he was fucking me straight on while I was sitting on the stool. My head swam with anticipation (and inebriation) as I contemplated W walking back in and seeing one of his All Time Favorite Fantasies fulfilled: me getting banged WAY out in the open. At the bar.

But it didn't quite work that way. Out of the corner of my eye, my W walked past us and I saw this gut-wrenchingly sad look on his face. I disentangled and found him in another room.

I would love to give you the dialogue in "dialogue" form, but I can't. Here's the operative portion of the exchange:

Me: What's wrong??

W: I thought maybe you'd like to *screw someone else* before we go.

Me: (thinking: umm . . . is he calling me a whore? In this environment? After everything we've worked for? I thought he'd like this. what's the problem? We just fucked this guy an hour earlier. Uh-oh. Oh, God . . . what's going on here? he's mad at me? Wait . . . AM I a whore? What am I doing?? I'm gonna go to hell for this. It's NOT natural. You're not supposed to fuck anyone you want. Oh, shit. I'm going to lose him. He's figured me out. Oh, God . . . Oh, God. I'm a fucking whore.)

Me: (silent)

Him: (leaves the room)

Me: (sits on the couch for a second)

Me: (gets up, stumbles to the closet, changes into street clothes, reenters the dance room)

Me: (attempts to solicit some advice/sympathy from regulars who know us and can talk to him)

Him: (listens politely to my minions on this issue and then leaves and ensconces himself near the exit doorway to wait for me)

Me: (gathers my things and joins him, warily)

Him: "I need the keys to the car."

Me: "Umm . . . I don't know where they, ur . . . well . . .
(fumbles through bags, then realizes the PURSE with the
keys is still inside, then walks away to retrieve it . . .)

And then we drove to the hotel in silence. I am hurt, looking out the
window and feeling so very sad that my blog will need to be deleted,
because W doesn't get it. I'm not a "whore" in the bad way. Sigh.
He never understood me. I knew I couldn't up this ante over and
over. I love him. I love him. I have to stop this madness. No more
fucking strangers.

We got back to the hotel and we undressed wordlessly. I climbed
into bed and slept/snored like a baby/fat man.

I awakened several times in the dark to him touching my
shoulder. He was making an effort to tell me he still loved me. I
drifted off each time feeling like we could make things work
tomorrow, but I couldn't believe he thought I was a whore. A
real whore – the kind that society says is bad. The kind that hurts
men and smacks them in the face. He'd called me A Whore.

So, you, reading this. Did you feel what I felt? Wait until I tell
you about the next morning. Valentine's Day.

It started with some snow.

Valentine's Day: How to Deal with the Whore

I awakened groggy from the drink, and sad about the night before,
to W walking quietly around the suite. (I learned later that he'd not
slept a wink the night before, but in this morning haze, all I knew
was that Early Bird was up and ready to roll.)

I rolled over and looked up at him standing next to the bed beside
the window. In the same fashion B had "sshh'd" me the night
before, W gave a **look** that said, "sshh . . ." and grandly pulled the
strings of the wood louvers to reveal . . .

SNOW!!!!!!!!!!

(I am a fanatic about snow. I'm like a little kid.)

There, right outside our window, was a Winter Wonderland.
The white was incredible. And it was still snowing . . . heavily. It
was silent. It was beautiful. I looked up at him with my sleepy face
and quietly whispered, "It snowed . . ."

"Happy Valentine's Day," he said. I grinned. The grin was genuine, and his was, too.

He left to get me coffee and I tooled around the place. I was nervous about the impending discussion of the night before. I figured he was being so nice because he felt like a jerk for his behavior. He came back quickly and we ended up on our tummies on the bed, gazing out the window at the sheer coolness of snow.

I stroked him absently at first, but then became more hot as he hardened and I needed his connection. I pulled down my bottoms and guided him into my pussy from behind, bending my left leg forward and sticking my ass in the air for him to see. We came quickly. I cried a little when I came.

We started to plan the day, but I, in typical fashion, needed closure from the night previous. W is not that way. He can leave it be until the "moment is right", which, translated, could be two years later. He always does return to an issue, but it's never quickly. I, on the other hand, need things to resolve rather fast (see previous entries . . . "Come" is relative, babies. It's probably all about resolution).

So I broached the subject. I was typically lawyerly, though this discussion was more emotional, as I wanted to give him an out, but needed an apology. I wanted to let him know that we'd misunderstood each other, and that I didn't "get" the swinger club thing. I'd been called a whore last night and that killed me, but I wanted him to apologize, acknowledge that we'd taken things too far.

As it turns out, he unbendingly, achingly, articulated his side of the story. W is very logical. He's very trusting. He's very loving. He believes in "good for goodness' sake". (I'm not kidding.)

He described what it was like to walk into the room and for the first time, see me breaking our basic rule – we don't play alone. He felt, as he put it, like he "really wasn't necessary".

Though I argued vehemently for a while, my soul took over and finally heard him. I had cheated. I'd broken The Rule. It was true. And behold, I was able to apologize. (I don't apologize often, and I only do so when I "get it". What's an apology if it is insincere??)

After a while of talking and understanding each other, we resumed the day's planning.

Here's what ensued:

1. A snowball fight.
2. Prolonged sushi lunch in a new restaurant that was funny and weird all at the same time.
3. Beautiful blue dangly earrings.
4. The best Valentine's Day we've ever had.
6. *Orgy Weekend: Part 4.* Unbelievably hot. You'll love it.

In the end, I wasn't a Whore, I was still Redwhore. The one he loves.

He just needed the "We", but I ran off with Bombay Sapphire for a while.

Things worked out. They always do. And my lesson was learned. W and I play together.

And I love it when that happens. You'll see on the next entry.

Orgy Weekend: Part 4

Thank you, darlings, for the kind emails. While I know you're dying for more description of the snowball fight and the blue dangly earrings, I thought I'd spend some time this morning giving you a peek at Saturday evening. I'll break these down into several parts.

Late Saturday Evening: Attire

I'm obsessed with clothes, particularly black clothes.

At last inventory, I counted 19 black dresses in my closet, most of which are entirely unsuitable for my work due to their revealing nature. Black works well for me for several reasons: the red hair is one. The hourglass figure is another.

This evening, I dressed in black patent stilettos, black stockings, a tiny black mini, and the most adorable little black shirt. The shirt is tight, long sleeved, with a deep scoop neck. The kicker is an inch-wide piece of vintage pink velvet that spans from each underarm across my cleavage, culminating in the center of my breasts with a little bow. It virtually begs you to untie your present and play.

Later in the evening, I changed into something less characteristic for me in celebration of Valentine's Day. Stockings and stilettos intact, I wore a red teddy that consisted of a push-'em-up-in-your-face bra and a thong. Beneath the bra portion is a tiny cutout of a heart shape. Over the teddy, I wore a sheer black little robe that was trimmed in fur on the collar, wrists and hem. The hem grazed the middle of my bottom, so it felt nice for me (and boys couldn't resist sliding behind me and rubbing their cocks on me and the soft fur).

So, we've established the costuming. Next entry will describe the first fuck.

Orgy Weekend: Part 5

Experience A:

It goes a little somethin' like this . . .

There's a man who we see consistently when we visit this club. He's probably early 50's, and it's obvious he's successful in life. He's very attractive and well-groomed, highly articulate, and very sure of himself in that good, mature sort of way. I've always enjoyed talking to him and playing with him because he instinctively recognized the first time that we met how much I want the come.

I have not a clue what his name is, and frankly, I don't care. I just like seeing him there occasionally and when it happens, he knows he'll get my pussy. And I know I'll get my come.

Tonight, he's in full form. When he sees my outfit, he gives my ass a look and simply smiles, then walks away in a very assured manner. I was engaged in a flirty conversation and just grinned and continued.

Later, I walked with W back to a room to watch several couples and groups having sex. One girl was getting banged from behind, a visual I find most fascinating and stimulating. We're standing in a dark area and I feel someone come from behind and begin to stroke his cock on my bottom. He rubs it around the fur of the robe, too. I look over at W and see that he's watching the man behind me appreciatively, and I really don't have to turn around to know it's the guy I described earlier.

As we're standing there, I begin to wiggle myself against him and encourage him to take it a step further. What I really wanted at that moment is for him to stick the tip in for a second, and then pull it out. I like the tease of a cockhead from behind me. And this guy is apparently a mind-reader . . . or an ass-wiggle-reader. He got it. He did it.

There's a bed next to us, and before we know it, W is lying on his back and I'm sucking him while my thong is pulled aside and the man is fucking me hard. I cannot describe to you how much he enjoyed this pussy. He was so into it (no pun intended). A woman can tell, by the way, when you're into it, versus just fucking it. (And there's nothing wrong with just fucking it, but GOD, there's *nothing* like someone having to stop repeatedly and breathe while softly rubbing your bottom with both palms, then swallowing deeply and pounding it twice before having to stop again.)

W is enjoying the show, and the blow. And sweet W got a nice view of the side because we were near a mirror. Before long, the man has gone a little soft, but bless his heart; he's still trying to fuck me hard. I turn my head and ask if he came. He has this sweet look on his face and whispers, "I'm sorry . . . it was just so *good*." My heart swelled and I told him that's *exactly* what I wanted . . .

As he extricates himself from the situation, I realize a crowd has gathered, so I turn around and ride W backwards, facing the group. I truly enjoy this position because I can control his cock while still letting him play with my ass. I'm juicing it up and enjoying feeling that hot slickness on his balls.

Unfortunately, some men reminiscent of actors in *Deliverance* approach and somehow come to the conclusion that I'm some sort of blow-up doll for them to manipulate.

It never ceases to amaze me how you simply must have a brain to be able to participate in parties like this successfully. Note that the man I described above gets me, has learned that I like his cock, and so he's aggressive in just the right way. On the other hand, I'll show you how one of the inbreeds behaved.

Me: (riding slowly on W's cock facing the room)
He: (walks forward and stands so close I can smell a rank cumin [yeah, the spice] on his shirt)
Me: (gently pushes him a little backwards and resumes grinding)
He: (moves forward and pinches my nipple. Hard)

Me: (less gently takes his hand away and places it on his
crotch . . . implying he should perhaps enjoy this in his own,
more private way)
He: (ignores his zipper and reaches for my nipple again)
Me: (has to quietly say the inevitable) "NO."

The word "No" is a powerful word in swing clubs. In all my years,
I think I've had to say it twice. Anyway, no hard feelings, it was
barely a blip on my radar screen.

But it does go to show you that there are some dumb men out
there. I mean, he could have come on my tits so easily and I'd have
never known he was intellectually deficient. I might have blogged
about it in that good way. And he'd have a nice memory to stroke
over later.

Oh, well.

Amidst the Busy Came Two Orgasms

W called this morning from his hotel room tired, cold and lonely.
Because I'm a chatterbox, I didn't realize that his "down" time-
frame was dangerously close to ending and he needed to head out
for a meeting within 15 minutes.

"But, sweetie!" I said. "I wanted to make you come . . ."

He murmured that he'd be happy to oblige me. I realized I must
be quick. I described to him a beautiful piece of porn that made me
come yesterday. It featured a young man stroking himself while
watching straight porn. He's standing next to a large mirror. When
he finally lost control, he squirted all over it.

I told W he must go to a mirror and look at that cock while he
stroked. I made him imagine that it was someone else's, and we
traveled serenely into nasty fantasies as his breath quickened and he
spurted all over the bathroom counter and mirror.

W loves looking at himself, which is a trait I normally have
misgivings about with other men. But he's always so fascinated
with the size of it, how hard it gets, how wet the tip gets, how nice
his balls feel when he grazes them. I give W a break on this because
his cock is a damned beautiful thing.

We disconnect because I've made him late, but I'm dripping

down my legs horny, so I revisit my favorite new pastime: gay porn. Good God, it's just so neat!

Here's something I find very funny . . . there are tons of vids of straight young soldiers who are quite obviously being told by the videographers that "the ladies are gonna LOVE this, boy . . . stroke that piece of meat . . ." There's always a straight porn movie playing, and the guy will be watching it while he's stroking. I wonder if the Marines I saw this morning ever figured out that they were placed on the **Absolutely Male** website. Ha. Fact is, *this* lady likes it.

Anyway . . . what sent me over the top was a vid of two guys sitting on a couch stroking while watching a movie. But the kicker was that one of the guys kept taking his eyes off the TV screen and sneaking a peak at the other guy's enormity. I exploded while telling him it's *really, really OK* to take a look.

A Mutual Crush

I frequently visit a little fuel station near my home. I like it especially because it has a nice wine selection and it sells my favorite Meritage for $3 cheaper than any other wine store in town. This is important for me, as I need "good" wine at least once a week or I begin to feel not pampered. (I remember the good ol' days when Coppola rocked my world. Sigh.)

There's this clerk. He's so compelling. He's maybe 23 and it's obvious that he's well educated by the way he talks.

Every time I walk in, he's so utterly charming that I find myself acting like a school girl. His body is cute and he has the most beautiful eyelashes I've ever seen. He's of French/Moroccan descent and has a delicious accent.

His lips are full and he always licks them when he sees me focus on them. He's very quiet, and he always gets a hungry look when I walk in. Apparently, I have been looking somewhat famished myself, because lately we've been giggling too nervously over my wine as we transact.

The other night, I popped in and was delighted to see he was working. (I think it must be a family business, because another man who works there looks exactly like him – so I never really know until I walk inside.)

As I placed the bottles on the counter, I happened to catch his eyes as he snuck a peek down at my breasts. I was wearing a sheer blue top with a thin, nude-colored bra. My nipples are perpetually hard anyway, but I fail sometimes to remember their impact on others.

We shared just a brief second, right then, when I looked down at them, too, and then looked back up and smiled. I lifted my eyebrow and pranced away, knowing he was watching my ass.

I love to flirt.

Nipples

One of my favorite friends in this realm wrote a great piece on the differences between 70s porn and how it's evolved over the years.

One of the subjects that comes up frequently between W and me is the beauty of natural breasts. I don't have a problem with fake ones, mind you, but I simply adore my breasts and thank the heavens above that, despite having children, they've not lost their spunkiness.

This morning, we made love with me in a little T-shirt that I had worn while a cute contractor was at my house yesterday. On my knees with just the T-shirt on, no panties, nothing else, W kneeled in front of me and I whispered to him, asking if he thought that contractor had wanted to touch them.

W fingered my nipples through the tee shirt with one hand while stroking his cock with the other. He squeezed them and bit them through the shirt. I occasionally commanded him to take his hand off his cock and use both hands to squeeze my tits so I could watch him bounce, pre-come oozing from the tip.

I finally pulled the T up and let him see them . . .

I fingered my clit while he panted and sucked my nipples until we both came – my hand stroking him until I saw the shots of warm come all over my belly and hands; my juice dripping down my legs as I exploded at the same time.

Nipples can be a glorious thing.

I Came To You, You Came For Me

You needed some voice. You needed a whisper. You needed your head to be held. You needed softness. You needed the sweet nasty. You needed to explore aloud the desires your cock was aching for. You needed my voice.

You needed to be commanded to think aloud. You needed to touch yourself through your pants and ask me to tell you more.

You looked at my mouth on a black cock. Sucking the tip. You watched him shove up inside my cunt, his blackness against my thighs, my black stockings contrasted against pink/white soft skin that bruises easily.

You took yourself in hand outside your pants and let me hear the slapping sound as you groaned and began to ask me what I would let you do. You wanted to suck his come from my pussy. You wanted to taste his come in my mouth. You wanted to spray yourself on my tits.

I told you I wanted you lying face down with your cock pushed between your legs so I could see the underside. I told you I'd spread your ass and lick it while someone else licked the sensitive, throbbing place that resides directly below your cockhead. I wanted your foreskin to be tongued underneath and around, around.

You moaned. You called me a whore. You exploded as you called me sweet, sweet, sweet.

I whispered goodbye, and wished you good dreams, deep sleep, and hung up the phone. I loved giving you that gift.

W Says Goodbye

I haven't been very clear about what's going on, but the last month has been painful. W and I have split up and it has been torturous. We're crafting a new kind of friendship, but the pain is real and raw. I can't go into details, but suffice it to say that life has changed considerably.

Long ago, early in the archives, you'll notice that the blog became "mine" instead of "ours". I always wanted him to post entries, but there was rarely time.

He writes to you now so you can understand a little more of what we had:

W: love letter to red:

You want to know what she lost. I cannot say. But I know what I lost. Guys, we all have this ideal. The perfect woman. Our holy grail. I found it. Only to have it slip from my grasp. What did I find? The perfect woman, the feminine ideal, is not what she is to you; it is what she is for you.

You wonder if it exists. Does the goddess exist in real life? Who is she?

She is beautiful. You don't even know why at first. You see her face and fall in love. The nose, eyes, hair, smile. It captures you in ways you never imagined. She radiates beauty and warmth and comfort. You look at her face and believe you can tell her anything.

Her body is compelling but you don't even notice right away. It draws you sexually but subliminally. Why is this like nothing before? Because she is red.

I loved her in ten minutes. She understands you in ways you never yourself could. She explores you. Your mind. Your self. She does it in minutes and finds parts of you that you had hidden from yourself.

Her body comes to life before you. It unfolds. Every single part is beauty you have never seen because it is shared with you. She opens herself. She is scared and vulnerable. But she so wants your adoration.

I adore her. Every naked inch.

Have you ever wondered what it is like to never want another? To never be tempted? To eagerly spurn anything in any circumstance put before you?

It is real. It can happen. I am not merely lovesick. You have read this blog and you know our lifestyle. Anything and everything was put before me and available. Men imagine having that.

But we crave much more. We want red.

Eight years. Her body was more beautiful on our last night than on our first. More desired.

That goddess does exist. She fulfills you and you want nothing in life but her touch. Her hand on your face. Her reach into your soul.

I cannot tell you why but I have lost her.

I want you men to know that she exists. It is not a dream. She can

*touch your soul and touch your body and make you see god. You will
believe she is god. And, truly, she is.*

*I want you women to know what power you have. Can red be the
only one? She was my one and only angel. You may have that divine
power of salvation, too. Try. Red so loves to try.*

*I told her this after only two months and now, eight years later, I
want it more: as I die, come to me, red. Let me feel your hand on my
face, let me taste your breath, look into my eyes with your love and
smile for me. Let me feel your tears splash on my cheek.*

And I will let go.

But We Come Back Together

It's always That One Reader who is faithful and earnest. I cate-
gorize the readership here (sorry – I do.) All, however, are very
helpful. You've been wondering for months what happened.

The **Critics** are wonderful, because I *need* this desperately.
They are the ones who are truly unafraid to call bullshit. This
is a wonderful thing that true friends can deliver.

The **Interested Observers** are neat-o, because they require
nothing from me. They occasionally just deliver an opinion, and I
learn from it, and we're all a happy family. They're the vast
audience that I consider as I type an entry.

The **Devoted Readers** are my babies. These are the people who
read the blog regularly and comment upon such in an act of love to
let me know they are reading regularly. They are the group that can
spur me to a change of opinion, or, in this case, spur me out of my
fear of rejection and write what is uncomfortable to write.

That One Reader, here you go:

So, I went through some depression. I'm just gonna talk girl-
friend-to-girlfriend.

It was hard. I drank into oblivion. I couldn't even look at porn. I
felt ugly and fat. I questioned my existence. It was gross.

He was almost suicidal, I think. He wrote these journal entries
that scared me. I'd read them and worry. But I still held my
ground. I needed to be independent.

I started to be present with the kids. I started to pursue the music
again. They responded and held me up for several weeks. By being

funny. By being authoritative. They were just *there*. It was a life raft.

W and I began to talk. We decided professional help was important. He's never been to therapy; I, on the other hand, believe all humans should be assigned a therapist at birth. Interestingly, he is the talkative one in these weekly sessions.

I've learned that I'm primarily in need of independence.

He's learned he's primarily in need of independence.

There's a lot of "life" in between. But we've been largely compatible for a long time, despite the lack of knowledge that we each primarily need independence.

This fact translated itself into a study, of sorts, into our ability to unite in a way that makes us both happy and fulfilled. The results have been fascinating for both of us. For example:

Weirdly enough, I have been a religious smoker for many years for the sake of enjoyment. I considered it my choice. For some reason, recently, the pleas of W and my children and friends started to make an impact when I was asserting my need for independence. I was able, for the first time, to hear them and start to get the message: there's a strong case I'll forfeit seven or so years from my life.

Another weird one – W started to realize he was controlling me. He realized I wasn't a given, and that I had opinions that were contrary to his moral values . . . i.e., I smoke. I say fuck (he had NEVER said fuck, ever). I'm impetuous. And he still loved me.

So, I stopped smoking for me.

W started loving me for me.

W said fuck for me (it was beautiful).

And I am learning a huge thing: it's time to start getting to know W and loving him for him.

So, that's where we are. It's just so sweet I can't describe it. But I have a prediction: I think W and I will stick.

Thanks for making me say it to all.

Just Add Water: The First Time After We Split

You walk up to the pool and I can see your hardness through the pants as I exit the water in my tiny bikini. I ask you if you're planning to change and open the sliding glass door. We're standing close. You strip off your pants and boxers. It pops out and I look at it. I had forgotten how big you are.

You hesitate to put on your bathing suit. You're staring at my body. My tits. My pussy. I turn around and walk back to the pool, teasing you with my bottom. You follow after with your suit on, cock straining the black material like a teepee.

You recline on a float. I hang on at your feet and swim you around, head even with your bulge. I move up to the side. I untie my top and throw it on the side. You watch my breasts float. You see the little nipples, pink and taut. Cold.

You grab yourself and squeeze. I take your fingers and make you squeeze the nipples, too.

I tease like this for what seems like hours.

We're finally in the bedroom. After so long. We have to be silent. A repair man has arrived and is downstairs. Your suit is off. I slowly peel mine off. You see the pussy. A small patch of red hair, smoothly shaven around the lips.

I'm literally dripping.

You're breathing hard. You lay back on the edge of the bed. I slip myself over you. I bend forward so we can both watch my pussy slide up and down, slowly.

You're astounded by how wet it is. How hot it is. I'm dripping all over you. It's sliding down your ass. I ride harder. You squeeze my nipples exactly how they need to be squeezed.

I come. A silent scream. I collapse on you. You flip me over. You slide in from atop. You fuck. Hard. You come while my tongue is slipping around yours.

And we look at each other and smile, breathing hard.

My inner thigh muscles are quivering as we make the salad later, preparing for the guests. You can't keep your hands off me. This could be so good if we let it be.

Just Add Water, Part 2

I need to offer a disclaimer that I'm not advocating anyone do anything at all, so Google "sex in the water" if you have any questions on safety or whatever; this doesn't take into account pregnancy, STDs, infections, nada – It's simply what **I** get to do.

Advanced Prep:

Find a secluded pool; explore the pool for the jet stream in the shallow end. Try out the jet to ensure its force isn't too soft to satisfy you. (Too hard is fine, since you'll be able to control it by how near or far your clit is from its stream.)

Practice for a moment or two to figure out your angle; most pools will allow you to adjust the angle of the stream, so figure out the angle based on how you feel with arms on edge of pool and bottom pointing outward.

Note: Your pussy needs to be able to take in and keep a cock without slipping out, so it's important to get that bottom up.

And then . . .

Wait a decent amount of time without sex with your partner so you approach it ravenously.

Wet yourselves completely after removing all clothes; your hair and faces must be wet.

Embrace each other standing, faces close in water that covers each of your shoulders. (Ladies, let him go as deep in the water as he can while still standing and head above water (duh).)

Wrap your legs around his waist (not crotch), and press your tits against his chest.

Kiss.

Kiss a lot.

Rub your pussy against his belly; don't give into the temptation to let the bouncing cock slide into you yet, Keep up the kissing – Point here is to get yourself as wet (lubricated) as possible, and to ensure the tease factor leads to a quickie, 'cause nearly all water sex is either a quickie or supplemented with a silicone-based lubricant, which I just feel is too contrived, but feel free if you'd like.

When you feel you want the cock inside you and you can't take it any more, wait.

Take his hands and make sure they're supporting your bottom. He'll want to lift you up and stick the tip in.

The moment he does that, kiss him hard and then move away toward the wall of the pool.

Back up against it and he'll follow, thinking he'll fuck you. But he won't.

Let him be oral here, but under NO circumstances do you let him lick your pussy. We're trying to preserve the natural lube as much as possible. If you like your nipples sucked, this is when to get it.

If you like to kiss, this is when to lay it on.

Get him to the jet.

Turn around and position your clit on it and help him guide himself into you.

The key here is to get it in and then keep it in; people don't understand that fucking under water is NOT about thrusting in and out.

Grind your pussy around it (preserving your natural lube) in the manner that continues to allow your clit to feel the water stream. My advice is to tell him to watch your bottom, since a) it will be moving around on him, which nearly all men love to see, and b) it will be as beautiful as it can be under the buoyancy of the water.

Tell him to let you know if he's ready to come. If this occurs, do NOT take the cock out. Simply stop moving and let the jet do its work. When it does, start to move again and come together.

It's powerful to guide yourself and a cock to fruition while buoyant and wet.

And so it goes.

Tasty Trixie or The Wandering Webwhore

Trixie

http://tastytrixie.com/blog

Friday 2 March 2001

Thanks to encouragement from my webwhore colleague, FuzzyBunny, you're going to have an opportunity to read this blog, an irregularly kept journal detailing some of the pertinent details in the life of a webwhore.

SCARY BUT TRUE!:

I like camming so much I requested a two-month leave of absence from my real "work". I have been there over five years and am BORED. I need to do something wild . . . bohemian . . . scandalous. So I've got two months to see if I can support myself (pay for health care, taxes, etc . . .) by "working" on a pay-per-view cam network. If I can make enough money camming (and other related ventures), I will quit my job. If I can't, I'll go back to the mundane uncreative life of a middle-manager in a manufacturing environment. Blech! If that happens I will probably not continue camming but will devote myself to pursuing an MBA and climbing up the corporate ladder. Oh well, at least I will have something fun to talk about at my 10-year class reunion which will be rearing its ugly head in a matter of months.

"So what did you end up doing with *YOUR* college education?" "Me? Well I juggle phone-sex with stroking my snatch in real-time on the internet!"

Thursday 29 March 2001

I finally broke down and actually paid to watch a girl on the cam network. I wanted to know the *secret* of how they're able to type AND maintain a guy's attention.

It was SO worth it. I only lurked there watching for about three minutes but I learned a lot.

She did things that I always feel stupid doing (ex. just typed and smiled without immediately jumping to spread her legs). After a few minutes, when she finally started lifting up her tank top I GOT SO HOT!!! It was *SO* sexy! I was thinking . . . ooooh yeah!!!! She had these little tits with tan lines and hard hard nipples and she was just smiling and rubbing them. I could see her looking at the camera AND glancing at herself on her monitor and it was *cute*.

Now I understand.

I will no longer sit there thinking, "Oh my gosh this guy has to be bored . . . I'm so boring, what can he *possibly* be getting from watching me juggle my breasts while I also am looking at myself and actually enjoying looking at me juggling my breasts??"

I think I finally get it.

Saturday 12 May 2001

CHANTILLY LACE AND A PRETTY FACE

Out walking today I smelled so many women in passing. Pleasantly smiling women with unpleasant overperfumed smells. Strong . . . overpowering . . . distracting . . . invasive smells. A cluster of three chatty middle aged women wearing slacks and high heels sinking into the ground while carrying flowers out of a reception hall. A sassy smoking white-haired woman at the crosswalk.

They all reeked of retro perfumes: Shalimar, Chantilly, White Shoulders, Vanderbilt . . . those strong powdery smells. Like odor-eating wetness-absorbing talcum. Designed to soak up, dry out. Maybe it's supposed to smell clean pretty pleasant polite feminine. But it reminds me of someone slapping a child's hands away, "dirty! Yucky! nasty!" Dry raw vulvas. For some reason that's what I always think of when I smell those kinds of perfumes. Vaginas, aged by self-hatred . . . unpleasantly abandoned . . . those perfumes always invoke a companion aroma in my imagination: the smell of stale neglected pussy caked with floury white powder, like dust swept under a carpet . . . like denial. Infected irritated brittle flesh confined and encased in a cell of synthetic fabric. To me it's the smell of sexual repression. The smell of ignorance. The smell of women who make sticky potato salad, carry handbags, protect their furniture with plastic slipcovers, and never leave the house without lipstick.

The one that really grossed me out was standing behind me in line at the grocery store. A lanky awkward 40ish woman wearing one of the old perfumes and assuring her overweight twenty-something son that SHE would pay for the flowers because they were ALWAYS buying grandma stuff. Her glasses were hung on a shoestring-like necklace and one end was accidentally looped across her face, trapped under the nose-bridge of her glasses. Under the perfume I caught a real NOT imagined whiff of sticky sweaty unwashed butt. That slightly cinammony sweet smell that I usually associate with unkempt obese people who haven't completely cleaned all of their crevices . . . not completely an unpleasant smell at first, but positively nauseating after a few inhalations.

Thursday 24 May 2001

I DON'T HAFTA

Ever since I quit my "real" job I have been reveling in the knowledge that I don't have to do anything. The recognition comes to me regularly sometimes just as a sassy childish celebratory phrase neenering through my being, and sometimes in response to unbidden irrational currents of anxiety that there's got to be something I'm forgetting to do . . . someplace I'm supposed to be at a certain time on a certain day. Then I realize, "I don't HAVE to do ANYTHING!" I DON'T have to do ANYthing. I don't have to DO anything.

The flip side of this freedom is the recognition of guilty wasted time, "I haven't DONE ANYthing!" I haven't gotten anything DONE!

Monday 25 June 2001

PLAY FOR ME!

One of the most poignant sad things said to me in the past few months came from my dad when he reminded me, "You would never play piano for me! The only time I ever heard you play was when I stood outside on the porch and listened. You'd always stop if you realized I was out there." I insisted that "never" was too strong a word, but he firmly insisted right back, "you NEVER played for me!" And I guess if that's what it feels like to him looking back on it, then that's "truth". That's what happened. It doesn't matter if a couple times I may have begrudgingly cranked out a tiny private piano performance for him because even if I did he doesn't remember it now.

It breaks my heart to finally see this piano-playing business from a perspective other than my own pressure-filled childhood viewpoint. At the time, I just wanted to be able to practice in peace . . . to not have to "perform" for anyone . . . to "please" no one but myself. In a tiny (by today's standards) 1200 sq-foot house with three bedrooms holding me, my 2 stepbrothers, my little sister, my mom and step-dad it was *hard* to practice without irritating someone or interrupting someone watching television or hearing requests for something more jolly. There was absolutely no peace and solitude (two things I *craved*). So if it happened that no one was home as I got older and I had a chance to just immerse myself in doodling around on the piano, the last thing I would want is my dad coming over and wanting to LISTEN. But now I can imagine how that must have felt to a father (who doesn't live with his kids) stopping by and quietly climbing the porch steps to see and hear his daughter playing piano with peace and comfort and love, but only because she doesn't know anyone's there listening and watching. I can imagine the moment when she stops and realizes and jumps to the door, scolding, "DADDY!!!"

When he brought it up he concluded by saying, "It was almost like you were ashamed of your playing." And he's right; I was. I hated being less than perfect. I couldn't enjoy the process in someone else's presence. I couldn't enjoy someone witnessing me unfinished, unpolished and less-than-completely capable.

It kills me how we do things to protect our vulnerabilities

without recognizing how our defenses hurt other people. How the process of concealing our imperfections so effectively distances us from being known by anybody.

It's funny because as soon as I moved away from home and stopped giving piano lessons and stopped playing for church I didn't have a piano for four or five years. I didn't play at all. And when my husband bought me a piano I vowed to myself that I would only play for myself. That I wouldn't wreck the enjoyment of playing by being pressured into putting on a little show for everyone. I don't know if it makes a difference. I have slowly started playing more here in my apartment, but I'm hypersensitive to the fact that people can hear me. I can hear the girl across the way playing *her* piano sometimes. Someone playing a violin above us. At other times they beat on drums. What would really makes me feel good is to be able to sing freely. Because it feels so good to sing. But I have a hard time opening my mouth up knowing people will be able to hear it. Knowing people can hear me singing makes me feel extremely vulnerable and self-conscious.

Funny that one of the most flattering feelings I've been given by a man was when one of the apartment boys (the crazy Irish one I made a mistake of sleeping with) stood outside my door and listened to me play piano for a good while before knocking. He's the only guy who's asked me to play for him. The only one. And I love that memory of him, his feet a soft dark creaking shadow on the floor seen under and barely heard through the crack at the bottom of my door. I let him be there . . . not sure if his presence was real or if I was imagining it because that's what I *wanted* . . . someone patient enough to recognize that I could only share some things at a distance and through a doorway.

When my dad mentioned that I "never" played for him I started thinking about this. And now I feel so anonymous and unseen realizing that every one of these guys (except the crazy Irish drunk) have gotten into bed with me with the piano standing about five feet away and they've never asked to hear me play. Never. These people who have called me amazing. Beautiful. Intriguing. Delightful. They never asked to hear me play. And I have not shared anything. And they have not seen or heard anything about me to make any meaningful compliment worth an iota of value based on any real knowledge of what/who I really am. Sure they've asked "if" I play. And maybe I was so cold and uninviting with my answer that they didn't press the point. I don't know. But it's a little bit sad to me that even while I recognize these things I am not comfortable changing them.

And now my dad is on oxygen and weighs 86 pounds. And I have to face the fact that he will never see me perfect. Finished. Complete. That even if he thinks he is proud of me, and I am sometimes proud of myself . . . I will not get to the point while he's alive of feeling that he has a good reason to be proud of me.

I wonder at my compulsion to withhold myself under the ridiculous self-defeating notion that I have to hide until I am fully realized potential instead of just a work in progress. I continue to operate under the illusion that I can and should be "complete" and perfect one of these days and that I can't allow myself to share me until/unless that happens. I look at my dad and see my destiny – that – I will probably dry up and blow away someday as a solitary dreamer full of grand illusions and unrealized potential.

MY LAST CHANCE TO WEAR THE CUTE-SUIT

It's so stupid and insecure, but sometimes I think the only reason I wind up fucking some guys is out of the fear that it could be my last chance to get laid. Seriously, for most of my young life I completely lacked opportunities to get laid. And if not for the advent of the internet I probably still wouldn't have sex readily accessible to me (unless it was within a monogamous relationship which I can't see happening with anybody I'd want it to happen with). Part of me can't forget how frustrating life was that way. When I don't have sex for a while I get really irritable and impatient and angry. So even though I don't really feel an urgent pressing desire for sex right at the moment and I have a lot better things to do with my time, I'm afraid to turn down an opportunity to see Mr Clean tomorrow night. I don't want him to think I'm no longer interested.

Sometimes I feel like I'm renting a cute-suit and so far the costume rental place hasn't called to tell me I was supposed to return it a couple years ago. It's like I can't believe I'm even remotely attractive and any day now I'll be forced to return to reality where I am an enjoyably weird nerd girl with a bitchy brainy funny personality but hold absolutely no sexual appeal whatsoever.

Tuesday 3 July 2001

TIT PICS 10 DOLLARS!

I often think about how much I'd like to carry around photos of my breasts and offer them for sale to anybody who stares at them in public. Really I don't mind (and actually I do enjoy) people giving them an appreciative glance or an irresistible gawk. But the blatant brazen stares (especially when accompanied by comments, honks, whistles or other sound effects) beg to be addressed. I just walked by a group of five guys in their late teens. One of them caught sight of my jugs bobbling somewhat boisterously by in my white shirt. I am not dressed like a working girl and just look like a generic nerd with a backpack. And I happen to have my breasts in a regular bra, unbound by any extra efforts to kill their natural bouncing. There is nothing about me that conveys "OOOH I'M TRYING TO SHOW OFF FOR YOU AND GET YOUR ATTENTION AND BE OBJECTIFIED". So when the boy who noticed them first pointed them out to his friends and they all turned to look I just wanted to fucking confront it. So I thought again about how nice it would be to have some pictures handy that I could sell, "Hey!! Wanna keep staring at my tits?? If you have $5 I'll give you a picture of them!!! If you have $10 I'll give you an autographed picture of my tits NUDE!!! And if you have $20 we can take a polaroid picture of you standing next to them!!!" Or I could make them pay homage to women in a way that they might find humiliating, "You wanna have a picture of my tits?? Shout out so that the whole park can hear you, 'Women are superior to men!' Scream it 25 times and you'll get the picture. If you say anything degrading at any time the offer will be null and void and you will not get your picture." When I fantasize about doing this I think about handing out a whole pamphlet about the controversies surrounding breasts in public (breastfeeding, etc.), how to politely appreciate breasts in public, sexual harassment, whether breasts are essential or accidental to femininity, etc. Maybe with some boxes that I could check off, "You have received this pamphlet because you were a) acting like a drooling dog and didn't seem to recognize that I'm a human being and not just a set of knockers walking by, b) subtly eyeing my body in a way that I found complimentary and enjoyed so I thought you might appreciate this (I'd probably give this group free pictures just for fun), c) appeared to be hypnotized by the swinging motion of my boobs so I wanted to snap you out of it and giving you this pamphlet seemed like a good way to interrupt your reverie."

Maybe I misinterpreted the stares from those boys though. They might have just been staring at the grease stain on my shirt where some taco juices dripped down my front and the stain never completely washed out.

Thursday 16 August 2001

ADVENTURES IN BABYSITTING

I survived my day of babysitting without the kids discovering my stacks of dirty magazines in the bathroom. I rekindled an appreciation for the disciplinary tactic known as "spanking", although I didn't use it since they aren't *my* kids (an utterance I whispered to many passersby witnessing their behavior in the grocery store and museum, "they aren't *my* kids!"). I didn't know whether to resolve to never ever ever bear children OR to resolve to raise my children (in the event that I have them) to be behaviorally superior to my friend's kids (and to so many other discipline-free children running rampant).

I surprised myself a little bit by being embarrassed over Ilsa's (the three year-old girl's) public masturbation. Today was the first opportunity I had to witness what my friend has been telling me about: Ilsa's love for lying down on hard surfaces with her hands pinned under herself . . . I've been celebrating her child's love for her body and hoping that her grandma doesn't break her enthusiasm. But there is definitely a time and a place – today in the museum was not the time and place. Her brother, Alex, is the one who pointed it out to me, "Look!! She's doing it again!" There she was, sprawled out on her belly on a wooden platform, rocking and rolling, and protesting Alex's tattling by insisting, "I can do it if I want!!!" I suggested she save it for private time when she's alone in her bedroom. She just moved to a higher platform. I told her to knock it off and not do that in front of me and her brother and everyone in the museum.

Still, her self-stimulating activities bode well for her future as a woman – I think it's great that in her development she has learned how to get herself off before figuring out how to wipe her own ass properly.

Thursday 6 September 2001

"SHE'S GOT A GOLD TOOTH / YOU KNOW SHE'S HARD CORE"

The other night one of my favorite smart and witty viewers made a troubled and befuddled comment that he never sees me showing my teeth in any of my pictures. He hit upon a really sensitive insecure spot with that observation.

My bean-skin tooth. I named it that in college when I saw a picture of me, my face, my smiling mouth and in it what appeared to be a hillbilly-quality blacked-out tooth. At first I thought the picture must have been taken after I ate a bowl of chili and a kidney bean skin laid on top of my most obviously crowded out set-back-from-the-rest tooth.

My bean skin tooth is the most eye-catching of my dental imperfections. A recessed shadowed tooth representing all of my insecurities related to my physical appearance. As vulnerable as my belly fat but less-loved and never delighted in. A subversive shard of exposed skeleton bearing witness to the fact that my family couldn't afford braces. It's like the black sheep of my family of facial features, a crooked little character pushing his siblings out of line. A bunch of kids trying to squeeze into a super small mouth-house . . . not enough room for everybody.

Part of why I can't look forward to Mr Clean's company is my bean skin tooth. That and a million other things that distinguish his world of physical perfection from my world of smelly animal physicality. The tooth sums up our differences – my discomfort with him, and his discomfort with imperfections. I haven't seen the guy in a couple of months even though there were lots of things I enjoyed about him. But it was hard for me to relax and completely enjoy our fuckfests when he was so anti-burp, anti-fart, anti-hair, anti-flab, running-to-the-bathroom-for-mouthwash before we kiss, PERFECT. Once we had a conversation about teeth. He had a big crush on Faye Dunaway in her younger days but no longer thinks she's attractive because her teeth seem to have gotten bad. OK, I'll give him that. Her teeth are looking pretty bad . . . not just quirky and human, but diseased. But when he said he thinks Nicole Kidman is ugly because she has "big gums" my lip curled with disdain at this bizarre standard of non-beauty. I pretty much started to say I didn't think I could feel good about myself in his presence when he interrupted to say, "You're a beautiful woman but don't you think you'd have a totally different smile if . . ."

If I fixed my teeth?? I would have a different smile? You're right, Mr Clean. I would. And I hate you for being right about that.

I told him it seemed pretty fucking vain to spend tons of money surgically or with braces altering a fully functional part of one's body. He didn't address the vanity point or the financial consideration, instead he simply said he couldn't understand *not* getting braces in a day and age when you can have clear braces and may not even have to wear them for very long. Harumph.

I've always been a little disturbed by people who are *too* perfect . . . I spend hours searching for a flaw. For something to love. How can you love a body or face that's flawless? It's disturbing. Unreal. Subhuman. Plastic. ANYBODY can be "beautiful" with enough money. So what's the point? There's a certain plastic beauty that I cannot desire applying to myself. Gross. Sometimes I look at pictures of movie stars and people with perfect teeth and am left cold. Disturbed. Like the poster with Mel Gibson and Helen Hunt for "What Women Want". I remember staring at that in the theater and their teeth . . . like dentures or something. Totally flawless and fake-looking. Gross! Bizarre looking at Mel Gibson's face . . . a reconstructed beauty. The guy was going to kill himself as a teen because his whole face was destroyed in a car accident or something. But now, after tons of plastic surgery, he's a sex symbol. Superficially scarless on celluloid.

Anyway, I told Mr Clean I would never go through such extensive efforts to alter my body. Or my bean skin tooth.

A few weeks after that discussion with Mr. Clean I picked up an issue of Oprah's magazine with a self-esteem theme. Very inspiring pictures of Oprah pre-makeup, going through a number of costume changes trying to look just right before her show – looking completely like SHIT. There was another photo feature showing women who showcase their most "imperfect" and/or unusual physical characteristics (like a long neck, nappy hair, etc.). Looking at this stuff I thought about my bean skin tooth and considered making an effort to accentuate it instead of trying to hide it. I thought about how stupid it's been for me to try to cover it up behind my upper lip thinking, "I might actually look pretty as long as no one can see my bean skin tooth". But the truth is, I'm not perfect. Why pretend?? By hiding it it's like I'm being ashamed of my imperfection which is the truth of my humanity that I'm supposed to treasure most of all. By hiding it I am not being true to myself.

I told my sister about these thoughts and she suggested that I get my bean skin tooth gold plated. *THAT* would really make a statement!! It would be *SO* Tacoma!! Then I discovered this site selling **tooth art**. Maybe a **tooth jewel** would be a good alternative to the gold plate?

But I don't want to be a comical caricature 24–7. I don't like the idea of having anything on my body that makes more of a statement than my voice. I don't want anything about my physical appearance to scream louder than what I say with my voice.

Saturday 22 September 2001

NAM VET NEIGHBOR NO LONGER

For the almost two years I've lived in the Bohemian Apartments I have shared the longest wall of my small scandal-filled studio with one neighbor, a kind grizzled Vietnam veteran named Tom. And now he is moving out.

From my noisy frolicking phone-sexy but self-conscious perspective I valued the fact that Tom always **insisted** he couldn't hear *anything* that happened in my apartment. I could count on Tom to mind his own business (except for making infrequent inquiries regarding my rotating line-up of male visitors, "It's just like a revolving door you've got there, isn't it?") and he could count on me to ignore his own noisy all-night drunks with a very annoying young male companion who laughs like a hyena. All night long. I never had to feel self-conscious worrying about what Tom would think about the noises emanating from my apartment . . . I never had to worry that he would tattle on me or hoot or whistle at me or tape cigarettes to my door after a noisy night of getting nailed.

But Tom's warm paranoid heart is moving out. Moving on. I will miss his kindly stuttered words and his insistence that whatever I did in my own apartment was my own business. I will miss his denial that any noises created in my apartment were audible in his, even right after thanking me for playing a Patsy Cline tune he heard my mom crank out on my piano the day before. I will never forget overhearing him kindly calming down a young woman who was insisting that nobody loved her and she had no reason to live. I will never forget his tearful thank you for the tacky shimmery Times Square Postcard I slipped under his door with a Christmas wish. I will never forget his suspicions that the crazy Irish drunk (apartment boy #2) had a sophisticated knowledge of phone systems and his wild-eyed whispered warning that I should NOT trust him farther than I could throw him . . . he could be tapping the phones or who knows *what*!!

I will never forget the time that I was in a corset bent over my table fucking my ass with a chubby red toy for a viewer at 3 a.m. with millions of lights and electronic equipment on when all of the power went out. My webwhore activities had caused a fuse to blow. Tom was the only other person to be affected (and the only other person awake in our century-old apartment building) by my fuse-blowing activities and he knocked on my door and reassured me, "Never fear, Trixie!!! I will go tell the manager." When our angry boyfriend-beating apartment manager demanded to know why the hell we were up at 3 a.m. anyway, Tom shushed me and stopped me from confessing any guilt or wrongdoing and deflected attention away from me by hammering her with questions, "You'll get this back on quick, right? Because see . . . I like ice cream. I have a gallon of ice cream in the freezer right now. There's nothing like getting a little bowl of ice cream every so often. You know, I like to go in and have a few spoonfuls when I feel like it . . . MMMmmmm, nothing like it, you know? Anyway, I have ice cream in the freezer and I just can't have it melting. So this *will* be back on right away, right?"

Dear sweet Tom who was in Saigon when I was born. I told him he's the best neighbor I could have ever asked for and I'll never get a better neighbor. He brought his hand to his heart and said, "You know, that touches me *right here*," his hand shielded his breast as though he were saying the pledge of allegiance, "*right here*. Thank you for saying that."

Bye bye baggy-pantsed booze-breathed kind-eyed alone-living father-to-many-who-never-visit. I will never have a better neighbor.

Tuesday 25 September 2001

SEX PREDATOR

I can't recall if I ever mentioned this before, but the guy (Dave) I lost my virginity to when I was 18 is now a registered sex offender. My sister found this out a few years ago quite by chance by punching in the zip code of our small hometown into an online database of level 2 and 3 sex offenders. And there he was. Anyway, I never did find out exactly what he did (online it just says he's a level 2 sex offender and his crime was a "sexually motivated felony").

Well, last night my mom called to tell me that she saw a community notice posted at the fire station warning residents of Dave's move within our town. Why the fuck doesn't he get out of our town?? God! You'd think he'd move somewhere where nobody knows him. WHY has he chosen to reside in this small town for the past six years since his criminal activities? The poster gives his address; he is living up the road from my mom and dad and grandma and grandpa (odd, because the last time I drove up that road all the way to the end I had the distinct feeling Dave was there). Eerie.

Apparently he was breaking into people's houses and climbing into bed with them. Apparently not raping them but hopping into bed and fondling them. A mother with her four-year-old son. An eleven-year-old kid. Who the fuck knows what else . . .

Are my weirdo-detecting sensors messed up? I used to think Dave was just being melodramatic when he told me that he was a bad person and did really bad things. As far as I know he started doing this shit long after we were doing our thing together. Who knows, maybe I turned him into a freaky pervert?

There's a part of me that is shock-resistant. That doesn't believe that some people are "worse" than others. Part of me believes that we're *all* capable of doing amazingly crazy, bizarre and violent shit. With Dave it always seemed as though he were trying to *prove* he was a freak, not that he really was. He believed he was *so* different. I believed he was just obsessed with himself and his perceived differences to the point where he lost all perspective. I remember him telling me about his step-dad coming in and sitting on the bed while Dave was sleeping. Or *pretending* to sleep. And his step-dad stroking his thigh while he "slept". That's it. That's all. Gross, but apparently that is all the sexual violation he suffered. I then shared with Dave things that had happened to *me* that were more violating. Not to discount his experience with nastiness, but to just let him know I knew what it felt like.

I remember a year later the subject came up and he had absolutely no recollection that I'd told him I too had been molested. His mind was so completely absorbed with his *own* experiences he just had no room for thinking about anybody else. The fact that he seemed to be missing the ability to empathize with others – that's the one time I recognized that Dave might indeed be different and bad. Well, I guess that and the time that he told me that he always felt like a million spiders were crawling all over him after we finished having sex.

Thursday 27 September 2001

SEX OFFENDER NOTIFICATION

I am looking at a community notification flier. With a picture of a guy with scary unrepentant predatory straight-staring eyes and a really freaky closely shaved haircut. I have another picture of him . . . and me standing next to him ten years earlier. Innocently average and handsome for a homecoming dance. Wow. The same guy. It's the same guy. The same guy I determined to have pop my cherry when I was 18 years old. My dad always told me I had a taste for shit.

I know it probably sounds bizarre but . . . I don't regret losing my virginity to him. Even though he tried to tell me afterwards that my mom paid him to have sex with me (which I almost believed even though I knew if my mom would have paid someone to sexually initiate me it wouldn't have been *him* – she tried to talk me into losing it to someone more "experienced" but I insisted that he was the fellow virgin with whom I intended to share this rite of passage). Even though it's nothing to brag about and the thought of having intimate memories revolving around this disturbing person should make me shudder and wish to forget . . . I don't wish I never knew him or did it with him. I can't explain it. My mom thinks I have a potentially dangerous fascination with people who are bizarre and live on the fringes bordering normalcy. I guess she's right.

I just want to try to understand. The dangerous part is that inside me there's an unshakable belief (delusion?) that we are all the same. It's an ideal I cling to for the sheer horror and soaring hope that it gives me. Or maybe that's the justification I use to pursue my macabre fascination and unusually high comfort level with freaky people.

This sounds off the subject, but I am feeling the need to read more Carson McCullers. I love her and her characters so much. *Reflections in a Golden Eye* is what I need to read right now.

I remember catching him in the alley when I was 16. And knowing but not really caring that he wasn't just walking to a friend's, the way he said. Knowing there was a different reason for him being in the dark alley where the inside of my sister's and my bedroom was visible through the wooden blinds.

I remember being 18 and finally having an unspoken fantasy come true. He knocked on our bedroom window. And I came out and we fucked standing on the cinder-block steps outside our back door while my mom slept inside and my sister wound up waking up and asking what was going on.

I remember being 19 (after he and I stopped talking and no longer fucked) and sleeping by myself in the detached garage we had converted into a bedroom. I remember all of the times I'd lay in the dark there listening to what I *knew* were human noises right outside my door. Whoever it was would enter stealthily enough to avoid setting off the motion detector. I wonder how many times I took a trip to the bathroom in the middle of the night and might have sleepily walked right past what must have been him. I remember I lay there alone once in the middle of the night, disconnected from the house and my mom and my sister. And this time he tried to open my door. It was locked. He knocked. He tried repeatedly to turn the doorknob. He wouldn't answer me when I asked who was there. He didn't say anything. I didn't know who it was. I always *wondered* if it was him but never really thought it was. It didn't line up right. I never thought he would be that weird with me. So silent and anonymous with me who was not a stranger. The rest of that night I laid there in bed scared to death and having to piss like a racehorse until the sun came up.

But today looking at this flier I realize it must have been him. It must have been him. Two years before he was convicted for sneaking into people's houses and touching girls he didn't know in their sleep. Criminal Trespass. Sexually Motivated Felony. Did he grab something to steal on the way *in* – or while he was running *out*?

I probably would have opened the door in the middle of that night if I'd have known it was him. If he would have said something. But I don't think that's the way it was supposed to work. I wonder if I knew him before he knew what he wanted. I wonder if he got caught and convicted before he knew what he really was going to do. Or if that was all there was to it for him. Supposedly that's pretty unlikely, statistically speaking. People like this (like what?) usually mature as criminal freaks, with their crimes escalating in severity and violence and seriousness and perversion as time goes on.

What would have happened if my door had been unlocked? What would have happened if I would have opened it? There is such a range of possibilities. Sad. Scary. Or fumbling to retain normalcy.

Oh, well. Who cares?? I'm going to Memphis.

But first I'm going to drive to the end of the road. In the twilight. And drive slowly looking in windows lit from the inside. Knowing that he's probably in one of them. A beastly self-centered miserable mystery.

And later tonight I will drive home to my safe city, so I don't have to sleep here less than a mile away from where he probably is. So I don't have to lie here and remember what it was like to imagine that someone was outside watching me. To imagine someone was close to my door. To tell myself I had an overactive imagination but then wind up experiencing the bizarre intersection of reality and paranoid suspicion.

DREAM COME TRUE

The past couple of days it's been hitting me that I basically am living one of my favorite "dream" lives: I get up whenever I want, I don't have a boss, I can wear pajamas all day, I have beaded curtains, and I usually get laid whenever I want to. I can eat as much top ramen and canned chili as I want, play my music as loud as I want, and pop popcorn in the middle of the night if I want. I can do damn near whatever I want. Since most of the things I want are inexpensive or cost absolutely nothing I can do . . . whatever . . . I want.

Sunday 11 November 2001

MOVING HELP

There's nothing like getting "help" from a man to remind me why I never want to be married to one or live with one or be tied to one in any practical manner. The Irish Think Tank is such an insecure insulting ass sometimes. He "helped" me start moving (I gave him step by step instructions on how to clean the cupboards and even then he fucked it up by not even wringing the sponge out so he's slopping water all over the kitchen, I almost fell on my ass and the once-clean floor became all muddy – some help! Then he got drunk and started hitting on all of my pretty neighbors. Then he moved the bookcase without bothering to take out the shelves. A passer-by had to bail him out of the stairwell – the helpful volunteer's fingers got smashed when the shelves loosened and all slammed as a heavy stack onto his digits.).

After a few hours of his "help" accompanied by lively insults he hurled at me, arguments over everything I suggested, and an unceasing stream of criticisms pertaining to my possessions, he announced that we should call it a night and WE could start up bright and early the next day. Let me tell you, all I wanted at this point was for him to fucking get away from me and let me start the next day in peace and quiet. We'd already spent the whole day together and I'd bought him dinner (as payment for the moving help) AND drinks at a different restaurant afterwards.

The Irish Think Tank was so rejected by my suggestion that I do everything I could by myself and then he would only really be needed for the three big things I had left that he completely came unhinged. He told me I was fucking stupid. I told him I really appreciated his help. For about thirty minutes he screamed at me, threw some of my stuff to the ground to accentuate his points, and finally stormed out in a huff. One of his parting comments was, "Well you shouldn't have any problem getting someone else to help you here since you've fucked every guy in this building!!" At that point I confronted him with his obvious underlying emotions of jealousy and rejection. Not only do I not have sex with him, but I don't want him to help me move. Oh WAH! Poor baby! At least that comment got rid of him.

Tuesday 29 January 2002

LUCKY ME

Ooooooooooooh . . . I feel like such a lucky girl! My houseboy is fucking delightful. He looks great on his yellow-rubber-gloved hands and knees scrubbing my floors AND he is a top notch pussy licker. TOP NOTCH! Never in my life have I been with a guy who knew so perfectly how to play with me EXACTLY how I want to be played with. He knows exactly how to tease tease tease and *barely* touch and stop and start PERFECTLY. It felt so good I almost cried. He never once pressed too hard. He understands the teasing art of humping. He understands legs together. He understands!!! This is the first person I've ever met who might possibly be more skilled at getting me off than I am at getting mySELF off!!

Yesterday was the first day in my new apartment where I actually allowed myself to completely enjoy just looking out the windows at the view without worrying about everything I had to get done. Since my house boy was accomplishing dreary housework under the gaze of my watchful exploitative husband-like perverse eye, I felt like things were getting done and I was just completely free to be a fiendishly bossy lazy bitch – drinking hot vanilla almond tea mixed with Kahlua, singing along with Tom Jones' *Sex Bomb*, and demanding that my houseboy spread his legs further and stick his ass up and out while he was washing dishes.

Wow – just thinking about all the fun we had yesterday I'm drifting off into the memory of it. . . . like the hot threatening hand-job I gave him while reaching around and grabbing him from behind and making him acknowledge with whimpers and pleas and "ohgodYES"s how much he'd love if I had a big hard cock to fuck him with. I loved watching us in my mirrored closet doors, both of us on our hands and knees with me hovering over his back with my black-bra clad tits heavy and round and rubbing on his back. I loved holding his head down and whispering menacingly, in his ear about how I'd make him suck my cock. I loved hearing him beg for me to let him come and finally permitting him to fill up my hand with hot spunk . . . and me feeding it to him and making him lick it up out of my palm. That's the first time I've ever talked to a guy like that in real life (and not just on the phone for "work") – what a huge thrill that was . . . gigantic!

And then to later wind up making out and kissing and rolling around and rubbing and being serviced with fingers and tongue for an extended leg-quivering time . . . coming from his fingers . . . him coming again while we rubbed our naked selves against each other without penetration . . . me coming from his tongue/mouth/ face . . . oh lovely LOVELY **LOVELY**!

I never anticipated that my ad for a houseboy would wind up providing me with so much fulfillment on so many levels. I am such a lucky lucky woman. MMmmmmm!!!

Sunday 3 November 2002

You wouldn't believe how many times a day I replay houseboy's come shots in my head. Come pulsing out of his turgid dick onto my thigh . . . creamy spooge puddling up in my muff . . . and now a replay from last night when we fucked in the tub. It was a surreal experience with the water sloshing around my ears and my face partially submerged, my head banging against the back of the tub. Eventually he pulled out and I raised my head out of the water to see his cock pointed at my face as he hovered between my legs . . . I looked just in time to catch ejaculate shooting straight onto my face and eyelashes.

Only the second time I've had come on my face. I think I'm developing a fondness for it.

Monday 26 May 2003

MOOD SWING

Last night we fell asleep listening to our favorite radio show, "This American Life". I finally woke up at the end of it and felt so completely happy and peaceful and safe snuggled up with houseboy – I felt a sense of groggy elation. Utter happiness and tranquility.

Then I blew out the candle burning next to our bed.

Within a couple of minutes somehow I was thinking about my dad again and found myself sobbing. Yes, I know it's Memorial Day . . . maybe that's where this is coming from. Yes, it will be exactly one year from now soon that he passed away. But I actually do think of him . . . well, all the time. Somehow both his loss and presence are constant companions. I probably just started bawling hard about it last night though because I am in PMS mode and couldn't hold back.

I watch him die over and over while I'm holding his hand. I watch him looking at me before he died . . . before I got the nurse off her lunch break . . . before I called my mom, my sister, and his twin. I remember how quiet it was when she shut off the oxygen. I remember more than that. Lots more that I replay over and over.

Maybe I still just worry too much about . . . things. Maybe I feel too much guilt to focus on letting go.

Maybe I just haven't reached the point where his life is full of more solid frequent memories than his sickness and death and the experiences associated with it. But that is the most recent thing, and it's hard.

Being a child and being on the other end of the spectrum ageing towards death have certain qualities. A ghostliness. Impermanence. Partial presence. A confused transitional state of being that's partially here, partially somewhere else . . . and not at all capable of fully expressing or comprehending that duality. They say confused things and don't realize until afterwards that they said them in the wrong place. Or they don't know why they said them. Only that they speak and feel and experience somewhere else too. Or maybe it's just underdeveloped (for the kids) and rotting (for the aging) brains not some otherworldly existence.

After the first time my dad almost died (four years before the real thing) he became a sort of ghost. Grandpa eased into that too in the years before he died, after his brother and sister passed away. They just weren't solid anymore. They went through the motions of being alive with us but they were faded. Voices thin and without body . . . as though half of the volume of their speech was being set aside. Like having the right speaker on your stereo unplugged and only the left one projecting.

I do not feel "grief" exactly for my dad or my grandpa. Maybe what I feel is grief for myself. With these two deaths I have aged too. Part of me is lost and belongs somewhere else. I feel initiated into that reverse process . . . growing up is over and I am starting to wind down too. I hope it's a long process but I feel it happening. Frequent thoughts of dead people send energy somewhere different from when you're thinking about the living people around you. It makes me feel like part of me is being sucked out – making me lose some solidity too and become ghostlier.

Another part of my own ageing that I feel aware of is how settled in I am with my liabilities. You stop caring about changing yourself. This is who I am. Deal with it. I'm my parents. Deal with it. I can be unpleasant and stubborn and irrational and immature. Deal with it because it's not getting better. After this many years I can't overcome myself. You give up on certain kinds of growth and start preparing for death. You store certain things up and you throw other things out. What will I take with me and what will I leave behind. In my family I don't think we are ever packed and ready when it happens, no matter how many years of warning we had. Maybe I'm just scared that I'll never be ready. I don't think my dad or my grandpa was. They had to try to resign themselves to it at the last possible moments but they were conflicted. I know they were.

Maybe I'm just fucking scared to death of losing the probable next two on the list.

Maybe part of me is too aware of the wait. We're all waiting.

Last night, while I was crying in the dark, the dog paced around then approached me. I remember when Daddy was in the hospital the first time. After the first few nights of sleeping at the hospital I finally came home to my house and there was a cat on the porch. For a few days this cat hung around . . . kept coming over. Never saw it before or afterwards. Never had cat visitors there. Just during this really hard time it visited and wanted in. So last night our dog led me downstairs and outside at midnight. I sat on the porch weeping while she lay in the dark listening.

When I finally got it out of my system and came back to bed, my head felt empty and good.

Friday 12 September 2003

DREAM

We had to escape (suddenly I was with another woman – I think it was Jessica Lange) so we took each others' hands and ran/glided over fields . . . over a sea, skimming the water with our feet . . . heading towards the sunset/sunrise . . . the horizon was flat and the grass and sea were very green and rich in contrast to the orange/peach sunset/sunrise.

We finally grew very tired and had to stop – we arrived in the back yard of a sort of farm and Jessica Lange was now a woman I know in real life. We chose a sort of outhouse or outbuilding to hole up in, hoping the owners of the farm wouldn't catch us. I was very hungry and didn't know if I could sleep without eating first. One of the walls of the outhouse/building was curiously absent so if the farmhouse people stepped outside, they'd see us huddled on the floor of their building. At this point it didn't matter to me because a) I knew it was a dream and b) I was now in possession of a short stubby vibrating tube of lip gloss, the kind with a roll-on applicator. The lip gloss was a thick gooey fake cherry or strawberry color and flavor. I rolled it over and around on my clit while huddled next to my companion. The lip gloss juice pulsed out of the tube as I rolled it around and made my pussy extra gooey, red, and obscene. The farmhouse woman was watching me too. I was embarrassed but reminded myself I was dreaming and kept using the lip gloss vibrator until I came.

Tuesday 4 November 2003

FLYING DREAMS

Over the past few months I've been having more flying dreams. Even though flight in my dreams almost always happens in response to threats to my life, I'm still so happy to be having these flying dreams. For one thing, flight is one of the biggest tip-offs to my dreaming mind that I'm dreaming . . . lucidity follows, and the flying is beautiful.

Last night's flying dream was set in an urban-gothic landscape. Fantastic tall but crumbling Gotham-esque buildings. Something about a seedy skin-trade . . . Saving strippers from the hands of a prostitution ring? I don't remember the specific story line, but at the point when things seemed most perilous when the bad guys were going to shoot me/us or crush my kneecaps by driving a car into a cement wall with me in between car and said wall . . . while the two slutty girls were shaking in their shoes . . . I became supercharged and realized not only that I could escape but that I was dreaming and could do whatever I wanted. I stepped up onto the guard rail of the parking garage and looked down from one of the highest skyscrapers in the dark foggy city . . . looked down down down on the tiny lit-up skyscrapers below me (this was a very very very very tall building we're talking about here, you know, looking dooooooooooooown as it was on other tall-in-their-own-right skyscrapers) . . . and I jumped smiling into the mist of the steamy city center's sky and I flew . . . did somersaults in the sky . . . wondered if I'd ever eventually hit the ground . . . but I never did. I just kept on flying.

Wednesday 10 December 2003

FANTASIZING ABOUT WARMTH . . . and other things

My mind is busy conjuring up radiant floor heating, a melt-into-comfort human-dog bed in front of the woodstove, a footbath under my desk, a gigantic bathroom with a chaise lounge, warm damp tiles, a womb-like bath, fuzzy heated robes. A hot spring in the middle of old-growth forest, a dense wet fog of warmth, a carpet

of moss and magical ferns with fronds of velvet and spores filled
with shimmering gold powder that clings to my damp skin when I
brush against them.

Feet that don't trip, the motivation and resources to buy people
Christmas presents.

God, it is so hard for me to be motivated to do anything but eat
and cocoon when I am cold. WebWhore Headquarters is just one
wall away from the woodstove but FUCK it feels farther.

I don't want to be cold. I want to be blanketed. Unobligated.
Stretched out. Pulsing all the way through my skin into my aura. I
want to be still but I can't seem to find the time to let go of "my
ideas" and unplug my mental switchboard.

I need to spend more time talking aloud to myself. I need to allow
myself to unhinge and empty.

Thursday 1 January 2004

I got to speak with my wanker last night who confessed to his own
penis responding to seeing pictures of **Tucker** in drag. I experienced tumescence myself upon hearing this . . . and about two
hours and forty-five minutes into the new year, found myself
sucking and fucking my boy-to-girlfriend wearing his new shiny
hair, garter belt, and stockings. I had the best orgasm while riding
him; he pinched my nipples just right, at just the right time, to send
radiant shivers throughout my body. It's funny how much more I
enjoy looking at HIM in garters and stockings and fondling him
than I do being the one dressed up, looked at and fondled. His ass
and legs are fucking hot – it arouses me so much just seeing his skirt
raised and lowered, raised and lowered over his ass and cock.
Caressing him with my eyes and hands brings me to an incompar-
able state of blessed-out peaceful relaxation and focused arousal.
He shaved more of his body hair to a point of near-hairlessness I've
never seen on him before; although I was sad to see the pit hair,
nipple curls, and scanty (but so beautiful) chest and collarbone hair
gone, feeling his silky hairless ass-cheeks in my hands made up for
the loss.

Thursday 29 January 2004

DREAMING OF PUSSY

I can still see the hot young teen pussy from last night's dream on display to me in a "hamburger shot" from behind.

In my dream I was a troubled young person (morphing between being a girl and a boy – for most of the dream I was a boy). The sky was drizzly and overcast (as it's been here the past couple of days). Lots of climbing on steep eroding hills with loose dirt and dead, strawlike, long, matted-down grass. I was somehow slipping away from my family. I was suicidal or something . . . they were trying to save me and I just wanted to get away. There were some people at a picnic, and lots of them were young girls. One who was a cross between Kirsten Dunst and the girl in *Thirteen* caught my eye because, as I mentioned before, she was lying on her side on the ground, looking over her shoulder smiling while her skirt was hitched up, exposing her pussy from behind. She didn't want to do anything with me, but I convinced her I could do a spectacular job of eating her pussy (in my dream I was absolutely FAMISHED for her pussy). All I needed to do was find a private place. I took her hand and we went running through dirt trails between a river and fields of dead grass with stunted leafless twiggy trees. I didn't want her to have to lay down someplace dirty or anyplace where someone would spot me eating underage pussy so it was difficult to find a good spot. I realized her feet were bare and I was anxious that she might change her mind with the delay so I scooped her up in my arms and ran, carrying her in my arms, ACHING to be alone with her pussy. After passing up a few acceptable but imperfect locations we wound up on a community college campus where I knew it would be next to impossible to find privacy. She sort of faded out of the dream at this point I think, as I focused on other anxieties.

A tractor and a crane – what was that all about?

Thursday 5 February 2004

FEMINIST GOOGLING

I'm excited because someone arrived at my website searching on Google for "year of roe vs wade" (which probably brought them to my herstory page).

It's interesting to think of my own life in terms of history. Is my life typical or atypical of my generation? Have I been molded by history . . . or have I defied tradition?

I find myself deriving pride and satisfaction from the belief that I have lots of sisters in history – now, in the past, and in the future. That I am related to long lost unknown grandmother whores, that I'm related to women all over the globe who continue to struggle in so many different ways by earning money for sex . . . and that I will be a crone to whores of the future. I'm awed by the knowledge that my own whore pride has reinforced the pride of other women . . . and that thread of pride will carry on and enrich the lives of future whores.

I wonder about the person searching for more information about the year 1973, the year of a small famous feminist victory and the year I, another feminist, was born. I wonder how many feminists see my life as another small victory . . . and how many might consider my life a defeat of feminist principles?

I am whore – hear me roar.

Monday 8 March 2004

Yesterday I took a call from my favorite wanker while Tucker went to the store to fetch me some marionberry pie. I took the phone to bed and used my "Hello Kitty" vibrator to stimulate my clit while we talked, but the batteries were wearing down. My wanker led me into talking about one of my favorite subjects (quantifying the number of anonymous cocks hardened by me and the amount of come spewed in my "honor") combined with fantastic notification systems for such events (something he introduced to me). I told him I would love to have an electronic panel that would display each time a penis hardened from stimulation I provided . . . just a little light for each erection pointed in my direction with no name attached to it at all. My wanker asked, "And what about that crucial moment when they lose control . . . does it also arouse you to know when that happens?" I added that it would be even better to have a little garden fountain statue like the little cherubic stone boy holding his teeny penis. But my statue would spurt man-sized loads of come every time someone anywhere ejaculated over me. I thought about how exciting it would be when doing group shows or having sex on the voyeurcams for my statue to get backed up and keep gushing come, jet after jet after jet splashing into a container.

Tucker came home while we were still on the phone, so I enlisted his service and asked him to go down on me while I continued talking with my wanker. My wanker dutifully began telling me about locker rooms of his youth and experiences with boys at camp while I tilted my pelvis back and forth in time to Tucker licking and sucking my clit. Within a few minutes I had a howler of an orgasm.

Sunday 28 March 2004

Wacky dreams from last night: I was a young person (who grew younger as the dream progressed) trying to get to Boston for school (at first maybe it was college and then it was boarding school). I wound up riding with a rich family – I felt very uncomfortable and out-of-place. The dad drove way too fast and they were such a happy family, even though the girls in the family couldn't control his reckless driving. The scenery was beautiful, the roads and off-ramps spiraling wildly down into tree-lined harbors with sparkling water. I was afraid we were going to fly right off the road, that he'd accidentally take a ramp that was incomplete. I was crushed against the side of the car in the backseat, there weren't enough seat belts.

Sometimes I was a girl in the family, and sometimes I was me, the outsider. He drove madly through gridlock, driving on the shoulder. At high speed we passed someone broken down on the side of the road. Long past this person the dad stopped and TURNED AROUND, using the shoulder to drive the wrong way on a four lane freeway back to the stranded driver. The girls in the family protested, and I felt especially uneasy considering there were police and firemen-types at the scene now, walking in the road's shoulder, investigating something. Two firemen in charcoal grey suits and masks were carrying a small stretcher with a sheet-covered lump on it. Two stiff baby arms jutted out dead and white from under each side of the sheet. Tiny baby palms faced up with plump paralyzed fingers curled up to the sky.

Later we were in a park with Bill Clinton and a young Chelsea Clinton for the opening procession for boarding school. A stone pathway snaked wildly through green grass. The size of the stones varied as did their elevation above the ground. All of the other kids and parents knew the routine. I had no parents and resisted following the serpentine pathway stone-for-stone, I wanted to just run ahead in the direction the path was leading rather than wasting time on the twists and turns everyone else scampered along just for the sake of ceremony. I thought, "The shortest distance between two points is a straight line!" Still I tried to fit in and to do what they were doing, but I was clumsy and heavy and kept falling off the path accidentally anyway.

Cumwhore Diary

Suzie

http://cumwhore.blogspot.com

Note: *When I started writing my blog, I had just ended a "relationship" with a man named Kevin. To call it a relationship is being very generous. In hindsight, Kevin was more of a fuck buddy than a boyfriend, someone who enjoyed the same sexual kinks and saw me as a safe, healthy, willing partner. As a result of ending things with Kevin, I began to ruminate about past relationships and to consider what I really did want from a relationship with a man. Hopefully this will help put some of the following ramblings into perspective.*

17 October 2003

I was once involved with a very nice, very vanilla guy whom I'll call Phil. Phil treated me like a queen. In the weeks that we were a couple, I don't think I ever opened a car door or had to wonder where he was or what he was doing. He was the type of old-fashioned guy who insisted on paying for dates, who wouldn't let my hand touch a doorknob if he was nearby. He had a great sense of humor and was a very attentive and generous lover. Professionally and in many other ways, we were made for one another. He understood when I worked late. He understood that when I said I was under pressure, I really *was* under pressure. He would rub my feet and run baths for me. He was a prize. I'm ashamed to admit that the only real complaint I had against him was that, sexually, he wasn't "rough" enough for me. I *enjoyed* our sex life – who doesn't like to be fucked? – but I always felt cheated, which wasn't fair to him NOR was it his fault at all.

I sometimes wonder what my life would have been like had I chosen Phil. Professionally, I would have had someone in my corner (which is nice) and personally, I would have had a very attentive and loving man to come home to (which is great) – but I know myself well enough to know that I would have ended up missing wild, uninhibited sex so much that I would have cheated on him OR I would have been so unfulfilled, sexually, that I would have ended up addicted to wild, uninhibited porn. I'm not Mother Theresa and I'm not a very good person but I think I did Phil a huge favor. He'll marry a lucky girl one day and I'll still be going to clubs and hooking up with guys who might fulfill me sexually but who don't really care about *me* at all. Kevin is a good example of that. Sexually he was willing to try anything but he'd sulk if I had to work late or if I was under a lot of pressure at work and didn't feel like clubbing. My life was only worthy of discussion, it seems, when it affected Kevin's ability to have sex.

As for swinging. I hate that term. It sounds very old-fashioned, very 70s. I can't think of a better term (or one more often used) to describe the consensual sharing of partners. The key difference between then and now is that now people are covered from head to toe in plastic. I'm sure in the 70s, people fucked without condoms and didn't give a thought to diseases, only to unwanted pregnancies.

The first time I went to a "swinging party" was when I was 22, while I was dating a guy I'll call Mike. He was my first wild lover. He would spank my ass while he pounded my pussy from behind and call me names during sex, both of which excited me to no end. He encouraged me to discuss my sexual fantasies and I divulged that I would like to suck him with another girl. I said that what would REALLY excite me is if I sucked his cock with another girl while people watched. His response was something along the lines of, "Lady, do I have a place for YOU!"

Mike had friends (couples) who were swingers and often had fully consensual parties at their home where people could watch, participate, not watch, not participate. In other words, the people at the parties were "into" that sort of thing but there was no pressure to perform or participate. Mike and I went to this party and I was expecting to walk in there and see . . . I don't know what I was expecting. I thought it would be a wild scene but most of the people who were having sex were in bedrooms, away from the crowd, but it was understood that if you felt like walking into a bedroom and watching, you could. There was a very casual and friendly atmosphere in their home and the hostess welcomed me and made me feel at ease without being "sexual" or "coy" about anything. I think my voice cracked a few times when I was asked questions (What do you do? How long have you lived in—?) There was such a palpable sexual charge in the house that I found myself getting wet out of nervousness more than sexual excitement.

Mike introduced me to a woman he obviously knew quite well. I'll call her Karrie. Mike asked if I wanted to go somewhere more private with Karrie and so we went to a corner of the room. Mike sat down on an armchair and took Karrie on one knee and me on the other. Karrie began to kiss him. I was jealous but I was very aroused. It was very sexy to see my boyfriend being kissed by someone else and knowing that this was all fine. I kissed Mike and then I kissed Karrie and before I could feel anything or stop myself, we were both working his cock. That was the first time I'd ever done many things: sucked cock in front of people, sucked cock with another girl and felt sexually aroused by the sight of another woman. Even now, I find it very erotic and sexy when two women suck a guy and they themselves touch tongues and co-operate in bringing him off. There were a few people watching and encouraging us until Mike stood up and shot on both of our faces. I don't remember wiping his come off my face. I do know that another man approached us, condom in hand, and asked if we would do him next. We did.

I felt so ashamed after it was over and the sexual excitement had died down but I masturbated a LOT when I remembered the experience (and altered it a little to erase the awkward moments). Mike and I didn't do this often, maybe twice more, but it set a pattern for me. When I meet guys now, it doesn't take me long before I'm fishing to see if they're into this sort of thing. If they're not, I lose interest quickly. I could live without swinging and exhibitionism if I had a dominant man in my life but I *know* that I couldn't live without both.

19 October

I feel like I'm leading a double life. I *am* leading a double life. My work acquaintances and my professional friends would tell you that I'm the most sober, hard-working, serious person on earth. And then there's the side of me that fantasizes about giving blow-jobs to several guys at once and being drenched in come. If there's only one thing about Kevin I'll really miss, it's the amount of come he was able to coax out of himself after a blow-job. I love that. The harder and longer it hits my face and tits, the better.

22 October

I went online earlier, thinking that perhaps I'd run into Sid or another online friend/acquaintance but instead I struck up a conversation with a complete stranger. We discussed BDSM for a bit and then he shifted the conversation from a detached, analytical discussion of domination and submission to telling me, in great detail, how he would dominate me if he had the opportunity. I always have sex on the brain but last night was worse than ever so when he started discussing how he would tie me to a wall and slap my entire body red and then anally abuse me while I screamed for him to be gentle, I was wet and masturbating. Then he typed out his phone number and told me to call him. I did.

I *never* had phone sex, outside of talking dirty to boyfriends. I've never crossed the line between fantasy (online) and reality (what could affect my personal or professional life) but I was so wet and horny and so desperate to hear a man's voice commanding my every move. I did *67 before calling his number, since I knew it would block my number, but as soon as I hung up the phone after masturbating myself into an intense orgasm, I felt the immediate pangs of guilt, shame and regret. What if my number wasn't blocked? What did I just do? I've been waiting for the phone to ring ever since I hung up: *Remember me?* I tried to convince myself that he was in all likelihood married and wouldn't dare call back – that *he* had more to lose by actually giving out his phone number than I had to lose by calling it – but I still can't fall asleep.

So was the phone sex worth it? Yes, it was. Nothing can compare to the sound of a man's voice directly in my ear, commanding my every move. It made me want to suck cock. It made me want to fuck. Every time he called me a slut or a bitch, my clit would pulsate harder and harder. I was so wet and so hot for his voice. With my eyes closed, I could feel him against my back. "Slap your pussy hard enough so I can hear it." I wanted to come I came. Now I feel guilty. I feel stupid for putting myself in such a dangerous position and I feel guilty because he probably WAS married and his wife was out of town.

So help me, I will *never* do that again.

30 October

I'm delighted to report that I have a date tomorrow night. "Ted" and I met several weeks ago through mutual friends and I was quite impressed by him. Unfortunately, he has been largely out of town since we met but he's in town for a while and asked me if I would be interested in going to a Hallowe'en party – small affair, lots of silliness, etc. He said, "Of course, you'll have to dress up. I know it's very late notice, but do you have a costume?" I wanted to burst into laughter when he asked that.

Yes, what *shall* I wear? My X-rated cowgirl outfit? My X-rated leather nurse's uniform? How about the cheerleader's uniform?

About Ted: without saying too much, he has a job that requires him to travel out of town a lot. That's something that bothered me when I first met him. He's not out of town just a few days a month – he's out of town so much that I'm surprised he even bothers to keep an apartment here in the city. He's intelligent and funny and has a voice that could melt butter. I think if this worked out and we had a relationship that was largely over the phone, his voice alone might be enough to keep me monogamous. I'm a little worried about seeing him again, if only because I'm afraid he will be dressed up in a really silly costume that might undercut his masculinity. Nothing worse than trying to bond with someone dressed as Mickey Mouse, right? I'm not expecting much to come from this but it *will* be nice to socialize and have some fun.

For the first time in a long while, I'm just feeling genuinely excited about something: a night of normalcy. Isn't that what most people try to *escape*!?

1 November

I can't believe I'm up and around so early.

I had a WONDERFUL time at the party last night. Ted was charming, funny, SEXY, and confident – all of the things that make me go weak in the knees with a man. The confidence thing is a HUGE part of what attracts me to a man. Ted has the air of someone who is absolutely sure of himself. What an aphrodisiac!

It was almost surreal how quickly and easily Ted and I hit it off and how easily the conversation flowed. *This* is why I tend to gravitate towards professional men: their jobs depend on them being quick, on being good talkers and showing confidence and style. When you spend as many hours on the phone as I do (and meet with as many clients as Ted does), you learn to adapt yourself to anyone's professional language. We talked about my job, his job, the places he's traveled, the people he's met, the places he has slept. He's positively dazzling. I commented that compared to his, my life must seem boring. Ted replied very seriously that while he loves to travel, he misses "home" and misses all of the things he could have if he were more settled. "I can't even have a plant," he said.

When the party was over, Ted drove me home and when we got there, I asked Ted if he wanted to come upstairs for coffee. I wish there were words to describe the smile he flashed at that moment. There were definite sexual sparks between us and as a result, my invitation was loaded with innuendo. I honestly *didn't* want to stop talking and that really *was* the main thing on my mind – but a fuck would have been OK, too. Ted told me that I was a "great girl" and that he wanted to take me out again, maybe for supper, but that he felt it best if we said goodnight in the car. "Believe me, I can't believe I just said that," Ted said with a chuckle. Neither could I!

Ted thanked me for a wonderful evening and said he would call me to arrange dinner plans, and then leaned in to kiss me. I'll be honest: I rarely get a sexual buzz from kissing. I love to kiss and I love to have a soft tongue in my mouth but I can't say that it's high on my list of erotic things to do. But when Ted kissed me, I felt a tremor go from my brain down my back, to my crotch and down to my feet. The kiss was *electric*. We made out for a long while and it felt like high school all over again, when the date is over and you want that person but there's nowhere to go to be alone, so you sit there in the car and kiss and touch and kiss until you feel like you're going to *die* from wanting that person. When Ted cupped my tits in his hands and squeezed them, I felt the electricity run through me from head to toe. "Are you SURE you won't come upstairs?" I asked. (Read: *I want to fuck you. I want to suck you. I have never wanted to be alone with a man as badly as I want to be alone with you right now . . .*) Ted pulled away and said, "Suzi, I *want* to go upstairs. I WANT to go upstairs. But not tonight. Not now." He kissed me again and walked me to my apartment door.

With every step we took, I kept hoping he would change his mind. He kissed me tenderly and let his hand run down my breasts. Then he put his hand on my crotch and gave my pussy a solid squeeze. He winked, turned and left.

And I went into my apartment, stripped down, put a hand down my panties and masturbated. I don't recall *ever* feeling so sexually aroused by a man. I've gotten excited by the prospect of fucking and sucking a man, but I can't recall a situation where just heavy kissing caused such shivers to run up and down me. Just writing about it now is making me wet. I can still feel his tongue poking between my lips. *Fuck!*

I can't stop squeezing my pussy. I wish I had a firmer grip so I could recreate Ted's hold on my pussy before he left last night. I masturbated last night and again when I woke up this. I'm thinking about it now and want to masturbate again. Even if our dinner tonight proves to be a disappointment, I'll content myself with a vivid, electric sexual memory that will carry me through the next few days. *Fuck!!*

2 November

I got fucked so well last night. I'm giddy with the memories of it.

Dinner with Ted was obviously fantastic. A lot of talk, laughter and a *lot* of sexual tension. By the time we finished our coffee, we were ready to head back to my place and fuck our brains out – which we did. We made out on my sofa like a couple of teenagers until I managed to get his jeans over his hips and assumed my favorite position: on my knees, in between his legs, sucking his cock. Ted had a nice thick cock – the kind I love to suck the most.

Thick enough to stretch my lips wide and yet short enough that I can deep throat it with ease. I looked directly into his eyes so I can mentally record the blow-job and relive it in perfect detail later, which I have done several times since last night, rubbing my clit raw at the memory of it.

Ted was a hard, passionate lover. I sucked him till he told me to bend over on the couch and show him some ass. He stuck his cock inside me and held onto my hips as he fucked me slow and hard, then fast and hard until we both came. We retired to my bedroom and kissed and did some juvenile heavy-petting until I felt Ted's cock responding again. We fucked again, this time in the missionary position with my legs spread wide to the sides. We managed to get a few hours of sleep before I woke up to the inexpressible delight of his hard-on pressed up against my ass. I started laughing out of sheer giddiness and soon he was joining in too. We fucked doggy-style with the two of us giggling throughout. It was the most exhilarating night of fucking I've had in ages. Fucking because I really dug the guy and fucking because it felt so *right*.

I felt no shame when I woke up this morning.

10 November

I had one of my infamous schizophrenic weekends. Ted called on Saturday and we chatted for a while before I nudged him towards some phone sex. Clearly he isn't all that into it. He said it makes him feel lonelier than he already feels. Once I cooed to him about how I would lick his cock and suck it and how wet it would be and how deep I would take it, I heard the unmistakable sound of him coming. There can't be a sexier sound than the wet sound of a lubricated hand on a cock, followed by the holding of breath and then the pure release of orgasm.

Ted guided me towards an orgasm and then said he had to hurry up and get ready for a dinner engagement. No sooner had I hung up with Ted than Kevin showed up. *Big* problem. I never should have let him in because I was still feeling horny and still soaking wet from the phone sex with Ted – and Kevin is a guy whose cock I know inside and out. I know the thickness of it, the length of it. I know how deep I can take it. I know how to lick and suck on his balls. I know where to kiss and where to lick and when to suck softly and when to suck hard. What came next is obvious.

Before I even understood the why of it, I was on my knees between Kevin's legs, giving him a blow-job. I'm sick of making excuses or trying to rationalize it: I just wanted to suck cock and I like Kevin's cock, so why not suck it? To be perfectly honest, it felt *good*. It felt good to have his cock in my mouth and to work it. It felt good because I know how Kevin likes to be sucked and I know just how much teasing he can take before I feel his hands grip my head and he begins controlling the situation. It felt good to work my clit with his cock in my mouth and cum with his cock in my mouth. It just felt GOOD to suck Kevin off and to feel his hands in my hair, pushing my head down onto his cock and then feeling him pull my head away and feeling his warm, sticky cum shoot all over my face. We cleaned ourselves off, Kevin picked up the DVDs he asked for and off he went.

There's no commitment between Ted and I yet, but I still felt guilty. For all I know, Ted has been fucking everything that moves on the West Coast but that doesn't make me feel any better. I'm just so sick of rationalizing everything that I do when all I *really* want is to have sex, suck cock, get fucked and not feel anything at *all* about it, other than that it felt goddamn great while it was happening and the afterglow is divine.

25 November

I finally caught up with Ted but we had to cut our conversation short. He was meeting some people for drinks and dinner and talked to me while he shaved and changed. The sound of his zipper unzipping or his buttons being buttoned or his tie being straightened – all of these things make me feel him in the room with me. "What are you doing now?" I asked. "Tying my shoes," he replied. "Put the phone near your feet so I can hear you," I said. Ted laughed, unaware of how serious I was. He promised to call me if he didn't get in too late and swore that he'd call my cell phone if he had privacy during his lunch break tomorrow. I felt so blue after we hung up. I rarely feel blue, but I feel blue right now.

I write mainly about Ted's and my sex life and I think that may give people the impression that ours is a sexual relationship with very little depth. The truth is that I'm starting to see more and more how Ted has influenced me in such a short time. I appreciate it that he doesn't give me pep talks all the time and doesn't use words like "strategize" and "mobilize" and "pro-active" around me {chuckle} but he HAS had a huge influence on me. When I complain about a problem or a person at work, Ted knows exactly how to focus in on the real issue. He asks me questions out of genuine interest and offers me sound advice because he cares. I cooed to him once, "Doctor, you helped me so much with my problem. How can I ever repay you?" Ted replied, "Fuck me tonight." And then the work stuff is over and we're back to having fun again. The dynamics between us just feel so right and so effortless. I know when it's time to drop a subject and I know when it's time to shift gears, and Ted instinctively knows when to do the same.

And I'm afraid to feel this way about him.

The truth of the matter is that I'm almost 30 years old and I don't think I've ever had a truly deep and lasting relationship. I've sabotaged every relationship I've ever been in. If the guy was vanilla and very kind and generous and loving, I'd dump him because he wasn't kinky. If a guy was kinky and a complete asshole, I'd dump him because he wasn't kind and generous and loving enough. Most of the men I've dated never lasted past the first date. I complained with Kevin that he knew little about me and didn't seem interested in knowing more about me and yet I have to ask myself, Did I even let him in? Did I make it easy for him or did I have a "Fuck me and shut up" attitude towards him that made getting to know me impossible? I'm sure there are men reading this who think a "Fuck me and shut up" woman would be nice to have, but would that *really* be good? You can be in a marriage with great sex but if there's no warmth, is it fulfilling? You can be in a relationship with someone who listens to you and hangs on your every word and yet doesn't thrill you in bed – is that fulfilling?

None of my past relationships have had potential. This thing with Ted . . . THIS has potential. How can I tell? Well, I'm quoting songs in his honor and singing them around the house, am I not? When you start singing cheesy love songs in someone's honor, you're in deep, *deep* trouble!

7 December

I'm so stunned by everything that has happened in the past two days that I hardly know where to begin. I had suspected for a long while now that Ted had definite Dom tendencies but this night confirmed every last one of those suspicions. I told Ted about giving Kevin a blow-job when we last spoke on the phone and Ted admitted he had had sex with an acquaintance of his during his last business trip. It was a difficult conversation to have – difficult to admit that those indiscretions made us jealous, which implies more emotion between us than we'd been willing to admit – but we did clear the air and Ted said we'd talk about it more when we were face-to-face.

When I met Ted for lunch yesterday, everything felt normal and right again. The conversation was easy. We went back to my apartment and no sooner were we in the door than I felt Ted's mouth on my neck and his body pressed up against mine. I can't *believe* how instantly my body responds to his touch. We went into the bedroom, undressing haphazardly, and I felt his hand on my bottom, caressing it, before he pinched one of my ass-cheeks so hard that I felt a sting of tears come to my eyes. I'm not a pain slut, yet I love the way my body reacts to pain. When I first feel it, I'm embarrassed and angry but when the sting of the pain subsides, I feel a very sharp, tantalizing "shivering" feeling that works its way up from my clit to my nipples to my head. Ted pinched my other ass-cheek hard and before the tremors could subside, he looked into my eyes. "So you like to suck cock, hm?" he asked. I nodded. "That's not an answer," Ted said. I told him in my most collected voice that I liked to suck cock. "Show me," he said.

I sat on the edge of the bed and took his cock into my mouth and worked it as lovingly as I could. I could feel the wetness of my pussy and the tremors in my clit as I worked his cock and felt so good that everything seemed normal between us again.

"Now call me Kevin," he said, "and suck my cock the way you sucked his."

I was stunned and confused and I told Ted that I didn't want to do that but he pushed his cock in my face and told me, "Don't say no to me. Now call me Kevin and suck my cock." I took his cock into my mouth again and tried to suck him but he would pull his cock out and say, "Look at me and call me Kevin." When I did as I was told, he would allow me a few more seconds of cocksucking.

"Did Kevin come on your face, Suzi?" he asked. I told him that he did. Ted held his cock in my face and told me that Kevin must have been very happy to have been sucked this way and how only a disgusting cunt would show her lover how she sucked another man's cock. I was stunned into co-operation. Everything felt unreal around me.

He told me to lie down on the bed and kneeled between my thighs, pressing his cock against my pussy. "Since you were nice enough to show me how you sucked Kevin's cock, I'll show *you* how I fucked Caroline," he said. He put his cock inside me and fucked me gently and tenderly. "Do you like this, Caroline?" he asked me. I managed to gasp out that I did, humiliated to be called another woman's name. He made love to me gently for a while before pounding me with long, hard strokes. "Now this is how I fuck *you*, Suzi," he said. He rammed his cock into me, rough and hard and angrily and then slowed his pace down to remind me of how he fucked that other woman.

It was humiliating and degrading to have him show me how he fucked another woman and to have him call me by her name but try as I did to steel myself against it, I found my pussy reacting to the images he put in my mind. Images of his cock inside another woman. Images of him on top of her, being slow and gentle. I imagined myself in the room with them. I imagined myself tied to a chair, helpless while watching him fuck this other woman. Ted smiled down at me and I imagined him fucking this other woman and smiling at me, tied to a chair, knowing there was nothing I could do to stop him from fucking her.

Ted pressed his thumb against my clit and rubbed it and teased it while he continued to take me with long, slow, hard strokes. I told him I was ready to come and he told me to say his name as I came – and I did. I felt my orgasm explode out of me. It was amazing to be looking into the eyes of a man I cared for so deeply and hear myself stammer out his name while I came. It felt so intense and personal. I've heard people say they were "dizzy with excitement" but I never believed such a thing was possible, and yet I DID feel dizzy with excitement after we had both come.

I didn't know what to say to Ted. I felt embarrassed. We had never discussed humiliation play (though I dropped a lot of hints) and I felt embarrassed for having responded so enthusiastically to it. I always imagined that I would pretend to need some "coaxing" into it but I couldn't help myself. That pussy-drenching response I have to being embarrassed and humiliated is too powerful for me. I can't resist it.

Ted and I discussed this afterwards and he once again reminded me of the woman he had dated in the past who was so enamored of him that she was willing to do anything he said. He said that he always wondered what it would be like to have that kind of control over a woman he actually cared for. I was silent for a long time as I thought this over and finally said, very carefully, "If we discussed it first – what you wanted to do to me – I think I would be open to it." Ted kissed me and said, "I'd like to mindfuck you and make you cry."

I don't expect ANYONE to understand why this would appeal to me as it does. I don't think anyone who has never craved being under a man's control as much as I've craved it could understand why a professional, intelligent, well-read, educated woman would dream of being subjected to pain and humiliation. And yet I do.

Ted went home last night because he had an early day today and it was just easier for him to go home than stay here. When I got up this morning and checked my mail, I found a one-line email from him saying, in effect, "I don't want any man to have any control over you except me." I'm shivering as I write those words just as I shivered when I read them. This sudden shift in our relationship fills me with such hope. To be loved by a man who isn't appalled by my "shameful" needs means a lot to me. I know I will get the usual barrage of "You are so naive" emails from people but I don't care. I don't expect anyone to understand. I only know that this is the first time in my life that I've been able – even after the arguments and the accusations – to envision a future with someone.

12 December

I came home from work last night and Ted ordered in some food as soon as I walked in the door. I had fantasized about "taking him" but he had other plans. As soon as he hung up the phone, he unzipped his pants, pulled his cock out and told me to get down on my knees and suck him. I started to lick and tease him and he told me that the take-out would be here in half an hour at the latest and that I had to make him come before it arrived. I smiled up at him and knew I'd be able to make him come in no time but as I sucked him, he ran his fingers through my hair and told me that he was going to come in my mouth and that I would have to hold the come in my mouth until the food arrived: "If you swallow, you'll be punished." I realized that I had a choice: either prolong the blow-job so I wouldn't have to have his come in my mouth for too long before the food arrived OR suck him hard and nasty (as I wanted to) and hold his come in my mouth for as long as I had to. I asked him what my punishment would be but he just looked down at me and shook his head. "That's none of your concern," he said.

I continued sucking him. I wanted to make the blow job last as long as I could but as always happens with me, I couldn't hold back. The feel of his hard-on inside my mouth and feeling it get harder with each lick of pleasure I gave him made me want to blow him like a whore and I found myself sucking on it like my life depended upon it. Ted put his hands on my head and stroked his cock with my lips until he came inside my mouth. "Show me," he said. I opened my mouth and showed him the pool of come on my tongue. He patted me on the head and told me to hold it in my mouth: "No swallowing, Suzi!" I sat on the sofa and watched the clock while Ted surfed the channels and periodically asked me to open my mouth to prove I hadn't swallowed his come. Finally, the buzzer rang and Ted let the delivery person in. "Go pay," he said, handing me the money. I gave him a confused, startled look and Ted laughed. "You don't have to say a word to him, do you? Just take the food, give him the money."

Finally, a knock on the door. I took the money, opened the door and felt silly for not being able to say hello or thank you to the delivery person. I handed the money over and when he began to give me change, I waved my hands to indicate that he should keep it. He looked puzzled by my behavior but wished me a happy holiday and left. Ted was behind me in no time. "Open your mouth again," he said. I opened my mouth and showed him the come that was still in my mouth, now mixed with the saliva I'd accumulated by trying NOT to swallow too much of his come with my spit. "Swallow," he said. I swallowed the come and he kissed me. "You're an obedient cocksucker," he said, and took me into the kitchen to eat the food.

Conversation at the table was normal: "How was your day? Did you bring work home again?" I could feel myself trembling inside as I ate but Ted ate and drank as if nothing unusual had occurred.

2 January

For a while now, Ted and I have been discussing the kind of D/s and role-play that we want to explore and I'm finding that Ted leans far more towards the sadistic than I do. This doesn't come as THAT big of a surprise to me but I still question sometimes if he's not going to become bored with my hard limits.

To be completely honest, I've never been much into pain. There are some pain-related activities that turn me on (hard spankings, face-slapping, hair-pulling, paddlings, nipple clamping, to name a few) and there are other pain-related activities that I have never tried but would CONSIDER trying with the right person (hard anal sex, whipping, caning, among others) and then I have a lengthy list of things I don't want to try under any circumstances. Ted has a few fantasies that fall into my NEVER pile. He has told me that these fantasies can remain fantasies and that if I'm never into them, it's OK with him BUT I can remember saying those same words to past lovers and not really meaning it.

My idea of really wonderful D/s play is psychological and emotional. Ted sent shivers up my spine once when he told me he wanted to "mindfuck" me until I cried. THAT is my ideal. I would love to be bound to a chair and teased for hours on end, left alone in a room to feel embarrassed, cold and even humiliated. Ted and I haven't really had the time for long, protracted psychological play and on the occasions when we've had hours at our disposal, his horniness has gotten the better of him and within 30 minutes of starting our play, he is ready to come and ready for me to be released so we can go out and do something. It's NOT unfulfilling because I enjoy my servitude and I LOVE feeling the depth of my submission to him BUT I would be lying if I said I wasn't wishing he would devote more time to the emotional and psychological side of playing. Sexual teasing is wonderful, but sexual teasing done while pushing me to my emotional and psychological limits is an experience that I find difficult putting into words.

This leads me to wonder if Ted really DOES grasp how important the psychological aspects of D/s are to me.

This leads me to wonder if I'm underestimating how important the sadistic aspects of D/s are to HIM.

Which has me feeling more confused than I should be.

11 January

I noticed in a chat room last night how often online submissives act like spoiled, petulant five year-olds. So many of them are your stereotypical attention-seekers who call themselves submissive, *defend* their submissiveness and yet top from the bottom at every opportunity. They deliberately anger people in the chat room and then coyly defy their Masters to "punish" them for their behavior. They make inappropriate comments and generally act like fools and then they sit on their Master's lap and coo about how devoted they are to him and how wonderful he is. Through it all, the Master does nothing to correct their submissives and demand that she stop making a fool of herself – and *him* in the process, since she's his responsibility and he looks weak and impotent in the face of her bratty behavior.

However, seeing this behavior make me think about an urge I've been fighting for quite some time now with Ted – the urge to *deliberately* push his buttons or break some of the (few) rules he has laid . . . down in order to see what his reaction would be and what punishment or discipline would come of it. I'm *aware* that I would be doing this deliberately and being aware of it has prevented me from actually pushing those buttons – but as I was watching the submissives deliberately provoking their Masters, I saw a bit of myself in that behavior.

But Ted has laid down a few very simple rules for me; I'll mention one only to make a point. Ted decided a few weeks ago that I wasn't paying enough attention to my skin. When the cold weather started, Ted insisted that I start moisturizing my skin. I told him I didn't see the point of it but before I could protest too much, he took out his Official List Of Rules and wrote it down.

So the next day, I started following this routine. It's not a LENGTHY routine but Ted oversaw it for the first couple of days to make sure I was doing it the way he wanted me to. Since that day, I've been following the routine because it pleases him.

One morning, I was washing my face and starting to put the lotion when it hit me that I didn't *feel* like doing any of this. I have nice skin; what's the point? I decided that since Ted was away on business, I'd skip the routine until he got back. It seemed so simple: he'll never know, will he? Yet that evening, when I removed my make-up and washed my face, I was conflicted about what to do. It's not the simple matter of whether or not to moisturize, but the bigger issue: if I stop doing things just because "Ted isn't around", then how serious is the commitment? If Ted has given me some very simple rules to follow and has promised that more would be added to The Official List, then how am I going to behave when the rules get harder? If I can't moisturize my skin for him, then what else *can't* I do for him?

I decided to moisturize and I mentioned it to Ted when he came back from his business trip. He was pleased to hear that I had followed the rule despite wanting to cut the routine short, but as we discussed this (and other rules), I had to admit that perhaps subconsciously, I wanted to disobey him just to see what his reaction would be. What kind of a punishment does "not moisturizing" warrant? A hard spanking? Deprivation?

I've obeyed his every rule and I've been every inch the submissive because the truth is, *I love to please him*. I love knowing that he's pleased with me and happy with my commitment to even the smallest things he asks of me. Ted said that he, as the Dom in the relationship, has often wondered what he would do if I disobeyed him: "What kind of punishment DOES 'not moisturizing' warrant?" Ted decided that he would probably deny me a week's worth of facials: "It seems fitting that if you don't want Lancôme on your skin, you don't want my come on it, either, right?"

So the punishment would suit the crime. It would also be poetic justice, which is nice.

Any tendency I may have towards bratty behavior and any urge I may sometimes have to deliberately disobey Ted or make him angry is squashed by the desire to make him happy and make sure he's pleased, but it was comforting to know that Ted has been thinking about this as well. He even admitted that he sometimes wished I would disobey just so he could have the pleasure of punishing me or disciplining me, but made me promise I would never do such a thing. I promised I would follow his rules and tell him if ever I broke one of them.

Just knowing I could suffer through a week without a comeshot to the face *should* be enough to keep me in line:-)

20 April

Note: I wrote this post in Word on 20 April but only got around to uploading it to Blogger today.

Last weekend was the first time Ted and I saw each other since he moved away.

I should backtrack a bit and tell you that Ted and I have been talking on the phone regularly since he moved but, with the status of our relationship so uncertain, the conversations have been overwhelmingly stilted and uncomfortable. Deep down, I know that Ted is resisting the temptation to tell me to quit my job and allow him to take care of us but he knows how much my career means to me and how hard it would be for me to give it all up. I'm much more honest and straightforward with him via email, where I don't feel as pressured to fill in the gaps of silence with meaningless chit-chat. It may take me a day to write one email – adding a line here, leaving it, going back to it to add another line or delete something, et cetera – but when I hit Send, I know that I've said everything I really wanted to say, as honestly and openly and fairly as possible. I did tell him that I've played with Kevin on a few occasions and, not surprisingly, Ted admitted to "a couple of quickies" with one of the women at his new office – something I find reckless and potentially dama-ging but won't lecture Ted about. On the one hand, I felt betrayed and hurt at the thought of Ted's cock inside another woman; on the other hand, the chances of us making our long-distance relationship work seem so slim that I couldn't care less. In other words, I don't know how the hell I feel.

Ted and I were originally supposed to see one another on Easter weekend, but those plans fell through. He called me last Wednesday and announced that he had purchased himself a ticket and would be landing late Friday evening. Against my better judgment, I was giddy with anticipation. Then I became angry. Was he taking a hotel room? Was he just assuming that it would be all right for him to stay at my place? What exactly were his plans? Did I have to pick him up at the airport? When he confirmed his flight time, I was irrationally angry with him, demanded answers – and of course Ted had made the arrangements that I knew he would make. He had taken a hotel room. He was renting a car. He would call me once he was settled in to his hotel room and make plans from there.

And so, on Friday night, at a little past 11 p.m., my phone rang – Ted telling me that he was at his hotel (a few blocks from my home, of course), had put his clothes away and wanted to take a shower: "And then I'd love to see you, if you're up for it." I told Ted that would be fine and told him I would go to the hotel.

I don't think that I can adequately describe just how strange and uncomfortable seeing him was. I was overwhelmed by in-stinct – to throw myself into his arms, to wrap my legs around him, to smother him with kisses, to play it cool, to be detached, to let him set the pace. The one true thing was realizing just how much I had missed him. Ted scooped me up into his arms and lifted me off my feet, repeating over and over again how much he had missed me and how wonderful it was to see me again. It had been a month since I'd last been in his arms and I have to confess, it felt like home. I know how trite that sounds, but it's true. It felt so perfect and so right to be in his arms again, and a month of pretending his departure hadn't hurt too much went down the drain. We hugged and kissed and settled in for hours of *really* catching up. Not the polite chit-chat from our phone calls, and not the admissions of "infidelity" carefully designed to hurt one another. We were honest but joyous and we talked till 3 a.m.

before going to bed together – no sex, but hours of deep, pleasing sleep.

I really loved being with Ted again. We spent Saturday shopping and eating and talking and on Saturday night, we made love. I rarely use that term to describe my sex life because most of the sex I have is "play" or "fucking", but when Ted and I went to bed on Saturday night, it was pure passion and affection and absolutely fulfilling. It was wonderful – almost too wonderful, as I've spent the last few days reliving it over and over in my mind, just as I did when Ted and I first slept together. It was slow, hard, intense lovemaking. The kind that makes you weak in the knees just to remember it.

I felt my heart break all over again on Sunday, when Ted checked out of the hotel and I reluctantly said goodbye to him as he headed back home. We made plans for me to fly out to see him at the end of the month. I'm going to ask Boss for an extra day off so I can make it a LONG weekend – from Thursday night to Monday night. I'll bring my laptop with me and I'll have ample time to get work done so there shouldn't be a problem.

I'm confused about everything again. When Ted moved away, I was ready to forget the plans I'd secretly made for a future together but after seeing him again and remembering how relaxed and at ease I am with him, it's hard for me to not fantasize again about the future I once thought we'd have together. When Ted was in my life, I placed a very high priority on our sex life and, I'll be honest, the fact that he was into D/s was one of the main reasons I *could* foresee a future with him. After being apart for a while and seeing him again, I see that sex is a small part of it. What really made me foresee a future with Ted are all the *other* things that are harder to find in a partner: trust, ease, intelligence, an innate understanding of what motivates me, et cetera. I could troll tomorrow in a bar and find a guy who'd be more than willing to push me to my knees, force his cock inside my mouth and treat me like a whore for the night – but what are the chances, really, of that guy being someone I'd be completely at ease with, with no desire or need to pretend anything or act differently or live up to a standard that I don't want to live up to?

The answer: *slim*!

We've spoken on the phone since he went back home and it

makes me miss him so much that I ache. My plan is to once again bury myself in work and my yoga classes and work off my sexual energy on the treadmill instead of with Kevin. I'm looking forward to seeing Ted again, even if that means having to go through the goddamned hassle of airport security and a two-hour plane ride during which I will no doubt sit next to the worst passenger that the airline can muster up. I'm trying not to get my hopes up that Ted and I somehow be able to make this long-distance relationship work but. . . .

~ sigh ~

10 May

I flew in to see Ted last weekend and still can't decide how I feel about it. I felt a twinge of envy all weekend long. I love my job and love the company I work for, but I was envious of Ted's new life – new job, new apartment, new people, new city, new challenges. I mentioned this to Ted and he reminded me that while I may *feel* envious, the truth of the matter is that I would HATE to have this much change in my life.

Ted and I had a great weekend. A lot of conversation and a lot of talk about the future. The agreement that we reached was that we would pursue our relationship but not commit to monogamy. I know that Ted is occasionally seeing someone ("a casual fuck," as he calls her) and I've enjoyed a few romps with Kevin; clearly, distance is making us more casual about the terms of our commitment to one another. That's fine. I still truly love Ted but emotionally, I'm not ready to deal with the *reality* that this may not work out. Ted is doing great at his new job and I've brought new business in to the company. Short of one of us getting fired or quitting, I doubt that we'll ever be together in the future. To be honest, it hurts AND it's OK. There's no ill will between us, no hard feelings, no regrets. I do find myself drifting into "could haves" every so often but it's less and less.

Obviously, what I miss most about being with Ted is the sex. As fun and daring and playful as Kevin is (and as able as he is to help me live out some of my "multiple partner" fantasies), I miss the

Dom/sub dynamic of my relationship with Ted. Sexually, I felt more secure and confident with Ted than I have with any other lover. Ted can tell me to do something in the middle of a crowded room and I'll do it, *knowing* that he made sure that whatever I did had the risk of discovery to it but not the actual *inevitability* of discovery. He knew my limits and knew which ones could and couldn't be tested, but more importantly he knew how to what extent those limits could be tested. He knew that I could quickly and spontaneously get soaking wet just by having him suddenly request a blow-job in the middle of a perfectly mundane situation, or requesting that I show him my pussy, not to fuck it but just to have a quick look at it before telling me to put my skirt back down or pull my pants back up: "We'll fuck later." Ted knew how to push every button unlike any other man I've ever known. He made me live in endless anticipation of the hard fuck that was coming later. For a woman like me, that means having a wet pussy almost all of the time. It was a thrilling way to live.

We've made plans for the last weekend of May, which is the only time that both of us weren't anticipating a very busy schedule at work. On Thursday night, Kevin called and asked if I was in the mood to play. Two of his friends (both of whom I know and one of whom I've fucked before) were in the mood for "some fun". On Saturday night, I went over to Kevin's to play with him, "Justin" and "John". I was used. I was told to strip for them as enticingly as I could. I let each guy finger my pussy. I had two cocks forced into my mouth. I sucked one cock and masturbated another while being fucked by a third. I sucked on a dildo while they drank beer and hooted at me. I was blindfolded and restrained when the three came on my body. After they came, the two friends brought me into the bathroom, stood me in the shower and hosed me down with the hand-held shower head, holding my pussy lips apart while flooding my "dirty cunt" with water, prying my mouth open while cleaning it out with water. They made me bend over in the bath tub while one held my ass-cheeks apart and the other washed my ass. It was hard and dirty and mean AND it was also exactly what I was in the mood for.

Monday morning, it was back into my work clothes and my job and the asexual Susan that everyone at work knows me as. If they only knew. I came home from work tonight, undressed and masturbated to mixed memories of Ted, at his place, sitting just out of reach while he stroked his cock and taunted me to "dare" move closer and suck it AND Kevin and his friends using me with complete disregard for my comfort.

Who can complain about a month in which *that* already happened? It can only get better from here, can't it? ;-)

Peep Show Stories

Pagan Moss

http://peepshowstories.com

A Conversation

26/1/04

A man walks into a peep show booth and picks up the phone.

"So how does this thing work?"

"You've never been to a peep show before?"

"No, it's my first time. To tell you the truth, I don't normally go to places like this."

"Well, you're in for a real treat. I love doing shows for new guys. I promise you won't be disappointed."

"So how much does it cost?"

"The show starts at $20.00 for ten minutes and just to let you know, the machine doesn't like the new $5.00 bills – the ones with the big heads."

"How about a $20.00 with a big head?"

"That'll work."

"So what do you do for $20.00?"

"I get naked for you and you get as comfortable as you like."

"So is there a slot or something where I put the money?"

"Actually, there's a bill acceptor to your left, next to the box of Kleenex."

"Oh, I see. Do I put my money in now?"

"Whenever you're ready, baby."

The bill acceptor makes a whirring sound and the shade begins to rise, revealing a young woman dressed as a school girl, sitting back on her Mary Janes.

"Hi, sexy. I like your suit."

"Thanks, you look very nice yourself."

"Let me stand up for you so you can get a better look. Do you like school girls?"

"Ah . . . well, sure."

"You like my white knee-highs and short plaid skirt?"

"Yes, they look very nice on you. How old are you, anyway?"

"Old enough. How old are you?"

"Old enough to be your dad."

"Mmm . . . I like older men, especially ones wearing nice suits. Are you just getting off work?"

"Yeah, something like that."

"I'm not wearing a bra under my blouse; I bet you can see my breasts if you look close. They're kinda small, but I have nice pink nipples."

"Yes, very nice."

"Would you like to see my panties? They're white and cotton and I've been wearing them all day."

"Actually . . . if it's OK with you, I think I'd just like to talk. I mean . . . no offense, you're very beautiful and I find you incredibly sexy, but I've got something I'd really like to get off my chest."

"Oh, sure, whatever you like. It's your fantasy, baby."

"Well, like I said, I don't normally go to places like this. I'm a married man . . . been married for 25 years."

"Wow, that's longer than I've been alive."

"Thanks, you really know how to make a guy feel old."

"I told you I like older men."

"I also have two daughters about your age."

"Sounds like the all-American family."

"Yeah, I guess you could say that."

"You sound sad. What's wrong?"

"I lost my job a month ago. I'd been working there for 20 years and those motherfuckers outsourced my job to India."

"I'm sorry, that really sucks!! But can't you find a job pretty easy? I mean, working 20 years and all."

"Not in this economy. The worst part of this whole thing is that I haven't been able to tell my wife."

"You haven't told your wife that you lost your job?"

"Nope, I've been waking up every morning pretending to go to the office. I never had a land line so I don't have to worry about her calling. If she needs to get a hold of me, she just calls my cell."

"Why didn't you tell her?"

"It's a long story, but basically, our marriage has been through a lot and I think this might be the fatal blow. I mean . . . I have a mortgage to pay for, college tuition, car payments. God, the list goes on and on."

"What do you do during the day?"

"Well, I look for jobs, of course. I have my phone. Some days I go to the library and other days I just sit in the park. It's all very sobering. I'm really tired, though. I can't go on like this any longer."

"So what are you going to do?"

"Well, I considered running away, but that obviously isn't the best choice for someone my age."

"You're right, that wouldn't be good. You really should talk to your wife. I think she would understand."

His cell phone rings.

"Oh shit, that's her. Today's her birthday. I'm supposed to be meeting her after work at our favorite restaurant. I'm going to take this, if you don't mind."

"I don't mind at all."

"Hi, honey . . . Yes, I'm just finishing up at the office . . . When do you think you'll be at the restaurant? . . . OK, I'll see you then . . . I love you, too.

"Well, I guess I better go. Thanks for the show and thanks for listening to my problems. You're a real sweet girl."

"I'm sure everything will work out. Are you going to tell her?"

"Yeah . . . sooner or later."

She watched as he left her booth, admiring the back of his suit. She cleared his remaining time and went back to reading her book.

Killer Heels

11/4/04

A customer walked in to inquire about the place. I kindly handed him the folder, which lists all the shows and prices. He surveyed the menu for quite some time, looking like he was having a hard time making up his mind. After a couple minutes passed, I kindly asked, "What kind of show did you have in mind, sweetie?"

"I know this is going to sound a little strange, but . . ."

"Yes?"

"Well, here. Why don't I just show you? It will be easier that way."

The customer proceeded to open a duffle bag which he had slung over one shoulder. He pulled out a clear plastic bag – the kind that people bring goldfish home in. He held it up for me to see.

I leaned forward to get a better look. "What's in there?" I asked.

"Crickets," he said, smiling.

"Crickets?" I asked, brow raised. "And what were you planning on doing with them?"

"I'm sure you've seen a lot here, so hopefully you won't think I'm too weird," he said with a snort. "It's not what I do with them, but what I was hoping you'd do to them."

"I'd love to help you out, but I don't do things with bugs. Although, I am curious about what you had in mind."

"I was hoping you could put on some spiked heels," he said, sizing up the meager four inch ones I had on now. "And then you could stomp on them."

The crickets hopped from one side of the bag to the other, their bug-eyes staring up at me.

"I'm sorry, but we don't stomp on living creatures here. It's against our rules." I started to walk away. "Thanks for coming in, though."

"Wait a minute," he said. "What if I had something that was small that looked like a bug. Nothing alive – just pretend. Could you step on that?"

"Will it make a mess? I mean, we just got new carpet."

"No, no, nothing like that. I don't have much else with me except for this notebook," he said, pulling out an old spiral pad. "But I was thinking that I could take some paper and wad it up like this." He demonstrated on a piece of paper he ripped out of the pad. He held up the wad for me to see. "We could just pretend these are bugs."

"Yeah?"

He set the wad of paper on the floor. "I can put them on the floor like this – maybe hide some. Then you'd come in just wearing maybe a bikini and some spiked heels. You'd see them on the floor and you'd act surprised, scared. Then you'd stomp on 'em. Maybe even scream a little. Could you do that?" he asked.

"I guess I could do that," I said "But that's considered a fantasy show, which means it's gonna cost you $100 for 30 minutes."

He took out his wallet. "You got a deal," he said.

He handed me the money and I filled out the paperwork.

"Follow me," I said. I took him to the room and gave him the spiel. "There's a hook on the back of the door for your clothes and there's oil on the table. Make yourself comfortable. I'll be back in a couple of minutes."

"Thanks," he said.

I left him to go about his insect-making while I went to the dressing room to change into my black string bikini and black seven-inch spiked heels, which were the tallest I had there.

A couple minutes later, I went back to the room and knocked. "Come in," he said.

I paused, preparing myself for what might lie on the other side of the door.

I slowly opened the door to find the customer sitting atop a towel on the couch, wearing nothing but his glasses.

Right away, I saw a couple of wadded up pieces of paper on the floor. I could sense his excitement in anticipating my reaction.

I walked toward the nearest wad, pretending not to see it. When I got right up to it, I screamed and stomped on the piece of paper, yelling: "A bug! I hate bugs! You filthy creature!"

The customer happily bounced on the couch, waiting for my next move. "I think there's another one over there," he said. He pointed to another piece of paper on the floor. "Get it!" he screamed.

I ran over to the other piece of paper and ground my heel into it.

"Oh, yeah, baby! Get it!" he cheered. "I think there's one hiding over there, too," he said, pointing to the other side of the couch.

I walked over to the other side of the couch and he leaned over the arm to get a better look. "There it is," he said. "Get it! Get it before it gets away!" he yelled.

"He's not going anywhere," I said, grinding my heel into the paper.

He started stroking his cock, saying, "Ooh, you do that so good, baby."

I saw that his cock was rock hard and I thought how interesting and somewhat disturbing it was that he was finding this all to be quite arousing.

There were ten paper wads in all and, by the time I got to the last one, he was dripping with sweat, his face fixed in painful delight. I could tell that he was going to explode upon the last stomp.

"I think that must have been the last one," I said, teasing him.

"No, no. There's one more. He's the worst one. He's big and black. He looks like a giant beetle. I saw him run over there. He's hiding from you," he said. He pointed to a silk fica in the corner.

I walked over to the plant. "Hiding, huh. It's no use, bug. I know where you are. Come out, or be smashed. It's your choice," I said. I looked around the fica for the wad of paper. He had slipped it halfway underneath the basket. "Are you sure he's here? I don't see him."

I looked back over my shoulder. He was working himself into a frenzy. "He's there. I think he's hiding under the basket," he gasped.

I lifted the basket and kicked the piece of paper out from underneath.

"There you are, trying to hide from me! You're not so clever now!" I said, shredding the last piece of paper with my heel.

The customer let out a huge moan. I looked over to see that his thighs were glistening wet.

The show was over.

As I walked the customer out to the lobby, he asked if he could tip me.

"What are you planning to do with those crickets?" I asked.

"I'm not sure," he said.

"I tell you what – don't worry about the tip. Just give me the crickets," I said.

"Deal," he said. He opened his bag and handed me the crickets. "You take good care of them," he said with a wink.

I held up the bag, wondering what I was going to do with them. "I sure will," I said.

Jade

27/4/04

It was Monday evening when I arrived for my first shift. I stepped out of the cab with a large duffle bag slung over my shoulder. I paused for a moment, looking up at the sign: Girls, Girls, Girls. I took a deep breath, opened the front door to the building and made my way up the stairs to the second floor. A young man covered in tats and piercings, wearing all black, looked up from a book as I approached the front desk.

"Hi, I'm Natalia," I said, smiling.

He scanned a clipboard on his desk and looked up at me, "You're the new girl?" he asked, brushing his long black bangs away from his face.

"Yeah, it's my first night."

"You're number 12," he said. He explained how I would need to type this number into the keypad mounted on the wall of the booth. I must have looked a little confused because he quickly added, "Jade is back in the dressing room right now. You'll be working with her tonight. She'll show you everything."

With that, he stood up. "Follow me," he said. "I'll show you to the dressing room."

I followed him as he disappeared behind a black curtain. I, too, passed through the curtain, which led to a dark corridor. There were video booths on either side. Some were occupied and the sounds of women moaning filled the air. He took a left at the end of the hallway and stopped in front of the first door. He took a ring of keys from his jeans pocket and unlocked the door.

He held the door open and gave me an indifferent smile. "Here you go," he said.

"Thank you," I said, stepping inside.

The door shut behind me and I stood there, scanning the room. There was a bathroom straight ahead and two large lighted mirrors, which hung over large counters on perpendicular walls. The place was dirty and in disarray, smelling strongly of stale cigarette smoke.

Jade was standing in front of one of the mirrors, getting ready. I dropped my bags. "Hi," I said.

"Hi, I'm Jade," she said, smiling. "Are you new?"

"Yeah, tonight's my first night."

"Cool," she said, looking back at her reflection. "You can put your stuff in an empty locker," she said. She pointed to the wall across from the row of booths.

"Thanks," I said. I picked up my bag and walked to the bay of lockers.

"You only get one, though, and you'll need to bring your own lock," she said, looking at me in the mirror.

I opened the first locker without a lock and found it was full of clothes. I opened another and found a dirty blanket inside.

"Yeah, some girls have more than one locker. They're not supposed to, though. I think the far left one on the bottom is free. It used to be Kitty's, but she got fired last week."

I opened the locker and to my utter delight it was empty. I opened my bag and started filling the locker.

When I was done, I looked over at Jade to see what she was wearing. It is a serious mistake to wear something similar to the girl you are working with – especially on the first night.

In the sex industry, it is never easy to be the new girl. Your presence seldom elicits feelings of excitement over prospective friendship, but rather evokes feelings of apprehension . . . unease. You are their rival.

Jade was wearing a black bikini, which appeared to be several sizes too small as rolls of white flesh generously flowed over the top of her bikini bottoms, practically devouring them. Jade was a larger woman – not just thick – but rather large-boned. Her shoulders resembled that of a linebacker and stuck out quite noticeably beyond her ample hips. She appeared to be in her forties, but had a Bettie Page haircut and a pierced nose, which might ruse prospective customers into thinking she was younger. She had a tattoo of a steer's skull on her upper right arm and a tattoo of a dream catcher on her upper left arm.

Jade had a pretty face when she smiled but, as soon as her smile dissolved, her mouth curled downward at the ends. Her eyes were big and dark, but empty. I sensed that life had not been so good to her and that she was not here by choice, but rather through mere desperation.

"I'm wearing black tonight, is that OK?" I asked, trying to be diplomatic.

"Fine with me," she said, applying her mascara.

"Cool," I said. I stripped out of my street clothes.

I sensed she was sizing me up out of the corner of her eye.

"Let me know when you're ready and I'll show you how to sign in," she said, climbing into her booth

I dressed and touched up my make-up and walked over to her booth when I was done. "I guess I'm ready."

"Which booth did you want?" she asked.

"I dunno . . . maybe the middle one," I said.

"Yeah, the middle one's good. It's easy to get tips through the tip slot in that one. Did you bring a blanket?" she asked.

"Yeah, I have one in my bag," I said.

She laughed and said, "I don't use one, but most girls do."

I opened the door to the second booth and laid out my blanket.

"Jump in and I'll show you," she said. She jumped into the booth after me.

She spent five minutes with me, explaining the different shows, what the girls charged, how tips worked, and how to work the keypad.

When she was done she said, "If you have any problems, let me know."

"Thanks," I said.

Jade went back to her booth and we both waited in silence.

An hour passed and no one came by. My legs were feeling a little stiff and I jumped out of my booth to stretch.

"Monday nights are slow," Jade said. "I normally don't work them, but I need the money. I have the new *National Enquirer*, if you're interested?"

"That's OK," I said, "I have a book."

Jade jumped out of her booth, too, and lit up a cigarette.

"You smoke?"

"No."

"Good for you."

She pulled up a chair in front of her booth and sat down, taking a long drag.

I grabbed a chair and sat down in front of my booth, too.

"Have you worked in the sex industry before?" she asked, exhaling.

"Yeah, I worked at the Lusty Lady."

Her face lit up. "Oh, I have an audition at the Lusty next week.

How do you think I'll do . . . I mean, do you think I stand a chance?"

I looked at her, knowing the Lusty and knowing the show directors. I knew there was no way they would hire her, especially in this job market.

"I know they're really tough over there," I said. "They make most girls audition at least twice."

She looked down. "That's what I was afraid of," she said. "But, I'm going through with it anyway. You never know . . ." she said, smiling.

"Do you have a boyfriend?" she asked.

"Yeah . . . how about you?"

"I'm married."

"How long?"

"A couple of months."

"Congratulations."

"Yeah," she said, the corners of her mouth turning downward.

"What's wrong?"

"He's missing."

"Oh, I'm sorry."

"Yeah, he's been gone for about a week now. I don't have good luck with men. My last husband died unexpectedly."

"Oh, that's horrible."

"Yeah, he died of a heart attack."

The lights on the main stage flashed on and off and Jade jumped out of her seat.

"It's mine," she said. "The first girl here gets the first stage. You get the next one," she said, running up the stairs.

I followed behind her and sat down on the top stair. I peeked around the corner, hoping to catch a glimpse of how the stage show worked. Jade stood on stage and adjusting her outfit and played with her hair while she waited for the window to open. The whir of the bill acceptor sounded and Jade rushed toward the window. The customer was in a one-way, but a light turned on above the window, signaling his presence.

"Hi, sweetie. Have you been here before?" she purred as she jiggled her large breasts in the window.

"No, first time here," I heard the customer say.

"Well, it's a $5.00 tip for topless and a $10.00 tip for full nudity.

We don't make any of the money that you put into the machine, baby."

I couldn't make out what the customer said next, but I could tell it wasn't good from Jade's reaction. She stood up and started walking toward me. I quickly got up and ran back to my chair.

"He wants you," she said, pulling the straps of her bikini top back over her shoulders. She walked past me with her head down and jumped back into her booth, slamming the door.

I went on stage and did the show for the customer. He tipped me $20.00.

After the show, I jumped back into my booth.

Jade's door swung open. "Did he tip you?" she asked.

"Yeah, just $5.00," I said.

"That guy comes in here all the time. He only gets shows with the new girls."

I knew she was lying and I felt bad for her.

The rest of the evening was slow. The customers that did come in all got shows from me and Jade was not happy. She seemed to have an excuse for each guy: "Oh, that guy hates me because I won't stick my finger in my ass," and, "I told that guy to fuck off because he wanted me to stick my whole hand up my pussy. Fuck that shit. I ain't no whore."

However, the customers she claimed to be assholes and freaks acted quite normal and well behaved with me.

At around 12.00 a.m. there seemed to be a rush of customers. I had shows pretty much back to back for the next hour of my shift. After my last show, I jumped out of the booth and saw that it was 1.00 a.m. I decided I had made enough money and started getting ready to go home. I walked past Jade's booth, which was open, and saw that she was playing a game on her broken cell phone.

"I'm going home," I said. "If you don't mind?"

"No, not at all. There's no use of two of us being here at this hour. After 1.00 a.m. it's pretty much dead anyway," she said.

"Well, it was nice meeting you," I said, holding the dressing room door open.

"Yeah, see ya," she said, her eyes glued to her game.

"Goodnight," I said, and left.

As the clerk cashed me out for the evening, he commented, "You did pretty good for a Monday."

"Really?"

"Yeah, it's usually just Jade and she's lucky if she gets house paid. She actually owes back rent. I don't know why she works here. I mean, no offense, she's nice and all, but she never makes any money. She'd be better off working at McDonalds," he said, handing me my money.

I thanked him and ran down the stairs to catch my cab.

I worked with Jade every Monday night for a couple of months. During that time, she started sharing stories of her life. She was quite a storyteller and, even though it was obvious she was lying most of the time, I always listened to every word. She once told me that her husband, who was Egyptian, was deported to Egypt. However, after only 10 days, he was quickly returned to the States. A couple days later, she said he flew down to Afghanistan to shoot a movie where he was killed when their set was bombed by terrorists. There was the story she told of her twin brother with whom she had a sexual relationship. She said he was a stripper and that he was murdered a couple of years ago. She also told me about her last wedding, which was a traditional Egyptian ceremony. Her and her husband were dressed in authentic wedding attire. She said she looked just like Cleopatra – make-up and all. She said that when the Egyptian priest asked if anyone objected to their marriage, a man jumped out of the crowd and approached her husband with sword drawn. She said that her husband also had a sword and a duel ensued.

Jade also had plenty of dark stories, which included being beaten and raped several times by various boyfriends, ex-husbands, friends of boyfriends/ex-husbands, and just friends. She said her most frightening experience was when her ex-husband asked her to sleep with one of his friends who was visiting. He told her his friend would pay her $500.00. She told me that the friend was ugly and smelled really bad. She said he looked like a scary Santa Claus. She told her husband no, but he proceeded to put something in her drink. She said her next memory was waking up on the bathroom floor naked, while the friend dressed. She was sore and wet down there and she knew she had been raped.

Every time I worked with Jade she made little, if any, money. Sometimes the customers were nice in passing on her shows, but there were those customers who were mean. They would stand in front of her booth just to roll their eyes, or to give her a dirty look. Sometimes they would go into her booth just to mess with her, asking her why she worked there because she was so ugly. I can't count how many times when it was her turn to do a stage show that she ran off almost immediately because the customer walked away, or wouldn't tip her. There were even times when customers flipped her off. Despite being rejected over and over again, Jade seemed to have an excuse for every situation. She was the queen of denial.

But then came the night when Jade broke down. It was a night I will never forget.

Jade had a regular who was very loyal to her. I'm not sure what she did for him, but he paid her very well, which probably sustained her existence there.

I came in one Monday night and found Jade singing while she was getting ready.

"You seem happy," I said.

"Yeah, one of my regulars is coming in tonight. He normally comes in Wednesday nights, but he told me last week that he would be coming in tonight. I guess he has some meeting downtown."

"Cool," I said. I got ready, too.

It was busy for a Monday night and it seemed like I had shows back to back for a couple of hours. Unfortunately, they were all basic shows, meaning all the money went into the booth – no tips. I finally had a break and ran to the bathroom. On my way back to my booth, I peeked into Jade's booth. She was reading the latest *National Enquirer*.

"Has your guy come in yet?"

"No," she said, her face buried in her paper.

I jumped back into my booth. About ten minutes later, a customer walked past my booth and smiled. He went into Jade's booth.

"Hi, baby," I heard Jade say in a sticky sweet voice. "I missed you. You ready for a show?"

I couldn't hear the customer's response, but a couple minutes later he came back out of her booth and gave me a wink as he walked past.

Jade's door swung open.

"What's wrong? Isn't he going to get a show?" I asked, leaning out of my booth.

"Yeah, he's getting money out of the ATM."

With that, she jumped out of her booth to freshen up her make-up and to adjust her outfit.

"Do I look OK?" she asked.

"You look great," I said, smiling.

"Thanks," she said. She jumped back into her booth.

A couple minutes later, someone ducked into my booth and immediately put money into the bill acceptor. I closed the shade to the hallway and peeked through the crack in the shade to see who was there. It was Jade's customer. Surely he must have made a mistake – gone into the wrong booth by accident. I waited as the shade lifted, expecting a look of embarrassment on his face at his misstep. However, the customer greeted me with a huge grin.

"Hi," I said. "Have you been here before?"

"Yeah, I normally get shows from Jade . . . your friend next door," he said.

"You're not getting a show with her tonight?" I asked.

"No, I walked past your booth and decided to get a show with you instead."

My heart sank. I knew if Jade found out, she would be devastated. This customer was all she had here. She counted on him. I hated him for putting me in this position and for hurting her.

I went through the motions of the show, but I couldn't help but think of Jade on the other side of the wall, playing games on her cell phone or reading her *National Enquirer*, eagerly awaiting her customer, wondering why he hadn't come back yet.

After the show, I told the customer that he should visit Jade.

"Not tonight," he said, shaking his head. "I'm late getting home to the wife. When do you work again?" he asked.

I reluctantly gave him my schedule and he left my booth.

I jumped out of the booth and found Jade sitting in a chair with her head in her hands. Her body shook and I knew she had heard us and that she was crying.

"What's wrong with me?" she asked. She looked up at me with streaks of black running down her cheeks.

"Nothing is wrong with you," I said. "You're beautiful."

She stood up and started to get ready to leave. The time was only a little past 11.00 p.m.

"Why do people hate me? Why can't I make any money here?

Everybody makes money but me." And with that, she totally lost it, crying uncontrollably.

I put my arms around her as she sobbed into my shoulder – the wetness of her black tears marked my bare skin. We sat there like that for a while. A customer walked by the window and smiled at me. I kicked the booth door closed. Jade finally composed herself, wiping the tears from her eyes.

"I'm sorry," she said. "I need to get another job. I can't do this anymore."

"If this job is making you feel this way, that's probably not a bad idea," I said, rubbing her back. "I don't think this business is good for anyone for too long."

I watched as Jade changed into a bright yellow sweatshirt and a pair of red and green plaid pants. She took a baby wipe from her bag and wiped the mascara from beneath her eyes.

Jade started to pack her bag. "Damn, I was really counting on that money." she said. The tears started to come again. "I don't have any money for bus fare and I don't have anything to eat."

I didn't have any cash on me besides the $40.00 tip her customer just gave me. I grabbed the $40.00 and handed it to her. "Here, it's all I've got right now."

"Thanks," she said, her upper lip trembling.

With that, she grabbed her bag and walked out the door.

That was the last time Jade ever worked at Fantasy and, for her, it was a good thing.

The other day, I was at the intersection of Bellevue and Denny, waiting for the light to change. I saw a woman standing on the opposite side of the street waiting, as well. The light changed and we both made our way across the street. As I got closer, I saw that it was Jade. Her face was soft and healthy-looking; her hair shone in the sun. She was nicely dressed and had a large book tucked tightly under one arm. We passed by one another without saying a word.

Sex in the Abattoir

2/6/04

I'd just been ripped from the nourishing teat of the Lusty Lady – kicked out of the litter you might say. But it was time; I had seen all

I could see in that place. And while many would have gone pale to see such things, my mind was like some kind of possessed machine, wanting to wrap itself around every possible scene . . . it was restless.

On my silent sojourn home, I passed the competition: The Champ Arcade. The Champ's fateful sign stared down at me and I felt as if it were drawing me in, seeming to recognize my predicament. I would have never given that place a second thought before that night. The Champ had a reputation. There were stories and the girls at the Lusty knew 'em all. There was the story about the girl who turned blue and died of a heroin overdose in the dressing room and there were stories of girls fucking customers every which way in the dark halls. The girls at the Lusty Lady were of the Indie Girl Finishing School variety and the Champ girls were more like the Switchblade Sisters.

Two weeks later, I found myself in the manager's office of the Champ, filling out my contract.

"Do you have your license?" the manager asked in a thick southern drawl. He was a young skinny guy, with a pockmarked face and long greasy hair. He wore skintight acid-washed jeans and a pinstriped button-up shirt, which hung open.

"No, I didn't know you needed one to work here. Is that a problem?"

"No, no. You can start today . . . just get it when you can," he said, flashing me a greaseball smile.

The manager showed me around the place. The dressing room was filthy and devoid of any comfort; it smelled like rotten cigarettes and garbage. The counters were littered with dead fast food bags and heaped ash trays.

The Champ was unlike any place I had worked before. The booths were actually themed rooms: one was decorated like a doctor's office, one looked like a French parlor, and another resembled a dungeon. And around the corner, men could go into a booth and watch a girl take a shower or a bubble bath.

At the end of the tour, the manager said, "Whatever room you like, you can have. The girl you were suppose to work with today called in and quit." After meticulously scrutinizing each room, I decided on the doctor's office, thinking it might help me forget how foul this place was.

The first day came and went and although it was relatively dead, I still left with over $200.00, which was more than I would have made at the Lusty – but then again – I wouldn't have had to spread my ass-cheeks either. But overall, it was a good day. I could do this, I thought.

The next day was busier. I had several business men during the lunch hour. It was getting so bad that the customers were complaining they were slipping on the floor and the janitor seemed to be conveniently absent. One customer refused to do a show in the booth.

"Can you do a show in the French parlor?" he asked. He spoke with a thick German accent.

"Sure, no problem," I said. "I'll meet you over there."

When I opened the door to the parlor, I could see his silhouette beyond the shade. I laid down on the bed in front of the window, waiting for him to put the money into the bill acceptor.

"Are you ready?" he asked.

"Yeah, baby. I'm ready for you."

A couple seconds later, the shade began to rise.

"Hi," he said. "I don't think I've seen you before."

"I'm new. Today's my second day."

"What's your name?"

"Natalia."

"Natalie."

"Natalia."

"Oh, Natalia. That's nice."

"Thank you."

He turned his head a certain way, which caught my attention. Something was familiar about him. It was as if I had seen that angle before. My mind raced, going through the archives, trying to make a match. He was an attractive young man with a muscular build. He had blond hair and piercing blue eyes. He wore a wedding band.

"I like your body," he said.

"Thanks," I said, moving across the bed like a lynx.

He started to touch himself through his slacks and I could see that he was hard. I slipped the straps of my bra off my shoulders and was reaching around back to undo the hooks when the match was made. It was Gunter and I hadn't seen him since high school – when he was a senior and I was a freshman. He was a foreign exchange student and we were on the same power lifting team. I'm pretty sure he wanted to fuck me back then. My body froze. I couldn't remove my bra but when I looked at him, I saw that he was starting to undo himself. I didn't know what to do. Should I tell him? No, I shouldn't. It will just make things weird. Besides, he probably won't come in again. But something took over – the voice of reason, maybe.

"Wait a minute . . ." I called out.

He looked up at me, startled. "What's wrong?"

"I think I know you."

He started laughing. "Really?"

"Yeah, my name's Cassandra. We used to work out together in high school."

A huge smile spread across his face. "Oh, my God!" he said. "Is it really you?"

"Yeah . . . it's really me."

"What are you doing here?"

"Working while I go to school. What have you been up to?

"I just got married."

"Congratulations."

"Thanks."

"You work down here?"

"Yeah, just a couple blocks away."

"On your lunch hour?"

His smile shrunk a little. "Yeah."

"You know, we don't have to do the show," I said.

He started touching himself again. "Actually, if you don't mind, I'd really like to finish the show."

"Sure, sure, of course," I replied, not believing my luck.

After the show, he asked for my schedule and said he would be back. However, things at the Champ didn't work out so well after all and I ended up quitting a couple days later – never to see him again.

A month later my Mom calls me up: "Cassandra."

"Yeah, Mom."

"Someone left a message on my voicemail, looking for your number."

"Really?"

"Yeah. He said his name was Gunter?"

"He called?"

"Yeah. He said he ran into you downtown the other day. He said he lost your number."

"Huh . . ."

"Do I know Gunter?"

"Yeah, Mom. I think you met him once. He was the German exchange student who was on my power-lifting team in high school."

"Oh, Gunter. Now I remember. He was such a nice boy."

Interview with the Moan

17/6/04

The shade of a peep show window opens, revealing a scantily clad young woman doing yoga stretches on stage. As soon as she sees the customer, she stands up and sashays over to the window.

DANCER: Hi, honey. You been here before?
Feeling self-conscious, the young man looks down at his foot as he traces a half-circle onto the floor with it.
CUSTOMER: No, first time.
DANCER: Well, baby, it's a dollar in the machine to keep the window up for a minute. I'll show you my tits for five and my pussy for ten.
CUSTOMER: What if I don't want to see you naked?
The dancer leans back and puts her hands on her hips – her eyes burn into his flesh.
DANCER: Whaddaya mean, you don't want to see me naked? You afraid of girls or somethin'?
CUSTOMER: Oh, no . . . no. I didn't mean anything by that. Gosh, no, you're beautiful. It's just that I'm a student and I have this project that I'm working on for a class.
DANCER: Oh, of course. You're here on research.
The customer produces one medium-sized tape recorder and a large microphone.
CUSTOMER: Yeah, I guess you could say that.
DANCER: What did you have in mind?
CUSTOMER: Well . . . I was hoping to record you moaning.
The dancer tilts her head in contemplation.

DANCER: Moaning? This is for a class?
CUSTOMER: Yeah . . . media arts.
DANCER: What college?
CUSTOMER: High School.

A huge smile spreads across the dancer's face. She puts her face down to the tip slot and whispers.

DANCER: High School? You know you have to be 18 to even step into this joint.
CUSTOMER: I know, I know. I had to show the guy up front my I.D.
DANCER: OK, you better not be lying or anything. I've got a business license, you know. If the City came down and caught me doing shows for underage boys, they'd probably have me locked up for child molesting or somethin'.
CUSTOMER: I turned 18 two weeks ago.
DANCER: Well, it's your lucky day. I don't normally allow customers to record my moan for anything less than fifty but, since it's practically your birthday today, I'm gonna give you a deal.
CUSTOMER: Whatever you could do, miss, I'd really appreciate it.
DANCER: First of all, please don't call me "miss". My name's Star.
CUSTOMER: Nice to meet you, Star. I'm Dan.
DANCER: Lovely to meet you, Dan. How 'bout I do the recording for ten dollars?
CUSTOMER: Does that mean I get to see you naked, too?
DANCER: Don't push your luck, kid. If you're lucky, I might flash you a nipple.

The customer reaches into his coat pocket, pulls out a wad of crinkled bills and begins counting. He then reaches back into his pocket and pulls out a handful of change.

CUSTOMER: How 'bout nine dollars, three quarters, two dimes, and one nickel?
DANCER: Oh . . . all right. You're lucky you're cute.

The crinkled dollars come through the tip slot one by one, followed by the sound of clinking change.

CUSTOMER: You got it all?
DANCER: Yeah, yeah. I got it ALL. Thanks.

The customer fiddles with the recorder, trying to get it ready. He puts the microphone up to the tip slot.

CUSTOMER: I'm ready when you are.

The dancer gets down on all fours and puts her mouth right up to the tip slot. She can see the customer's belt through the hole, along with the microphone. She moans loudly and lasciviously, giving the whole place a show. After the final crescendo, the customer turns off the recorder.

DANCER: Did you get it all, baby?
CUSTOMER: Yeah, thanks. This is gonna be awesome.
DANCER: You have fifteen seconds left. You wanna see my tits?
CUSTOMER: Sure.

The dancer pulls up the top of her bikini, revealing young, round breasts. She gives them a quick shake.

DANCER: Do you like them?
CUSTOMER: Yes, they're beautiful.

The shade starts to fall and the customer waves goodbye. The dancer yells through the slot as he leaves the booth.

DANCER: Maybe you can think about them when you're listening to that tape later.

The dancer leaves the stage and jumps back into her booth, thinking about the young man she just left and hoping that a customer will be along soon, inquiring about the toys in her window.

Some Know

29/6/04

He exits the theatre and walks past my booth on the way to the bathroom every day. He never gets a show; he prefers to watch the girls do the nasty on the big screen. He has white hair and pink skin like paper. His frame is large and he walks with dignity like a World War II vet. The clerk says he's been coming in for years, showing up in the morning and leaving at night. He's the most faithful soul in this place.

He is open-minded for his age – never complains about the tranny porn they play on Wednesday nights.

One day he comes into my booth and asks me how much for a show.

When I tell him, he puts in a twenty.

I joke that I see him every day.

He says he's been trying to cut down.

He asks if I work out of here.

I tell him I've been tempted, but . . .

He says he'll pay me two hundred dollars for an hour.

I ask him what he wants me to do.

He tells me he's got diabetes real bad – can't risk an infection.

I tell him I'm sorry to hear that.

He says he was thinking just a private dance – maybe a hand-job.

I ask him what the special occasion is.

He says he's going away – to a place where these places don't exist.

I think how nice that would be.

He slips me his number and a five-dollar tip through the slot.

I take off my top and shake my tits.

He smiles and claps his hands.

I take off my panties and show him my bare pussy.

He clutches his chest.

I dance around the booth, flashing him pink here and there – but not too much. He lived through the war; I don't want to kill him now.

For his sake, the curtain falls.

He tells me goodbye and to call him.

I smile and tell him I will.

I lie . . . again.

The next day, I wait for him to walk by. I have my lines ready to go, but he never shows.

I don't worry at first. But then one day turns into many.

He never misses a day, let alone two weeks. His absence is surely out of death or disconcertion.

Sadly, it is to be the former. Nothing spreads faster than the news of death and suddenly everyone was talking about it.

I heard it from the janitor. He said someone found his body a couple of days ago. He didn't know how long he'd been dead – just that he died alone in his sleep.

Swan Lake

30/6/04

He stumbles through the front door with his derelict hair and clothes covered in filth, like he does every Friday night. He sits down and waits in silence – his wiry beard resting on his chest. When I come out to greet him, the whole place smells of cheap alcohol. He looks close to death and I think maybe he'd be better off stinking in the waiting room at Harborview. But this is his therapy – probably one of the only things still keeping him alive.

As I walk over to him, he starts to stir. He looks up at me and I sense he's searching, trying to remember if I'm the one.

I reassure him. "Hi, sexy. It's good to see you. Did you miss me?"

He smiles, remembering. "Yeah, I did."

"I missed you, too," I say, getting the paperwork ready.

He looks like he couldn't afford the video booths at the local peep show, let alone the ninety-dollar fantasy show he gets here. But he always pulls out a wad of cash and with one eye trying to focus, counts out five twenty-dollar bills.

"Keep the change," he jokes. "It's the State's money, anyway."

"Thank you," I say and I take him down the hall to the same room I've been taking him for the past three months – the one the other girls don't like to use. They claim he smells.

As soon as he steps into the room, he starts stripping, leaving a trail of clothes from the door to the couch. I tell him I'll be back, but he never answers. He's in his own world, standing naked before a mirrored wall, sizing up his reflection.

When I come back, a couple minutes later, he's still there, admiring his flesh.

"Do you have your music tonight?" I ask.

"Yeah," he says. He pulls out a CD from his bag and hands it to me.

I walk over to the CD player and put it in. "Hmmm . . . Tchaikovsky . . ." I say, pressing play.

The music fills the air.

He sits down on a towel spread out on the couch. "I thought you'd like it," he says. "You seem like the type."

"Funny," I say. "I was thinking the same thing about you."

I sit down on the chair, which he places right in front of him. I always sit in the chair like some kind of pseudo psychiatrist – a witness to his madness. Maybe it wasn't such a bad use of the State's money after all.

We spend the first part of the show with our eyes closed, exchanging energy – the way he and his sister used to do when they were kids. He showed me how they did it, sitting face-to-face, the palms of their hands and the soles of their feet almost touching.

"Can you feel the energy?" he asks.

"Yeah, baby, I can feel it," I say.

We sit that way for a while, exchanging energy. I think I'm getting the raw end of the deal.

He suddenly stands up as if drawn by the music. He faces the mirror and starts stretching and doing side bends.

"What do you think of my body?" he asks.

My eyes take a gander at his portly hirsute physique. "It looks good!" I say.

He stands sideways and sucks in air. He places one hand over his stomach, attempting to flatten the bulge.

"I just need to lose this," he says, turning this way and that, assessing the goods. "Then I'll be happy."

He turns around to look at his ass and clenches his cheeks.

"You should feel this," he says, poking his ass with his finger.

"Yeah, looks tight . . ." I say.

He starts dancing to the music. I step back and lean against the wall, watching him leap, promenade and plie – his fingers soft and graceful.

"Wow, you're really good at that," I say.

"I used to do ballet when I was a kid."

"I can tell."

He digresses, standing on his tippy-toes, flexing his calf muscles at me.

"Check 'em out," he says, poking again at his flesh.

"Very nice," I say.

"You should feel them," he says. "Seriously, you won't believe it."

"I believe you; I can see them from here."

"Come on," he says. "You gotta feel how hard they are."

I knew he was harmless. I'm sure he hadn't been touched by a girl for a long, long time. I felt it was the least I could do, just a small token of humanity. I walk over and poke his calf with the very tip of my finger, withdrawing it quickly.

"Wow, just like a rock!" I say.

Satisfied, he sits back down on the couch and wipes the sweat from his brow with a towel.

I stand right in front of him and start flexing my leg muscles. It's what he likes and it's one of the strangest things anyone has ever asked of me.

He starts stroking his placid cock, staring at my legs. His cock starts to grow in his hand.

I tell him he's sexy. He seems to agree with me.

He strokes and strokes like he's working toward something – something that's gonna take him a while. I wonder if he'll be able to do it, or if maybe the alcohol's gonna win out tonight. His eyes start rolling back into his skull and he struggles to bring them forward, blinking and shaking his head, trying to focus again on my thighs.

I tell him I want to see him do it tonight; I want to see it real bad.

He nods and keeps at it, while Tchaikovsky blares in the background.

I run my hands over my thighs, telling him how strong they are. That seems to do it.

His face twists up in agony and his whole body curls up in a ball, like he's been punched hard in the stomach.

I fetch him a hot towel and wait for him outside the door while he recovers. The drunkards are never to be left alone as they often find their way out into the hallway, stumbling about in the dark like lost children.

I hear him hum as he puts on his clothes. The music stops and I knock on the door.

He steps out of the room and we walk down the hallway in silence. In the lobby, I tell him I had a great time. He smiles, curtsies, and stumbles out into the street.

I wonder how he'll manage.

I grab the cleaning supplies and put on a pair of latex gloves. I walk back to the room and his smell hits me in the face. I empty half a can of Lysol, trying to kill the stench.

One of the mistresses walks by the room and looks in. "I don't know how you deal with that guy," she says, holding her nose. "You couldn't pay me enough."

I thought about what she said as I scooped up the soiled towels.

The Recipe

3/8/04

It was around Christmas time and the men were coming in in droves – their arms full of brightly colored packages and bags, brimming with well thought-out (or hastily picked) gifts for wives, sons and daughters. And if the holiday crowd wasn't enough to keep the girls sweating and smiling, there was also a deluge of horny men displaced by the sudden closure of the popular peep show down the road. As delighted as the girls were at the prospect of more customers and the money, which surely accompanied them, the rumors swirled.

There was talk about the girls at the other joint and how they had been turning dirty tricks – doing more for less money. The girls knew they had their work cut out for them when the new guys scoffed at the prices: "Forty for masturbation? You've got to be kidding me. The girls at the other place were doin' it for $20.00." But the girls banded together, deciding not to budge. They circled the wagons around their sexual prowess, knowing this was the last peep show in town, and the men ended up caving in, knowing they couldn't assuage their hunger elsewhere. But the price war wasn't the only battle to be waged. Many of the new customers expected the same types of shows that the other girls were doing. They weren't looking for masturbation or toy shows . . . they wanted a piece of you. We were like little lambs, resting in our fattening pens. We sat innocently, waiting for the wolves . . . waiting for our slaughter.

It was a couple of days before Christmas and I was working with Tulips – the new girl. She stood 5'2" and weighed about 200 pounds – a regular butter ball. She had greasy white skin, dotted with red crusted spots. Her hair was long, thin and covered in more grease. Her face was round and trollish with a forehead like a slab of marble. She often donned a peach-colored nylon housecoat, along with a pair of white fluffy slippers.

Tulips wasn't just new to our scene – she was fresh to the business. She claimed to be a 40-year-old feminist who believed there was nothing wrong with the naked body. It was something that was beautiful – it provided pleasure and pleasure was healthy. She was bubbling with enthusiasm, claiming she hadn't gotten any in a while and was looking forward to getting off. I thought to myself – this woman might stand a chance. She wasn't a beauty – more resembling a dirty housewife than the sexy girl-next-door type – but, for enough men, there are more important things than beauty.

Tulips was horny and eager to please, often acting more like a customer service representative than a shrewd business woman. Money didn't seem to be her motivator as she was happy to make house and bus fare to get home – maybe make enough to order food like the other girls. She just wanted to be included with the girls, even if she didn't look like them.

It was around noon and the lunch crowd started to file in. Tulips was dancing on stage when a customer came into my booth. He was short, fat and bald and wore thick black-framed glasses. He wore a plaid button-up shirt and pleated khaki slacks. He picked up the phone.

"Hi, what's your name?" he asked.

"June. What's yours, big boy?" I shot back.

"Gary," he said, nervously.

"Don't think I've seen you here before, Gary. You new?"

"I used to go to the other place, but they closed it down."

"Well, you're lucky, Gary. This place is so much better."

"Yeah?"

"What gets you off, Gary?"

"Well . . . I'm into something a little different."

"Are you a naughty boy, Gary?"

"Yeah, I am. I used to see this girl at the other place. She was real good. I was actually hoping she might have come over here, but I haven't seen her around. We had this arrangement that worked out pretty good for both of us. I'd give her a list of things to eat for a week and then I'd come back to pick something up," he said with a wink.

"What did you pick up, Gary?"

His face turned real serious. "She went to the bathroom in a bag and gave it to me."

"She peed?"

"No, the other one."

"Oh . . ."

"Trust me, I made it worth her while. I'll make it worth yours, too."

"Hmmm . . ."

"If I like what you got, I'll come in at least once a week."

I wasn't interested, but morbid curiosity has a way of creeping in. "So what would I have to eat?"

"Just fruit and vegetables."

Hm, I was a vegan, but no. "Sorry, I don't think I'm gonna be able to help you out."

He seemed prepared for rejection. "That's OK, I understand. You workin' with anyone else tonight?"

I was reluctant to respond, feeling I would be offering her to a pariah. "Yeah, she's a new girl. Her name's Tulips."

"Tulips," he said with a smile. "I like that name."

He thanked me for my time and left the booth. A couple seconds later, the door to Tulips' booth opened and closed. I pressed my ear against the wall of the booth. I could hear their introductions, but when the conversation got down and dirty, their voices trailed off in silence. I sensed Tulips was either stunned silent, or was whispering her response – not wanting anyone else to know of their deviant pact. A few minutes later her booth door flung open.

"He didn't get a show?" I asked.

"No, he's just checking the place out," she said. "He likes big girls and said he'd be back next week."

The next day during lunch time, Tulips decided to forgo her customary trip to the closest fast-food joint. She'd normally return, clutching a couple of grease-soaked, brown paper sacks. But today, she gingerly pulled out a packed lunch from the refrigerator and walked directly back to her booth. I couldn't keep myself from sneaking a peek at what was inside the bag. I wanted to see if she was preparing herself for him. I strolled up to her booth and looked inside. Tulips was leaning over a large spread of freshly cut vegetables and sliced fruit.

"Wow, looks healthy," I said.

"Yeah, I'm tryin' to lose a little," she said, patting her belly.

The days went by and Tulips stuck to her diet – her dedication was a painful display. But she had lost ten pounds and was bathed in a healthy glow.

At the end of the week, her customer finally came back to claim his prize. When Tulips saw him go into her booth, she quickly closed her door. I pressed my ear against the wall. After the initial exchange of pleasantries, the conversation grew silent, like last time. After a couple of minutes, Tulips jumped out of her booth with something plastic and shiny in her hand, and locked herself in the bathroom. I could only imagine the horror taking place in there. After some time, I heard a flush and then the water turn on, and then off again. The door opened and Tulips walked out of the bathroom, carrying a small black plastic bag. She opened the dressing room door and stepped just outside – holding the door ajar. She started talking to someone, but I couldn't make out the conversation – just some laughing at the end. Tulips came back into the dressing room without the bag.

As Tulips walked past my booth, I searched her face for any sign of regret. But there was nothing different. Her face still had the healthy glow – she looked better than ever.

Tulips kept at it – eating her veggies and fruit – and delivering the goods at the end of the week. Each week, she looked better, dropping weight right and left. It finally got to the point where she was getting looks and shows from other customers, too. She even started sneaking trips to the store downstairs to cash in on her employee discount, picking up sexy little outfits – the housecoats slowly disappeared.

I kept waiting for the day to come when she couldn't take it anymore, thinking she might be passive-aggressive, but that day never came. I finally asked her, "So how are you liking it here? You seem to be really getting the hang of it."

"Yeah, I love it here – the girls, the customers – everyone's so nice. I finally feel beautiful."